Whole-Body Cryostimulation

Paolo Capodaglio

Editor

Whole-Body Cryostimulation

Clinical Applications

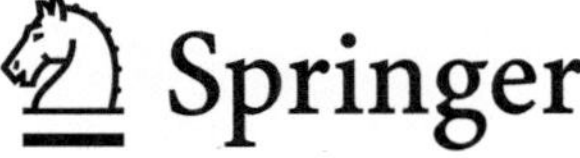 Springer

Editor
Paolo Capodaglio
Research Laboratory in Biomechanics
Rehabilitation and Ergonomics
IRCCS Istituto Auxologico Italiano
Piancavallo (Verbania), Italy

Physical and Rehabilitation Medicine
Department of Surgical Sciences
University of Torino
Turin, Italy

ISBN 978-3-031-18547-2   ISBN 978-3-031-18545-8   (eBook)
https://doi.org/10.1007/978-3-031-18545-8

This Springer imprint is published by the registered company Springer Nature Switzerland AG
The registered company address is: Gewerbestrasse 11, 6330 Cham, Switzerland

Paper in this product is recyclable.

Foreword

As the Chairman of the Working Group of the International Institute of Refrigeration (IIR) on "Whole-Body Cryotherapy/cryostimulation," it is my great pleasure to introduce the book entitled *Whole-body Cryostimulation. Clinical Applications*, organized by Professor Paolo Capodaglio from the University of Torino and the IRCCS Istituto Auxologico, Italy.

The topic of the book is of great interest and is going to be published at the time the IIR Society needs to have in one place the collection of the whole information of this very important subject concerning Whole-Body Cryostimulation (WBC) as the topic is developing fast and the applications being multifold.

For his challenge, Professor Paolo Capodaglio has been able to gather the big names of the field—almost all of them belonging to our Working Group and the remaining going to join it very soon—in order to summarize the up-to-date knowledge of the topic and the expanding application possibilities in clinical conditions.

The book entails in a pleasant way the basic science behind the physiological adaptations when a subject is exposed to very cold temperature and how exposure can enhance health both in healthy persons and patients.

All the chapters of the book are interesting and informative and many different kinds of people will—I am sure—enjoy the reading such as users (regular or future users) of cryochamber and cryosauna devices, stakeholders, clinicians from different disciplines, practitioners, scientists, researchers, and students.

I also hope this book will stimulate scientific thinking, collaborations between the different authors of this book and newcomers, in order to be able to propose in the near future large multi-centric research works concerning cryostimulation under the realms of the IIR Working Group on WBC.

Laboratory Mobilité, Vieillissement, Exercice (MOVE)   Benoit Dugué
Faculty of Sports Sciences, University of Poitiers
Poitiers, France

Introduction

Can cold-based therapies become an effective adjuvant therapeutic option in treating different pathological conditions? It was back in 1978, that Whole-Body Cryostimulation (WBC) as we know it today emerged for the treatment of patients affected by rheumatoid arthritis. The progressive technological evolution of cryochambers has made them a favourite for athletes on a worldwide basis. Despite this extensive use in Sports Medicine and growing medical literature, clinical applications have not fully taken off: in the USA, they are still clouded by FDA's safety concerns, whereas in Europe clinical interest is brewing, with Poland being the only National Health system reimbursing WBC to treat chronic pain, and Italy, where the Ministry of Health has very recently (May 2023) given the green light for its clinical use in rheumatological conditions, fibromyalgia, muscle recovery, obesity, and mood disorders.

The discoveries of the 2021 Nobel prize winners for Physiology and Medicine, David Julius and Ardem Patapoutian, on a family of temperature receptors, in particular TRPM8, seem to strengthen the rationale for a therapeutic use of cold. Cold is a stress factor for the body that can induce an insulative autonomic response aimed at reducing heat loss (peripheral vasoconstriction), enhancing thermogenesis, and modulating the nervous impulses allowing adaptation to the external environment. Similarly to physical exercise, which challenges and trains our cardiorespiratory and musculoskeletal systems, WBC acts as an allostatic load to train our homeostatic systems. The beneficial effects on well-being and, as emerging, on metabolism, are partially related to the acute response but mostly become evident when exposure is repeated. They are related to the activation of the central nervous system and the consequent neurohumoral responses that drive a cascade of changes in the endocrine, circulatory, neuromuscular, and immunological systems which is, at present, only partially exploited for therapeutic use.

Growing scientific evidence supports a safe clinical use of WBC as an adjuvant treatment in many conditions of rehabilitation interest, from orthopaedic to neurological, metabolic, and autoimmune. We can now safely provide defined doses of cold to the body and measure its acute, short-, medium-, and long-term effects at molecular, physiological, clinical, and functional level. We know today that energy homeostasis is maintained by the mutual interaction of glucose, lipid, adipose tissue, and bone metabolisms. It is therefore not surprising that WBC shows a wide range of effects on different organs and systems of the body. The perception of WBC as a therapeutic option has changed from a conventionally intended symptomatic therapy to an adaptive treatment able to positively affect the body at many different levels, enhance the homeostatic responses, boost metabolism, modulate pain, mood, sleep, and autonomic balance. This novel view is favouring the shift from WBC as a symptomatic treatment for pain in inflammatory conditions to an adjuvant therapy for endocrine diseases affecting the metabolic sphere and dysautonomic conditions. This volume gathers the cutting-edge research on the evidence-based clinical benefits of repeated exposures of the whole body to extreme cold for a short time and reviews its current clinical use, the potential new clinical applications, and future research directions.

Research Laboratory in Biomechanics   Paolo Capodaglio
Rehabilitation and Ergonomics
IRCCS Istituto Auxologico Italiano
Piancavallo (Verbania), Italy

Physical and Rehabilitation Medicine, Department
of Surgical Sciences
University of Torino
Torino, Italy
p.capodaglio@auxologico.it; paolo.capodaglio@unito.it

Contents

Part II Applications in Clinical Conditions

Part I

Introduction

Prolonged or Repeated Cold Exposure: From Basic Physiological Adjustment to Therapeutic Effects

Jacopo Maria Fontana, Benoit Dugué, and Paolo Capodaglio

Basic Physiology of Cold Exposure

Biophysical Factors

All homeothermic animals, including mammals, maintain high body temperature in the range of 36–42 °C and can regulate their internal body temperature within a range of approximately 1 °C, despite wide fluctuations in the temperature of their surroundings [1]. The summed effects of internal heat production and heat transfers between the body and its surroundings reflect the internal body temperature. If the body produces more heat than it dissipates, body tissue accumulation is positive and deep body temperature increases. On the contrary, if heat production is less than that dissipated to the external environment, heat accumulation will be negative and deep

J. M. Fontana (✉)
Research Laboratory in Biomechanics, Rehabilitation and Ergonomics, IRCCS Istituto
Auxologico Italiano, Piancavallo (VB), Italy
e-mail: j.fontana@auxologico.it

B. Dugué
Laboratory Mobilité, Vieillissement, Exercise (MOVE), University of Poitiers, Poitiers,
France
e-mail: benoit.dugue@univ-poitiers.fr

P. Capodaglio
Research Laboratory in Biomechanics, Rehabilitation and Ergonomics, IRCCS Istituto
Auxologico Italiano, Piancavallo (VB), Italy

Physical and Rehabilitation Medicine, Department of Surgical Sciences,
University of Torino, Torino, Italy
e-mail: p.capodaglio@auxologico.it; paolo.capodaglio@unito.it

© The Author(s), under exclusive license to Springer Nature
Switzerland AG 2024
P. Capodaglio (ed.), *Whole-Body Cryostimulation*,
https://doi.org/10.1007/978-3-031-18545-8_1

body temperature will decrease [2]. The heat balance equation describes these relationships between production and loss as follows:

$$M + R = C + E + K + S$$

where M represents metabolic heat production (the metabolic rate generated internally by food digestion and to maintain the core temperature), R is the power absorbed in the form of radiation (minus that lost through radiation from the body), C is the power lost (usually if the body is warmer than its surroundings) through convection, E is the power lost through evaporation of sweat, K is the power lost through conduction (gained if the environment is warmer) and S is the heat storage representing the heat gain by the body if positive or the heat loss from the body if negative. S represents the 'steady state', since its value is negligible compared to the other quantities (which is a healthy state for a mammal). Depending on the environment, therefore, R, C, G and S can have negative values. All units are in Wm^{-2}.

When exposed to environments colder than body temperature, dry heat loss mechanisms (conduction and convection), as well as radiation, allow heat to flow from the body core to the environment. Wind increases convective heat loss from the body surface, the so-called wind chill effect, while immersion in water allows greater convective heat transfer than exposure in air at the same temperature, water having a much higher heat capacity than air causing higher conductive and convective heat loss. Heat loss between the body and the environment can be limited by clothing, which may provide more or less insulation depending on the material and width or, when wet, supply significantly less insulation than when dry. Thus, environmental characteristics, in addition to temperature, influence heat loss and gain and the resulting physiological effort to control and protect body temperature [3].

Acute Physiological Responses to Cold

The core temperature of humans is ~37 °C. Approximately 60% of the total body energy produced is in the form of heat used to maintain body temperature within certain limits, even when the surrounding temperature is low. During cold stress, changes occur in the endocrine, circulatory, neuromuscular and immunological systems. Our body has two mechanisms that help maintain core temperature during cold exposure and reduce or restore heat loss: (1) vasomotor responses to reduce dry heat loss to the environment and (2) metabolic responses to replace heat lost to the environment through heat production, or thermogenesis. The combination of these mechanisms is called thermoregulation (Fig. 1.1) [4–6].

Primary Thermoregulatory Responses to Cold: Vasomotor Responses (Peripheral Vasoconstriction and Vasodilation)

The skin's extensive blood supply helps regulate temperature: dilated vessels allow heat loss, while constricted vessels retain heat. In addition, the skin regulates body temperature through its blood supply, thus contributing to body homeostasis. The dermis is characterised by the presence of more cold receptors (10 times more) than heat receptors [7].

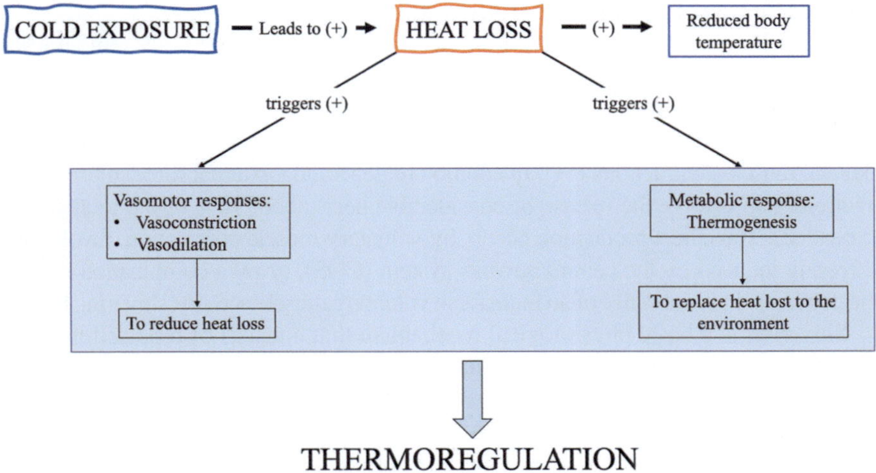

Fig. 1.1 Acute physiological response to cold

Peripheral vasoconstriction is the principal mechanism to reduce heat loss elicited in humans after being exposed to cold. Specifically, the homeostatic autonomic responses of thermogenesis and vasoconstriction are elicited [8] through the strong changes primarily in skin core temperature that stimulate cold receptors and the thermoregulatory centre in the hypothalamus [2, 3]. This somatosensory pathway transmits the afferent signals from the skin to the median subregion of the preoptic area (POA), in the anterior hypothalamus, from which efferent signals arise causing cutaneous vasoconstriction and/or shivering thermogenesis. Cutaneous circulation represents the key point in thermoregulation.

Upon exposure to cold, vasoconstriction causes a shift of blood from the skin vessels to the deeper veins and from the periphery to the core of the body and the heart region, increasing preload and central arterial pressure and reducing heart rate (HR) [3, 8]. This causes a reduction in heat transfer between the body core and external tissues, such as skeletal muscles, subcutaneous fat and skin, effectively increasing the insulation of the body envelope without, however, preventing heat dispersion across the exposed body surface, which is faster than it is replaced.

During vasoconstriction there is an activation of the sympathetic system accompanied by the release of norepinephrine. The latter is known to modulate pain, along with other compounds, such as the release of endorphins and slowing the conduction velocity of sensory nerve fibres and, in particular, slow-conducting C-fibres that deactivate sensory receptors and their connections with proprioceptors. Cryogenic temperatures cause autonomic balance alterations induced by changes in peripheral and central blood volume [9]. Furthermore, in athletes, vasodilatation can also occur about 4 min after exposure to the WBC and lasts for several hours after exercise, while basal skin temperature returns after about 14 min [10], suggesting a hunting response (the process of alternating vasoconstriction and vasodilation in extremities exposed to cold), the strength of which could be influenced by many factors, such as the temperature of the WBC or the frequency of exposure.

Metabolic Heat Production: Thermogenesis

Our body has various ways of limiting heat loss and defending body temperature. Metabolic heat production, or thermogenesis, is the mechanism, whereby the body can increase heat production in order to replace heat lost during cold exposure.

The major source of the metabolic heat produced to protect against cold stress are skeletal muscle contractions [11]. In addition to generating external force, muscle contractions also involve the release of considerable heat (about 70% of the total energy expended). Thus, heat production occurs by voluntary muscle contraction, involuntary shivering induced by the central nervous system (CNS), or by a combination of both mechanisms. In the absence of an increase in voluntary muscle activity, shivering begins.

Shivering is a basic physiological mechanism that consists of repeated involuntary rhythmic muscle contractions during which most of the metabolic energy expended is released as heat and little external work is performed; it can begin immediately or after several minutes of exposure to cold and is initiated by a decrease in skin temperature. Lowering the core temperature provides the greatest stimulus for shivering, with a ratio of T_{core} to T_{skin} contribution of 3.6:1 [12]. Shivering usually starts in the trunk muscles, then spreads to the limbs [13] becoming maximal at an internal temperature of ~34–35 °C and ceases at ~31 °C [14]. The severity of cold stress (such as exposure to air or water and the magnitude of the change in core temperature) can influence the intensity and duration of the shivering response. As shivering intensity increases and more muscles are involved, whole-body oxygen uptake (VO2) increases, requiring greater systemic oxygen transport resulting in increased cardiac output (CO), heart rate (HR) and stroke volume (SV). CO increases mainly due to increased SV, which appears to be the result of an increase in central blood volume associated with cold-induced peripheral vasoconstriction, with limited variation in resting HR under cold exposure [15]. Furthermore, depending on the volume of blood redistributed in the chest during exposure to cold and changes in preload, a decrease in HR may even occur.

In people who shiver it is possible to reach metabolic rates of 200 W or more. As the intensity of shivering increases and more muscles are recruited to shiver, the whole-body metabolic rate increases, typically reaching about 200–250 W during resting exposure to cold air, but often exceeding 350 W during resting immersion in cold water. A shivering metabolism of 763 W has been recorded during immersion in water at 12 °C [16].

Another mechanism of heat production is non-shivering thermogenesis. In fact, some animals, including humans, respond to cold exposure with increased metabolic heat production by non-contractile tissues without any muscle contraction being involved [17].

This mechanism depends on the specialised adipose tissue known as brown tissue (BAT), which is rich in mitochondria, has high oxidative capacity and abundant expression of electron transport chain components and uncoupling protein 1 (UCP1). UCP1 dissipates the mitochondrial proton motive force (Δp) generated by the respiratory chain and increases thermogenesis releasing energy directly as heat instead of channelling it into formation of the energy carrier ATP.

Since it was discovered that adult humans have functionally competent BAT, several studies have investigated its function in energy metabolism. Early studies identified active BAT in adult humans upon an increased uptake of the glucose tracer, fluorine-18 fluorodeoxyglucose (18F-FDG), from the circulation following acute cooling. A number of studies using positron emission tomography/computed tomography (PET/CT) with 18F-FDG after cooling have shown that adult humans may have an active BAT that is activated by exposure to cold. However, not all individuals have a cold-sensitive BAT, revealing a loss of a potentially important metabolic function in a large portion of the population [18]. Furthermore, adult BAT activity increases in the postprandial period and is related to the absorption of circulating fatty acids and glucose [19], suggesting a cold-independent, although still regulated by the sympathetic system, role of BAT in promoting metabolic homeostasis. Substantial glucose uptake from supraclavicular BAT demonstrated that a large portion of the glucose absorbed during cooling is subject to anaerobic metabolism and released as lactate [20]. However, glucose is not considered to be the main substrate for BAT thermogenesis in adult humans. Although the uptake of non-esterified fatty acids (NEFA) in BAT during cold activation was associated with BAT thermogenesis [21], no estimation of the extent of oxidative metabolism can be performed since the PET tracer 14(R,S)-[18F]-fluoro-6-thia-heptadecanoic acid (18FTHA) (a long-chain fatty acid analogue) is trapped in the mitochondrial matrix. However, it can be estimated that during cooling, BAT dietary fatty acid uptake was two fold higher than in the neck subcutaneous white adipose tissue (WAT) and three fold higher in skeletal muscle [22]. Interestingly, extensive BAT recruitment was found in patients with pheochromocytoma, a catecholamine-producing tumour in the adrenal gland characterised by high circulating endogenous levels of norepinephrine [23]. In addition, massive BAT infiltration, and glucose uptake, of the visceral adipose tissue depots of these patients was reported suggesting how human visceral adipose tissue holds an unprecedented potential for brown adipogenic differentiation, while no browning was observed in the subcutaneous adipose depots [24]. Similarly, adenosine, a by-product of norepinephrine production released locally by BAT, has been shown to have a physiological effect higher than the effect of cold, highlighting its importance in BAT activation [25] (Table 1.1).

Table 1.1 Physiological effects of cold

Haemodynamic	Peripheral (cutaneous) vasoconstriction and/or shivering thermogenesis
	Shift of blood from the periphery to the body core, increased preload and central arterial pressure, reduced HR
	Reduction in heat transfer between the body core and external tissues
	Increased insulation of the body envelope preventing heat dispersion across the exposed body surface (which is faster than it is replaced)
Neuromuscular	Decreased nerve conduction velocity
	Decreased muscle spasticity
	Increased pain threshold
Metabolic	Increased heat production by voluntary muscle contraction, involuntary shivering induced by the central nervous system or both
	Increased heat production by non-contractile tissues: Mitochondria of BAT increase thermogenesis releasing energy directly as heat instead of channelling it into formation of the energy carrier ATP
	Increased CO, HR and SV
	Increased whole-body basal metabolic rate

The Therapeutic Use of Cold: A Centuries-Long History

Cryostimulation, coined to refer to the use of cold exposure among healthy participants (e.g. athletes), is a relatively recent physical treatment based on the positive effects of cold immersion, whereas the term 'cryotherapy' is restricted to the therapeutic use of cold in the management of injuries, disorders and painful conditions, a centuries-old practice. Cryotherapies vary depending on the medium used to achieve the desired purpose: to remove heat, reduce internal and tissue temperature and alter blood flow. They include the use of ice, water or cold air. The ancient Greeks already used cold water for medicinal purposes and analgesic benefits, as well as for relaxation and socialising, as documented by Hippocrates in the 4th century BC [26]. The same procedure appears centuries later, with the first records of human temperatures in health, disease and experimentation in the early 20th century [27].

Whole-Body Cryostimulation

Although the use of cryotherapy methods with cold water and ice for recovery from exercise has long been known, the application of extremely low air temperatures (below -100 °C), typically administered in the form of vaporised liquid nitrogen or refrigerated cold air, is a relatively new technique.

The first whole-body cryostimulation (WBC) chamber was built in Japan around 1978 by Dr. Toshima Yamaguchi, who conducted pioneering work on the treatment of rheumatoid arthritis and pain management in general [28].

Yamaguchi's initial work on the effects of exposure to WBC reported a rapid decrease in the temperature on a person's skin and a reduction in subjective assessment of pain due to an increased release of endorphins. Eighty percent of patients achieved complete relief of symptoms and chronic pain problems. His results were first presented in 1979 and helped promote the use of WBC worldwide. It was not until 1984 that WBC was brought to Europe by Prof. Reinhard Fricke, who established a cryostimulation medical protocol for hundreds of patients with multiple sclerosis and arthritic conditions [28].

Despite the popularity of WBC for the treatment of various diseases, only in the last decade has its use been extended to the world of sports for exercise recovery.

Local or whole-body cold exposure has been used for a number of years in the context of sports and medicine to relieve pain and inflammatory symptoms through cold-induced analgesia [9]. Cryostimulation is in fact an innovative technology that is growing significantly and it is mainly known by the main public for its use in sports medicine after physical exercise (training and/or competition) to reduce effort-related pro-inflammatory responses, to relieve exercise-associated muscle soreness, damage, fatigue and inflammation, and to enhance muscle post-exercise recovery. Two types of cryostimulation are available today in the market: partial body cryostimulation (PBC), in which the subject's body, but not the head (which must stay above the gaseous environment to preserve breathing), is exposed to cold, and total body cryostimulation, in which the whole body is exposed to cold air (WBC). In PBC, cryogenic fluid is injected and vaporised around the body in a cryosauna, while in WBC, cold production is based on vapour compression cycles with refrigerants and/or cryogenic fluids, mostly liquid nitrogen, in a cryochamber.

WBC cryochambers can be: static cold chambers and forced convection chambers based on wind chill. Cryochambers are more sophisticated than cryosauna tanks, but they prevent the problems of anoxia through the use of indirect injections into the chambers, and the entire body is in a cold environment for treatment.

In contrast to the extreme temperatures claimed by device manufacturers, the temperature decreases after -110 °C cold air recorded on the skin (-8 °C to -14 °C), muscles (≈ -1.1 °C) and core (≈ -0.3 °C) are quite moderate. Notably, these differences are smaller in magnitude than those measured after application of ice packs or after immersion in cold water (between 8 °C and 15 °C) [29], a result that, given the laws of thermodynamics, reflects the lower capacity of air to transfer heat compared to ice or water (heat transfer coefficient being 0.024 k, 2.18 k and 0.58, respectively) limiting PBC/WBC capacity to extract cold from the body.

However, in the case of PBC/WBC, this reduction in heat extraction is partly offset by the fact that a much larger body surface area is exposed compared to other cooling techniques.

Regarding the cryostimulation temperature, the manufacturers state that temperatures range from -110 °C to -195 °C in cryosaunas, from -60 °C to -160 °C in static cold WBC technologies and from -40 °C to -60 °C in forced convection WBC technologies [30, 31]. However, studies on the actual temperatures recorded inside the different devices during an exposure showed a range from -10 °C to -42 °C in cryosaunas and -34 °C in a forced convection WBC chamber [32], while no studies reported temperatures in a static cold WBC chamber during the exposure. Thus, it appears that in a closed system such as the cryochamber, cooling is more homogeneous, inducing a greater reduction in average skin temperature over the entire body, while the cooling effect of cryosauna is less pronounced because, being an open system, the gas rises by dispersing into the surrounding environment. Moreover, in cryosaunas the cold temperature is not homogeneous and the coldest areas are located at the bottom of the cabin [33].

The average change in skin temperature can be summarised as follows: ~ -8 °C in a cryosauna after a 3-min exposure is (mean skin temperature after exposure between 22 and 24 °C); ~ -11 °C in a static cold WBC chamber (mean skin temperature after exposure between 18 °C and 20 °C); and ~ -14 °C in a forced convection WBC chamber (mean skin temperature after exposure between 16 °C and 18 °C) [30, 31]. The duration of exposure depends on the protocol used, but can be the same among different devices. The 1-min exposure is commonly administered as the first exposure to subjects enrolled in protocols involving more than one.

General Physiologic Effect of Partial/Whole-Body Cryostimulation

Cryostimulation primarily refers to a device that can rapidly cool the entire body by applying a strong temperature gradient between the inside and outside of the body. The body's general response to cryostimulation follows the physiological processes of the body subjected to cold temperatures indicated in the previous paragraphs. Review of recent studies allows for objective verification of the efficacy of this approach and evaluation of physiological responses in the context of cryostimulation confirming how heat stress induced by cryostimulation causes changes in the endocrine, circulatory, neuromuscular and immunological systems, as it provides an allostatic load on the body's homeostatic systems which, elicit homeostatic autonomic responses of thermogenesis and vasoconstriction [8]. Specifically, the postcryostimulation physiological response mimics that which may occur after exercise to reduce the development of oedema and in reducing inflammation: vasoconstriction resulting in a decrease in the amount of blood in and around muscles and in some organs [34], and decreased fluid diffusion in the interstitial space [35]. In the context of recovery after physical exercise, a WBC/PBC exposure helps recovery by lowering muscle temperature causing reduced muscle enzyme activities, metabolism, inflammation and secondary degradation after hypoxia (lowering ischaemia/reperfusion problems) [30]. The release of norepinephrine from the ends of sympathetic nerve fibres has an impact on pain, and this may explain the analgesic effect of WBC which contributes in relieving the pain symptoms. Besides such mechanisms, cryogenic temperature reduces the conduction velocity of sensory nerve fibres and impulsion in the slow conducting C fibres disabling the sensory receptors as well as their connections with the proprioceptors. In addition, it seems that there is a decrease in the production of pro-inflammatory and oxidative substances, whereas the anti-inflammatory and anti-oxidative compounds are produced in larger quantities [36, 37]. At distance from the cold stimulation, an increase in the parasympathetic cardiac control may also happen, as a compensatory mechanism downregulating the blood pressure [38, 39], even during the night [40]. Changes in muscle, skin and core body temperature, with a maximum drop of core temperature after 50–60 min, and the autonomic and thermal reactions to cryostimulation have been observed even up to 6 h after WBC exposure [32, 39, 41, 42]. Such changes may result not only in lower fatigue sensation but also in mood improvement with positive impact on depression and sleep quality and quantity [43] (Table 1.2).

Source of Variability in the Physiological Response to WBC

Individual characteristics and inter-individual differences, such as body size, BMI, cardiorespiratory fitness level, gender and amount of subcutaneous fat and fat mass, are the primary source of variability in the physiological response to cold as well as WBC [2, 44].

Table 1.2 Symptoms that may benefit from WBC and goals of the treatment

Symptoms	Goals
Pain	Decrease pain and inflammation
Stiffness	Decrease spasticity, pain, inflammation Increase range of motion
Oedema Inflammation Muscular soreness Muscular fatigue	Decrease oedema, inflammation and oxidative stress Reduce effort-related pro-inflammatory responses Promote tissue healing Mimic exercise physiological response Relieve exercise-associated muscle soreness, damage, fatigue and inflammation Enhance muscle post-exercise recovery
Depression Fatigue Disturbed sleep	Enhance homeostatic autonomic responses of thermogenesis, vasoconstriction and vasodilation Increase the parasympathetic cardiac control Increase release of endorphins Reduce fatigue sensation Improves mood, depression and sleep quality/quantity

Anthropometry, Body Composition and Sex

During cryostimulation, the interaction between the cold environment and the body occurs primarily at the skin level from which the heat is transferred to the surrounding environment.

Skin temperature has been shown to decrease significantly after WBC, accompanied by a decrease in core and muscle temperature [41, 45]. Metabolic rate and heat production are also significantly reduced in participants with overweight, compared to lean participants, during light air cooling (15 °C) and a warm-up period after cooling [46]. Consistent with the relationship between BMI and cooling, differences in the degree of skin temperature cooling have been reported between high and low BMI in individuals following WBC [47] with a medium positive correlation between BMI and the decrease of the mean body temperature after WBC. Other studies examined the impact of WBC on skin temperature. Klimek et al. reported that in women, thigh surface temperature remained decreased for 75 min after WBC in women and 90 min in men [48]. Hammond et al. study showed that skin response of individuals to WBC appears to depend upon anthropometric variables and sex, with females demonstrating higher levels of both adiposity and cooling than males [49]. Moreover, a significant relationship was observed between body fat percentage and ΔTsk in the combined dataset and between fat-free mass index and ΔTsk in males. The study of Polidori et al. seems to confirm the higher capacity of cooling in females since for achieving the same cold-induced response, the required duration of cryostimulation is longer for males [50]. Along with skin temperature, several papers showed the decrease in muscle and core temperature but with little attention paid to sexual dimorphism (such as adiposity and menstrual cycle), morphological and protocol differences.

The effectiveness of cryogenic stimulus is directly related to individual fat mass percentage and initial fitness capacity. WBC has important anti-inflammatory/antioxidant effects that may counteract the decreased activity of antioxidant enzymes found with increased body fat and central obesity [51]. This could explain the fact that WBC exerted an antioxidant effect only in normal-weight subjects, whereas subjects with obesity had higher basal levels of oxidative stress than their lean counterparts, and their total oxidative status and antioxidant capacity did not change after 20 sessions of WBC [52].

Cardiovascular System and Cardiorespiratory Fitness Level

In addition to changes in surface body temperature, WBC also affects the cardiovascular system. The decrease in HR after exposure to cryogenic temperatures is followed by an increase in SV and stroke index (SI). In contrast, systolic (sBP), diastolic (dBP) and mean (mBP) blood pressure values, cardiac indices (CO, CI) and total peripheral resistance (TPR, TPRI) do not vary in response to WBC [53, 54]. However, the range of changes in the above parameters suggests that WBC could cause an increase in preload without affecting afterload of the heart [53]. However, Lubkowska and Suska (2011) reported a significant increase in sBP and dBP as a form of whole-body stress response to cryostimulation [55]. Interestingly, women and men seem to have the same cardiovascular responses to WBC [56].

Globally, even if the findings are not always in line, WBC appears to yield an anti-inflammatory effect that is highly correlated with the fitness level in individuals with obesity.

Not several studies focus on fitness level specifically, being many performed on just athletes (which should have a high fitness level) or healthy individuals not characterised in that matter.

Ziemann et al. compared the results obtained in participants with low (LCF) and high cardiorespiratory fitness (HCF). The authors reported a significant decrease in tumour necrosis factor alpha (TNFα) concentration in subjects with obesity after ten 3-min WBC sessions at -110 °C from their baseline values, which were elevated, most likely due to low-grade systemic inflammation. This result was correlated with cardiorespiratory fitness since the difference was more pronounced in LCF as compared to HCF [57].

In HCF and LCF subjects with obesity, 10 sessions of WBC increased Interleukin-10 (IL-10) and the rise was sustained 24 h after the last session. Interestingly, baseline values of IL-10 were already significantly higher in the LCF group, suggesting that elevated IL-10 concentrations could be a component of the enhanced defensive response to low-grade systemic inflammation.

However, the results are not always as expected. Dulian et al. confirmed the anti-inflammatory effect of WBC in people with obesity, reporting that the decline in C-reactive protein (CRP) levels was similar in both the low fitness (LFL) and high fitness (HFL) level group with obesity regardless of the number of sessions (either 1 and 10) [58]. A similar decrease was also observed in well-trained athletes exposed to 5 sessions of WBC for up to 96 h after exercise [59]. However, WBC did not induce significant changes in men or menopausal women with obesity, regardless of their body mass (high or normal) or comorbidity with metabolic syndrome reproducing the results obtained by Śliwicka and colleagues who did not show significant changes in CRP levels after 10 WBC treatments in 20-year-old men without obesity, regardless of their fitness level [60].

Physiological Adjustments to Prolonged or Repeated Cold Exposure to WBC

Chronic exposure to cold, regardless of the type of exposure (prolonged, serial, intermittent, etc.), results in changes in physiological responses called adjustments, not to be confused with the adaptation process. In contrast to physiological adjustments to heat, chronic exposure to cold can produce three different patterns of physiological adjustments: 1) habituation, 2) metabolic adjustments and 3) insulative adjustments. Habituation is distinguished by physiological adaptations characterised by attenuated responses compared to an unacclimatised state. Metabolic acclimatisation is characterised by an increased thermogenesis, whereas insulative acclimatisation is characterised by enhancing the mechanisms that maintain body heat. The rate of acclimatisation depends on changes in skin and core temperature and the duration of exposure. Heat exposure usually involves the whole body producing overall systemic adjustments, while cooling often involves smaller regions (head, face, hands, feet, etc.) keeping the rest of the body protected from cold stress [2]. Therefore, local or regional adjustments in physiological responses may be more readily experienced with chronic cold exposure than with chronic heat exposure.

Habituation

Habituation represents the most common physiological adjustment to repeated exposure to WBC. A significant increase in plasma norepinephrine has been found after a single session of WBC at $-110\ °C$, while this increase decreases after several exposures [38, 61, 62], as per the lower autonomic response recorded compared to the first day. These observations suggest not only a reduction in sympathetic activation but also a lower amplification of heat shock over time and a consequent increase in treatment dose from one cycle to the next to delay habituation [63]. Furthermore, the first cold exposure (both PBC and WBC) may trigger an initial psychological stress response that disappears or subsides with new or subsequent exposure suggesting that the degree of habituation developed in response to cold exposure might be related to the severity of the stress, such as the duration of the exposure.

Metabolic Adaptations

The increase in metabolic rate upon cold exposure has long been known. Cold exposure increases resting energy expenditure (REE) by activating shivering and the non-shivering thermogenesis in tissues including WAT, BAT and skeletal muscle. Moreover, cold exposure increases lipid catabolism and WAT trans-differentiation into BAT thermogenesis in order to increase thermogenesis [64–66]. In humans,

BAT increases free fatty acids (FFA) uptake, metabolic rate [67, 68] and cell number [69] to maintain the body temperature in response to cold. Moreover, cold-induced BAT activation could enhance glucose uptake and improve whole-body glucose disposal and insulin sensitivity [70–72]. The increased oxidative metabolism in BAT directly contributes to augmented REE upon cold exposure [65]. However, there is still little evidence that cold acclimatisation produces sufficient enhancement of the thermogenic response to cold (shivering or non-shivering) to provide any meaningful thermoregulatory benefit for cold exposed humans [2]. After acute cold exposure, the REE significantly increased in healthy people with detectable BAT levels [73]. However, no increase in REE was observed in individuals with obesity exposed to a short-term acute cold due to the small number of BAT activations (Hanssen et al. 2016) or in people living in the deserts of Australia and southern Africa exposed to repeated nocturnal cold exposure [74, 75]. Similarly, cold-induced thermogenesis was not changed in people sleeping in a room at 19 °C for 1 month [76].

Only one obesity study has shown that single or multiple sessions of PBC significantly induced REE increase in women with normal weight and with obesity, although it showed different efficacy as those with obesity were less responsive than controls with normal weight [77].

The explanation could be: the lower amount and lower activity of BAT (metabolically active adipocytes that can increase REE), which has been found to be inversely related to BMI and lower in subjects with obesity than in lean subjects [70, 78]; lower free fat mass that is known to be critical for non-chill thermogenesis [65]; lower skeletal muscle mass that is responsible for heat production and energy expenditure through mechanisms such as proton leakage and substrate synthesis and degradation [65]; a dysfunctional WAT, which, through altered insulin signalling [79], lipid oxidation [80], mitochondrial function [81] found in obesity, can affect muscle metabolism and its substrate oxidation, reducing its thermogenic capacity in response to cooling; the poor thermogenic activity of WAT.

Some studies suggest that exposure to WBC may induce at least a short-term improvement in metabolic profile that could fuel more complex preventive strategies, including physical activity and pharmacological interventions, by improving peripheral insulin sensitivity as well as brown adipose tissue (BAT) mass and activity [82], counteracting the risk of developing insulin resistance (IR), type-2 diabetes mellitus (T2DM) [79] and the inflammatory state associated with obesity [8]. Moreover, WBC seems to affect the expression of myokines and adipokines suggesting a more systematic use of WBC as a possible therapeutic strategy in individuals with metabolic diseases [9].

Among the advantages of cold exposure in the form of WBC, in the literature we can find a shift in the hormones fibroblast growth factor 21 (FGF21) and irisin [58, 80]. FGF21 is a potent, extracellularly acting metabolic regulator, involved in the regulation of lipid, glucose and energy metabolism. FGF21 promotes glucose uptake in fat, whereas in the liver, it stimulates gluconeogenesis and decreases lipolysis. Its expression is selectively increased in the liver by fasting, by overfeeding in the pancreas, by exercise in muscle and by cold exposure in BAT enhancing the core body temperature and decreasing the respiratory quotient. Irisin is a hormone secreted from skeletal muscles in response to exercise and mediates the beneficial effects of exercise in humans, such as weight loss and thermoregulation, playing a role in boosting thermogenesis in humans, thus mediating part of the exercise-induced weight loss. An increase of irisin causes the browning of WATs thus improving adiposity and glucose homeostasis since it stimulates the activation of p38 and ERK signalling, enabling UCP-1 expression in adipocytes [81]. Moreover, studies have shown that irisin possesses protective properties against obesity, IR and non-alcoholic fatty liver disease (NAFLD), showing in some of these metabolic alterations a correlation with inflammatory markers, which suggests that irisin may regulate the inflammatory response and the expression of inflammatory genes or even reduce oxidative stress in macrophages and endothelial cells [83]. Interestingly, Dulian and collaborators noted an increase of irisin level in response to 10 sessions of WBC in inactive men with obesity, which was also positively correlated with subcutaneous fat tissue [58].

Chronic and acute WBC exposure leads also to an improvement in glucose homeostasis indicators together with an improved amino acid profile, suggesting an increased metabolism of branched-chain amino acids (BCAA) in skeletal muscle during WBC. In one study, these changes were accompanied by a decline of serum myostatin concentration which, in addition to regulating muscle cell growth, seems to inhibit glucose uptake, therefore contributing to systemic IR and metabolic deregulations such as obesity, T2DM and ageing, when at elevated levels [79].

Overall, the use of WBC induces at least a short-term improvement in metabolic profile supporting its preventive role and, when combined with physical activity and possibly pharmacological interventions, could be effective against the risk of developing IR and T2DM.

Insulative Adaptations

Insulative adaptations are represented by the enhanced heat preservation mechanisms and a lower skin temperature when exposed to cold with unchanged metabolic rates and core temperatures. Thus, with insulative acclimatisation, cold exposure elicits faster and more pronounced cutaneous vasoconstricton resulting in lower thermal conductance of the skin than that observed in the unacclimatised state. As a result, the decline in skin temperature is greater in the acclimatised than unacclimatised state. Perceptual and affective adaptations to repeated cold stress have received little attention. One study only addressed thermal sensation and thermal comfort ratings associated with WBC (and winter swimming in ice cold water) in women. The results showed that thermal sensation and comfort became habituated at an early stage of trials, during the first exposure, with cold sensation being less intense already after the second exposure [84]. This may be due to the short exposure times without significant core cooling with concomitant autonomic effector responses and/or psychological factors.

References

1. Ivanov KP. Modern theoretical and practical problems of homoiothermia and thermoregulation. Ross Fiziol Zh Im I M Sechenova. 2006;92:578–92.
2. Castellani JW, Young AJ. Human physiological responses to cold exposure: acute responses and acclimatization to prolonged exposure. Auton Neurosci Basic Clin. 2016;196:63–74.
3. Young AJ, Sawka MN, Kent BP. Physiology of Cold Exposure. National Academies Press (US); 1996.
4. Lim CL, Byrne C, Lee JK. Human Thermoregulation and Measurement of Body Temperature in Exercise and Clinical Settings. Ann Acad Med Singap. 2008;37(4):347–53.
5. Charkoudian N. Mechanisms and modifiers of reflex induced cutaneous vasodilation and vasoconstriction in humans. J Appl Physiol. 2010;109:1221–8.
6. Cheshire WP. Thermoregulatory disorders and illness related to heat and cold stress. Auton Neurosci Basic Clin. 2016;196:91–104.
7. Romanovsky AA. Skin temperature: its role in thermoregulation. Acta Physiol Oxf Engl. 2014;210:498–507.
8. White GE, Wells GD. Cold-water immersion and other forms of cryotherapy: physiological changes potentially affecting recovery from high-intensity exercise. Extreme Physiol Med. 2013;2:26.
9. Fontana JM, Bozgeyik S, Gobbi M, Piterà P, Giusti EM, Dugué B, Lombardi G, Capodaglio P. Whole-body cryostimulation in obesity. A scoping review J Therm Biol. 2022;106:103250.
10. Bouzigon R, Dupuy O, Tiemessen I, De Nardi M, Bernard J-P, Mihailovic T, Theurot D, Miller ED, Lombardi G, Dugué BM. Cryostimulation for post-exercise recovery in athletes: a consensus and position paper. Front Sports Act Living. 2021;3:688828.
11. Horvath SM. Exercise In a Cold Environment. Exerc Sport Sci Rev. 1981;9:221.
12. Frank SM, Raja SN, Bulcao CF, Goldstein DS. Relative contribution of core and cutaneous temperatures to thermal comfort and autonomic responses in humans. J Appl Physiol. 1999;86(5):1588–93. https://doi.org/10.1152/jappl.1999.86.5.1588. Accessed 16 Jan 2023
13. Bell DG, Tikuisis P, Jacobs I. Relative intensity of muscular contraction during shivering. J Appl Physiol. 1992;72:2336–42.
14. Castellani JW, Young AJ, Ducharme MB, Giesbrecht GG, Glickman E, Sallis RE. American College of Sports Medicine. American College of Sports Medicine position stand: prevention of cold injuries during exercise. Med Sci Sports Exerc. 2006;38(11):2012–29.
15. Muza SR, Young AJ, Sawka MN, Bogart JE, Pandolf KB. Respiratory and cardiovascular responses to cold stress following repeated cold water immersion. Undersea Biomed Res. 1988;15:165–78.
16. Golden FS, Hampton IF, Hervey GR, Knibbs AV. Shivering intensity in humans during immersion in cold water [proceedings]. J Physiol. 1979;290:48P.
17. Himms-Hagen J. Nonshivering thermogenesis. Brain Res Bull. 1984;12:151–60.
18. Carpentier AC, Blondin DP, Virtanen KA, Richard D, Haman F, Turcotte ÉE. Brown adipose tissue energy metabolism in humans. Front Endocrinol. 2018;9:447.
19. Schrauwen-Hinderling VB. Carpentier AC (2018) molecular imaging of postprandial metabolism. J Appl Physiol Bethesda Md. 1985;124:504–11.
20. Weir G, Ramage LE, Akyol M, et al. Substantial metabolic activity of human Brown adipose tissue during warm conditions and cold-induced lipolysis of local triglycerides. Cell Metab. 2018;27:1348–1355.e4.
21. Din MU, Saari T, Raiko J, et al. Postprandial oxidative metabolism of human Brown fat indicates thermogenesis. Cell Metab. 2018;28:207–216.e3.
22. Blondin DP, Tingelstad HC, Noll C, Frisch F, Phoenix S, Guérin B, Turcotte ÉE, Richard D, Haman F, Carpentier AC. Dietary fatty acid metabolism of brown adipose tissue in cold-acclimated men. Nat Commun. 2017;8:14146.
23. Klímová J, Mráz M, Kratochvílová H, et al. Gene profile of adipose tissue of patients with Pheochromocytoma/Paraganglioma. Biomedicines. 2022;10:586.

24. Søndergaard E, Gormsen LC, Christensen MH, Pedersen SB, Christiansen P, Nielsen S, Poulsen PL, Jessen N. Chronic adrenergic stimulation induces brown adipose tissue differentiation in visceral adipose tissue. Diabet Med J Br Diabet Assoc. 2015;32:e4–8.
25. Lahesmaa M, Oikonen V, Helin S, Luoto P, Din MU, Pfeifer A, Nuutila P, Virtanen KA. Regulation of human brown adipose tissue by adenosine and A2A receptors - studies with [15O]H2O and [11C]TMSX PET/CT. Eur J Nucl Med Mol Imaging. 2019;46:743–50.
26. Tsoucalas G, Sgantzos M, Karamanou M, Gritzalis K, Androutsos G. Hydrotherapy: Historical landmarks of a cure all remedy. Arch. Balk. Med. Union. 2015;50:430–2.
27. Lamotte G, Boes CJ, Low PA, Coon EA. The expanding role of the cold pressor test: a brief history. Clin Auton Res. 2021;31:153–5.
28. Allan R, Malone J, Alexander J, Vorajee S, Ihsan M, Gregson W, Kwiecien S, Mawhinney C. Cold for centuries: a brief history of cryotherapies to improve health, injury and post-exercise recovery. Eur J Appl Physiol. 2022;122:1153–62.
29. Bleakley CM, Bieuzen F, Davison GW, Costello JT. Whole-body cryotherapy: empirical evidence and theoretical perspectives. Open Access J Sports Med. 2014;5:25–36.
30. Bouzigon R, Grappe F, Ravier G, Dugue B. Whole- and partial-body cryostimulation/cryotherapy: current technologies and practical applications. J Therm Biol. 2016;61:67–81.
31. Bouzigon R, Arfaoui A, Grappe F, Ravier G, Jarlot B, Dugue B. Validation of a new whole-body cryotherapy chamber based on forced convection. J Therm Biol. 2017;65:138–44.
32. Savic M, Fonda B, Sarabon N. Actual temperature during and thermal response after whole-body cryotherapy in cryo-cabin. J Therm Biol. 2013;38:186–91.
33. Bouzigon R, Ravier G, Dugue B, Grappe F. Thermal sensations during a partial-body Cryostimulation exposure in elite basketball players. J Hum Kinet. 2018;62:55–63.
34. Charkoudian N. Skin blood flow in adult human thermoregulation: how it works, when it does not, and why. Mayo Clin Proc. 2003;78:603–12.
35. Banfi G, Melegati G, Barassi A, d'Eril GM. Effects of the whole-body cryotherapy on NTproBNP, hsCRP and troponin I in athletes. J Sci Med Sport. 2009;12:609–10.
36. Lombardi G, Ziemann E, Banfi G. Whole-body cryotherapy in athletes: from therapy to stimulation. An updated review of the literature. Front. Physiol. 2017;8:258.
37. Banfi G, Lombardi G, Colombini A, Melegati G. Whole-body cryotherapy in athletes. Sports Med Auckl NZ. 2010;40:509–17.
38. Louis J, Theurot D, Filliard J-R, Volondat M, Dugué B, Dupuy O. The use of whole-body cryotherapy: time- and dose-response investigation on circulating blood catecholamines and heart rate variability. Eur J Appl Physiol. 2020;120:1733–43.
39. Zalewski P, Bitner A, Słomko J, Szrajda J, Klawe JJ, Tafil-Klawe M, Newton JL. Whole-body cryostimulation increases parasympathetic outflow and decreases core body temperature. J Therm Biol. 2014;45:75–80.
40. Douzi W, Dupuy O, Tanneau M, Boucard G, Bouzigon R, Dugué B. 3-min whole body cryotherapy/cryostimulation after training in the evening improves sleep quality in physically active men. Eur J Sport Sci. 2019;19:860–7.
41. Costello JT, Culligan K, Selfe J, Donnelly AE. Muscle, skin and Core temperature after −110°C cold air and 8°C water treatment. PLoS One. 2012;7:e48190.
42. Costello JT, Baker PRA, Minett GM, Bieuzen F, Stewart IB, Bleakley C. Whole-body cryotherapy (extreme cold air exposure) for preventing and treating muscle soreness after exercise in adults. Cochrane Database Syst Rev. 2015;2015(9):CD010789.
43. Rymaszewska J, Ramsey D, Chładzińska-Kiejna S. Whole-body cryotherapy as adjunct treatment of depressive and anxiety disorders. Arch Immunol Ther Exp. 2008;56:63–8.
44. Gordon CJ, Fogarty AL, Greenleaf JE, Taylor NAS, Stocks JM. Direct and indirect methods for determining plasma volume during thermoneutral and cold-water immersion. Eur J Appl Physiol. 2003;89:471–4.
45. Selfe J, Alexander J, Costello JT, et al. The effect of three different (−135°C) whole body cryotherapy exposure durations on elite Rugby league players. PLoS One. 2014;9:e86420.

46. Ooijen AMJC, Westerterp KR, Wouters L, Schoffelen PFM, van Steenhoven AA, van Lichtenbelt WDM. Heat production and body temperature during cooling and rewarming in overweight and lean men. Obesity. 2006;14:1914–20.

47. Cholewka A, Stanek A, Sieroń A, Drzazga Z. Thermography study of skin response due to whole-body cryotherapy. Skin Res Technol. 2012;18:180–7.

48. Klimek AT, Lubkowska A, Szyguła Z, Frączek B, Chudecka M. The influence of single whole body cryostimulation treatment on the dynamics and the level of maximal anaerobic power. Int J Occup Med Environ Health. 2011;24:184–91.

49. Hammond LE, Cuttell S, Nunley P, Meyler J. Anthropometric characteristics and sex influence magnitude of skin cooling following exposure to whole body cryotherapy. Biomed Res Int. 2014;2014:628724.

50. Polidori G, Elfahem R, Abbes B, Bogard F, Legrand F, Bouchet B, Beaumont F. Preliminary study on the effect of sex on skin cooling response during whole body cryostimulation (−110 °C): modeling and prediction of exposure durations. Cryobiology. 2020;97:12–9.

51. Manna P, Jain SK. Obesity, oxidative stress, adipose tissue dysfunction, and the associated health risks: causes and therapeutic strategies. Metab Syndr Relat Disord. 2015;13:423–44.

52. Pilch W, Wyrostek J, Piotrowska A, Czerwińska-Ledwig O, Zuziak R, Sadowska-Krępa E, Maciejczyk M, Żychowska M. Blood pro-oxidant/antioxidant balance in young men with class II obesity after 20 sessions of whole body cryostimulation: a preliminary study. Redox Rep. 2021;26:10–7.

53. Zalewski P, Klawe JJ, Pawlak J, Tafil-Klawe M, Newton J. Thermal and hemodynamic response to whole-body cryostimulation in healthy subjects. Cryobiology. 2013;66:295–302.

54. Bonomi FG, De Nardi M, Fappani A, Zani V, Banfi G. Impact of different treatment of whole-body cryotherapy on circulatory parameters. Arch Immunol Ther Exp. 2012;60:145–50.

55. Lubkowska A, Suska M. The increase in systolic and diastolic blood pressure after exposure to cryogenic temperatures in normotensive men as a contraindication for whole-body cryostimulation. J Therm Biol. 2011;36:264–8.

56. Westerlund T, Oksa J, Smolander J, Mikkelsson M. Neuromuscular adaptation after repeated exposure to whole-body cryotherapy (−110°C). J Therm Biol. 2009;34:226–31.

57. Ziemann E, Olek RA, Grzywacz T, Antosiewicz J, Kujach S, Łuszczyk M, Smaruj M, Śledziewska E, Laskowski R. Whole-body cryostimulation as an effective method of reducing low-grade inflammation in obese men. J Physiol Sci. 2013;63:333–43.

58. Dulian K, Laskowski R, Grzywacz T, Kujach S, Flis DJ, Smaruj M, Ziemann E. The whole body cryostimulation modifies irisin concentration and reduces inflammation in middle aged, obese men. Cryobiology. 2015;71:398–404.

59. Pournot H, Bieuzen F, Louis J, Fillard J-R, Barbiche E, Hausswirth C. Time-course of changes in inflammatory response after whole-body cryotherapy multi exposures following severe exercise. PLoS One. 2011;6:e22748.

60. Śliwicka E, Cisoń T, Straburzyńska-Lupa A, Pilaczyńska-Szcześniak Ł. Effects of whole-body cryotherapy on 25-hydroxyvitamin D, irisin, myostatin, and interleukin-6 levels in healthy young men of different fitness levels. Sci Rep. 2020;10:6175.

61. Leppäluoto J, Westerlund T, Huttunen P, Oksa J, Smolander J, Dugué B, Mikkelsson M. Effects of long-term whole-body cold exposures on plasma concentrations of ACTH, beta-endorphin, cortisol, catecholamines and cytokines in healthy females. Scand J Clin Lab Invest. 2008;68:145–53.

62. Mäkinen TM, Mäntysaari M, Pääkkönen T, Jokelainen J, Palinkas LA, Hassi J, Leppäluoto J, Tahvanainen K, Rintamäki H. Autonomic nervous function during whole-body cold exposure before and after cold acclimation. Aviat Space Environ Med. 2008;79:875–82.

63. Yurkevicius BR, Alba BK, Seeley AD, Castellani JW. Human cold habituation: physiology, timeline, and modifiers. Temp Austin Tex. 2022;9:122–57.

64. Vallerand AL, Jacobs I. Rates of energy substrates utilization during human cold exposure. Eur J Appl Physiol. 1989;58:873–8.

65. Palmer BF, Clegg DJ. Non-shivering thermogenesis as a mechanism to facilitate sustainable weight loss. Obes Rev. 2017;18:819–31.

66. Huo C, Song Z, Yin J, Zhu Y, Miao X, Qian H, Wang J, Ye L, Zhou L. Effect of acute cold exposure on energy metabolism and activity of Brown adipose tissue in humans: a systematic review and meta-analysis. Front Physiol. 2022;13:917084.
67. Ouellet V, Labbé SM, Blondin DP, Phoenix S, Guérin B, Haman F, Turcotte EE, Richard D, Carpentier AC. Brown adipose tissue oxidative metabolism contributes to energy expenditure during acute cold exposure in humans. J Clin Invest. 2012;122:545–52.
68. Leitner BP, Huang S, Brychta RJ, et al. Mapping of human brown adipose tissue in lean and obese young men. Proc Natl Acad Sci USA. 2017;114:8649–54.
69. Klingenspor M. Cold-induced recruitment of brown adipose tissue thermogenesis. Exp Physiol. 2003;88:141–8.
70. Yoneshiro T, Aita S, Matsushita M, Kayahara T, Kameya T, Kawai Y, Iwanaga T, Saito M. Recruited brown adipose tissue as an antiobesity agent in humans. J Clin Invest. 2013;123:3404–8.
71. van Marken Lichtenbelt WD, Vanhommerig JW, Smulders NM, Drossaerts JMAFL, Kemerink GJ, Bouvy ND, Schrauwen P, Teule GJJ. Cold-activated brown adipose tissue in healthy men. N Engl J Med. 2009;360:1500–8.
72. Virtanen KA, Lidell ME, Orava J, et al. Functional brown adipose tissue in healthy adults. N Engl J Med. 2009;360:1518–25.
73. Chondronikola M, Volpi E, Børsheim E, et al. Brown adipose tissue improves whole-body glucose homeostasis and insulin sensitivity in humans. Diabetes. 2014;63:4089–99.
74. Scholander PF, Hammel HT, Hart JS, Lemessurier DH, Steen J. Cold adaptation in Australian aborigines. J Appl Physiol. 1958;13:211–8.
75. Wyndham CH, Morrison JF. Adjustment to cold of bushmen in the Kalahari Desert. J Appl Physiol. 1958;13:219–25.
76. Lee P, Smith S, Linderman J, Courville AB, Brychta RJ, Dieckmann W, Werner CD, Chen KY, Celi FS. Temperature-acclimated brown adipose tissue modulates insulin sensitivity in humans. Diabetes. 2014;63:3686–98.
77. De Nardi M, Bisio A, Della Guardia L, Facheris C, Faelli E, La Torre A, Luzi L, Ruggeri P, Codella R. Partial-body Cryostimulation increases resting energy expenditure in lean and obese women. Int J Environ Res Public Health. 2021;18:4127.
78. Pfannenberg C, Werner MK, Ripkens S, Stef I, Deckert A, Schmadl M, Reimold M, Häring H-U, Claussen CD, Stefan N. Impact of age on the relationships of brown adipose tissue with sex and adiposity in humans. Diabetes. 2010;59:1789–93.
79. Kozłowska M, Kortas J, Żychowska M, Antosiewicz J, Żuczek K, Perego S, Lombardi G, Ziemann E. Beneficial effects of whole-body cryotherapy on glucose homeostasis and amino acid profile are associated with a reduced myostatin serum concentration. Sci Rep. 2021;11:7097.
80. Lee P, Linderman JD, Smith S, et al. Irisin and FGF21 are cold-induced endocrine activators of Brown fat function in humans. Cell Metab. 2014;19:302–9.
81. Zhang Y, Li R, Meng Y, et al. Irisin stimulates browning of white adipocytes through mitogen-activated protein kinase p38 MAP kinase and ERK MAP kinase signaling. Diabetes. 2014;63:514–25.
82. Hanssen MJW, van der Lans AAJJ, Brans B, Hoeks J, Jardon KMC, Schaart G, Mottaghy FM, Schrauwen P, van Marken Lichtenbelt WD. Short-term cold acclimation recruits Brown adipose tissue in obese humans. Diabetes. 2016;65:1179–89.
83. Chen Z, Yang L, Liu Y, Huang P, Song H, Zheng P. The potential function and clinical application of FGF21 in metabolic diseases. Front. Pharmacol. 2022;13:1089214.
84. Smolander J, Mikkelsson M, Oksa J, Westerlund T, Leppäluoto J, Huttunen P. Thermal sensation and comfort in women exposed repeatedly to whole-body cryotherapy and winter swimming in ice-cold water. Physiol Behav. 2004;82:691–5.

Adaptive Endocrine and Metabolic Effects

2

Giovanni Lombardi

Introduction

Metabolic and endocrine responses to whole-body cryotherapy (WBC) represent one of the most widely investigated aspects in cryostimulation settings, together with the inflammatory responses. The established, although not univocally defined, metabolic effects of short-term exposure to extreme cold support the use of this therapeutic strategy, as an adjuvant of the standard pharmacological treatments, in several dysfunctional or pathological conditions in which a deregulated metabolic response, either primary or secondary to an inflammatory disease, exists.

Despite the richness of the literature, most of the studies are rather observational and 'limited' to the description of the response. On the other hand, the knowledge about the biological mechanisms behind these responses is quite limited. Therefore, in order to provide a better contextualisation of the observations made in humans exposed to WBC, there is the need to recapitulate what is already known, starting from the genetic inheritance that makes possible this adaptability and moving to the main concept of adaptation to cold.

G. Lombardi (✉)

Laboratory of Experimental Biochemistry and Molecular Biology, IRCCS Istituto Ortopedico Galeazzi, Milan, Italy

Department of Athletics, Strength and Conditioning, Poznań University of Physical Education, Poznań, Poland

e-mail: giovanni.lombardi@grupposandonato.it; lombardi@awf.poznan.pl

P. Capodaglio (ed.), *Whole-Body Cryostimulation*, https://doi.org/10.1007/978-3-031-18545-8_2

Human Adaptation to Cold: A Matter of Fact

During his evolution, human beings have moved from the area of origin toward higher latitudes and colonised Asia and Europe but, also, faced up to climate changes that brought the environment to pretty extreme conditions.

Among the human ancestors, Neanderthals occupied different regional niches across a large territory from southern Spain to southern Siberia. Although not all Neanderthals lived in cold environments, much of Neanderthal anatomy and physiology are cold-adapted. Similarly, although living in harsh, cold regions represented a relevant push to adaptation, recent analyses suggest other forces like genetic drift and developmental plasticity are a better explanation for some aspects. Besides body shape (i.e. the ratio between body surface and volume, in favour of the latter) and broad, short nasal morphology that clearly represented either adaptation or advantageous features that helped adaptation to cold, also specific metabolic features characterised this ancestor. Investigators have attempted to estimate Neanderthal total energy expenditure (TEE, kcal/day), which consists of basal metabolic rate (BMR, kcal/day), thermic effect of food (TEF), physical activity levels (PAL) and thermoregulatory costs. It is likely Neanderthals had extremely high TEEs, and they experienced all around increased metabolic costs for each component of TEE as a result of inhabiting, navigating, and extracting energy from cold, harsh environments. These high TEE estimates correlate well with the morphological features (short stature, broad noses, large, broad chests) since they conferred larger oxygen intake capacity, which would have supported the high energy demand. Further high BMR was driven by high thyroid hormone levels and the high TEE was supported by a protein-enriched diet (up to 35%) and high PAL (up to 3.0). Interestingly, by comparing Neanderthals and anatomically modern humans, it emerged that our ancestors were inefficient in terms of locomotion and, therefore, in combination with the high PAL, the resulting high energy expenditure likely served as a key source of heat production [1].

From this background, it seems evident that several genetic traits that were induced by (or accompanied) the adaptation to cold are still part of the genetic heritage of modern humans. Therefore, cold exposure has the potential, driven by the neurohumoral activation, to profoundly affect homeostasis and, therefore, to induce multiple metabolic responses aimed to restore it.

Metabolic and Endocrine Adaptation to Cold

Adaptation to cold may occur, in humans, through acclimatisation or acclimation. The adaptation includes, besides genetic and morphological changes, several physiologic and behavioural responses. Acclimatisation and acclimation have been widely studied in several different contexts, from indigenous populations, to polar or ski expeditions, sporting activities, military training, in urban people, or under controlled conditions involving exposures to cold air or water. Divergences in results represent a common motif in this research area, but the main cold adaptation responses have been identified in insulative (circulatory adjustments, increase of fat layer) or metabolic (shivering or non-shivering thermogenesis) responses and they can result into a positive (enhanced) or negative (blunted) adaptation. The pattern of cold adaptation is dependent on the type (air, water) and intensity (continuous, intermittent) of the cold exposure. In addition, several subject-specific variables (e.g. age, gender, body composition, exercise, diet, cardiopulmonary fitness and health status) affect the responses to cold. Habituation of thermal sensations is the first response to cold stress, immediately followed by the cardiovascular one. Metabolic and endocrine responses intervene thereafter. Adaptation is more effective with prolonged duration or higher frequency of the cold stimulus, while if the stimulus is discontinued, adaptation will gradually disappear. Noteworthy, some of the responses can even be harmful and predisposed to cold injuries (e.g. habituation to cold sensation) [2].

From a metabolic point of view, cold exposure elicits heat production in order to offset heat loss.

Insulative Response

Peripheral vasoconstriction reduces skin temperature, effectively reducing heat loss at expense, however, of the nutritive blood flow to the extremities, putting viable tissue in danger. This is saved by the 'hunting response', that is, alternation of vasoconstriction and vasodilation, that reduces heat loss, but also protects the extremities [3, 4]. Counter-current heat exchange occurs when blood is shunted to deep vessels of the extremities and heat from deep arteries transfers to veins to warm cold venous blood returning to the heart to maintain core body temperature. With insulative acclimatisation, thermal conductance at the skin is lower during cold exposure than observed in the non-acclimatised state due to a more rapid and cutaneous vasoconstrictor response: as a result, the decline in skin temperature (T_{skin}) during cold exposure is greater in the acclimatised than non-acclimatised state. An example was given by the thermoregulatory responses of Aborigines from Australian outback who were measured, while they slept naked outdoors in 5 °C cold air, and compared to responses of non-acclimatised European control subjects exposed to similar conditions. BMR of non-adapted European subjects increased, while the Aborigines' BMR remained unchanged as ambient temperature fell, while their core temperature (T_{core}) and T_{skin} fell more than in the Europeans, evidencing a lower thermal conductance. Ama diving women of Korea, who dove daily without protective suits in water at 27 °C in summer and 10 °C in winter, exhibited greater insulation than non-divers. Interestingly, the enhanced insulation of the diving women did not appear to be the result of a more pronounced vasoconstrictor response to cold. It was speculated that the insulative acclimatisation exhibited by the Ama divers represented development of an improved counter-current heat exchange mechanism in the peripheral circulatory system. However, studies to confirm that speculation are not available [5].

Healthy young men, never exposed to significant cold, were exposed to 90-min immersions in 18 °C water, 5 days/week for 8 weeks. At the end of the cold acclimatisation programme, they showed physiological adjustments consistent with hypothermic habituation (i.e. blunted thermogenic response to cold) and others more consistent with the development of an insulative acclimatisation: a more pronounced rise in blood norepinephrine concentrations and a greater decline in T_{skin}, suggesting the development of a more pronounced cutaneous vasoconstriction, in response to cold [6]. These findings were later confirmed by other researchers [5], and insulative adaptations have also been demonstrated in adult and young children undergoing CWI [7, 8]. Interestingly, during resting CWI, T_{core} declined in acclimatised swimmers, whereas exercising while CWI did not cause any decline in T_{core} [7].

Metabolic Response

In humans, skeletal muscle contractile activity accounts for the greatest portion of cold-induced thermogenesis. Thermogenesis is initiated by voluntary behavioural modifications consisting in increasing physical activity (e.g. exercise, increased fidgeting) or shivering. Shivering is due to small muscle contractions, which result in a metabolic rate increase although only a minimal, inefficient increase in body heat production and, as such, it is not an optimal long-term physiological solution to cold exposure [9]. However, in the case of robust musculature, as for Neanderthal, it is possible that the shivering-produced heat could be more efficient [1]. Shivering starts either immediately or after several minutes of cold exposure, and is triggered by the decrease in skin temperature, but the greatest stimulus is provided by the fall in core temperature (with a T_{core}/T_{skin} ratio of 3.6:1 [10]). Maximal shivering is obtained at T_{core} = 34–35 °C and ceases at T_{core} = 31 °C [11]; it usually starts in the torso and moves to limbs. Shivering usually begins in the torso muscles and then spreads to the limbs, and intensity and extent depend on the severity of cold stress [12]. The greater is the shivering intensity increases, the more are the muscles recruited to shiver the greater is the increase in whole-body metabolic rate increases: 200–250 W during exposure to cold air, greater than 350 W during cold water immersion (CWI) up to 763 W recorded during immersion in 12 °C water [5].

Non-shivering thermogenesis, that is, the increase in cellular metabolism without increased muscle contraction, is associated with brown adipose tissue (BAT). BAT is a multi-vacuole, mitochondria dense tissue in which, thanks to the high expression levels of uncoupling protein 1 (Ucp1) the electron transport chain is not coupled to ATP synthase complex and, therefore, the potential energy accumulated within the electron gradient straggling the inner mitochondrial membrane is dissipated into heat [13]. It has been well established that rodents increase metabolic heat production in BAT in response to cold exposure. Despite the initial thought that only hibernating animals and human infants had BAT, and that once human infants, who lack the ability to shiver, burned through their BAT depots, they were unable to deposit more [14–16], more recent works has found BAT among adult living in cold and temperate climate [17, 18]. Particularly, using positron emission tomography

(PET) and computed tomography (CT) scans along with the tracer 18F-fluorodeoxyglucose, it has been discovered that adult humans do indeed have active BAT that becomes active upon cold exposure. In human adults, BAT is located along the major deep blood vessels and more superficially in the neck, supraclavicular tissue, and thoracic and abdominal paraspinal sites [19]. Measuring oxygen consumption and surface temperatures over the supraclavicular region (control) and sternum (non-BAT region) under room temperature and mild-cold conditions revealed that individuals with greater BAT activation also experience a greater increase in metabolic rate [20]. A decade discussion is open about the effective possibility that physical exercise increases BAT amount and activity, through the PGC-1α-induced release of the myokine irisin from the skeletal muscle membrane protein FNDC5A, that acts on white adipocytes where it induces the expression of Ucp1 and, in turn, drives a metabolic shift from white to brown (likely, beige or bright) [21, 22]. The metabolic buffering properties of BAT during prolonged cold exposure suggest that it may have been an efficient heat producing organ in Neanderthals. Furthermore, if the positive correlation between exercise and BAT is established in humans, this could imply an additional thermoregulatory advantage to Neanderthal high PALs [1].

BAT activation rate is negatively correlated with body mass index (BMI) and % body fat [14, 15] and women appear to have more BAT than men [19]. However, there is no evidence that BAT thermogenesis may provide enough heat to limit the decrease in T_{core} during acute whole body cold exposures [5].

It has been suggested that prolonged or repeated exposures to cold can enhance the thermogenic response: a pattern called metabolic acclimatisation [23]; either exaggerated shivering or development of non-shivering thermogenesis could account for a more pronounced thermogenic response to cold during metabolic acclimatisation.

Populations of the circumpolar regions (e.g. Alaskan Inuits, Native Americans, Alacaluf) experience higher BMRs than subjects from temperate areas, and this in turn hesitates into a warmer skin temperatures and less shivering under cold exposure [23], although the maintenance of high BMRs also during warm periods attributes this adaptation to other factors such as diet [24–26]. Ama diving women experienced a substantial increase in BMR between summer and winter, compared to non-diving women of the same communities who, instead, maintained constant BMRs through the year. This observation strongly suggested that acclimation was an effect of chronic cold, and not of diet or other lifestyle factors [27].

Other than these cross-sectional observations, there are longitudinal studies (i.e. with subjects repeatedly exposed to cold) that suggest that a metabolic acclimatisation to cold can develop in people living in temperate climates. In his paper from 1961, Davis [28] reported that men exposed to 12 °C, 8 h/day, for 31 days experienced an enhanced non-shivering thermogenesis in response to cold and decreased shivering.

Similarly, it has been demonstrated the development of non-shivering thermogenesis as a result of cold acclimatisation during winter, through indirect calorimetry to derive BMR and electromyography (EMG) activity of the pectoralis major to measure shivering, in 17 young men during 80-min exposures to 16 °C, once in the summer and once in winter. BMR during exposure was 0.15 kcal/min higher in winter than in summer, while EMG activity was similar [29]. Increased non-shivering thermogenesis in brown fat stores was also described in 17 healthy young men and women, during a cold chamber acclimatisation programme (10 consecutive days, 6 h/day, 15 °C air) [30].

Metabolic Response to Cryostimulation

As a physical treatment, cryostimulation has gained, in the last two decades, wide popularity thanks to its anti-inflammatory and analgesic effects. Less studied but relevant, as well, are the metabolic effects, some of which strikingly related to the anti-inflammatory ones. This novel view is favouring the shift from WBC as a symptomatic treatment for pain in inflammatory conditions as an adjuvant active therapy for endocrine diseases affecting the metabolic sphere. The exposure to extremely cold air, although brief, causes a thermal stress that first affects the derma: the high amount of cold receptors (ten fold higher than heat receptors) dispersed in the skin accounts for the quick and massive circulatory, neuromuscular, immune and endocrine responses all aimed at restoring the homeostasis. The stressful allostatic load first induces an insulative autonomic response aimed at reducing heat loss (peripheral vasoconstriction) and enhancing thermogenesis (via the activation of the hypothalamic thermoregulatory centres) [5, 31].

Activation of cold receptors in the skin triggers the sympathetic nervous system (SNS) that induces the insulative response. The efferent sympathetic nerve terminals release noradrenaline (NA) that activates α-adrenoreceptors expressed by the smooth muscles of the peripheral vasculature and induces vasoconstriction. The net result is the displacement of blood from the cutaneous district to the deepest compartments. The higher cardiac preload determined causes the transitory increase of arterial pressures, reduces heart rate [31]. Together with other cold-modulated mediators (e.g. endorphins), NA modulates pain and decreases the conductibility rate of sensory fibres and of their connection to proprioceptors [32, 33]. From a vasomotor point of view, also the recovery from cold is a relevant aspect since, after the cessation of the stimulus, a reactive vasodilation takes place and the resultant increase in peripheral blood flow (as higher as four fold) helps the washing out of the catabolic wasting materials. Further, the post-stimulation activation of the parasympathetic branch of the nervous system decreases blood pressure, an effect that lasts hours after the end of the stimulus [34–36]. Interestingly, changes in muscle temperature (T_{muscle}), T_{skin} and T_{core} reach a maximum after 50–60 min from the application and the autonomic reactions can last up to 6 h after the exposure [34, 37–39].

Other than the vasomotor-mediated insulative reaction, the metabolic response to WBC is relevant to determine the effects of the treatment. In particular, non-shivering thermogenesis prevails, and it is driven by muscle contraction [40]. Metabolic activation of muscles in turn affects the fate of the energetic substrates both in the muscle itself and in other organs (i.e. adipose tissue) [41]. However, there are several variables that affect the net response to the cold stimulus: body size, BMI, fitness level, amount of subcutaneous fat and gender [5, 42, 43].

Effects of WBC on Metabolic Indexes

According to the observation made in two decades of research, repeated exposures to WBC determine several benefits that are more or less directly related to an improved (or potentially improving) metabolic profile. In general terms, the principal effects that have been reported are improved inflammatory, metabolic [31] and antioxidant profiles [44], improved peripheral insulin sensitivity, enhanced BAT volume [45], decreased adipose tissue volume [46] and enhanced endorphin secretion [47]. Besides the anti-inflammatory effects, that, however, have relevant impacts on metabolism (i.e. low-grade inflammation (LGI) and metabolic inflammation), the main hypothesis is that WBC activates the same molecular pathways as physical exercise and, therefore, WBC is considered as an exercise-mimicking activity. Similarly to exercise, WBC is supposed to be beneficial in patients affected by dysmetabolic conditions, and it would be likely effective in the treatment of obesity and diabetes [48].

Effects on Body Composition

Repeated WBC exposure induces changes in body composition, mainly associated with reduction or redistribution of fat; however, the results are sometimes contrasting. The principal confounding variables intervening in these studies are represented by dietary and physical intervention.

Ten sessions, and even more 20 sessions, caused a significant reduction in waist, hips and abdominal circumferences, waist/height ratio, triceps and abdominal skinfold thickness as well as improvement in body mass, BMI, absolute total body fat and leg fat in healthy postmenopausal women, overweight women and postmenopausal women with metabolic syndrome. In this latter group, WBC also induced a significant reduction in the percentage of the total, trunk and android fat [46]. Similarly, 20 WBS sessions caused improvements in fat mass, body fat %, hips and waist circumference and BMI class I obese males [49]. The same group demonstrated a significant reduction in subcutaneous fat tissue thickness class I obese subjects [44, 49]. Contrasting results were obtained, instead, by other researchers: according to Ziemann and colleagues, 10 WBC were not sufficient to elicit any change in body composition in men with class I obesity [50] as well as 40 WBC sessions, combined with intensive training, in subjects with BMI > 30, did not determine changes in body weight, waist/hip ratio, BMI, fat mass, skeletal muscle mass and subcutaneous fat mass [51].

The comparison among these studies is made further less effective by the lack of control groups. However, it is possible to hypothesise that subcutaneous tissue in obesity may represent a key variable in the response to cold stimulation: with its insulating properties it could limit heat loss and, therefore, it can slow down the increase in BMR [52].

Effects on Lipid Profile and Energy Metabolism

According to the results from the WBC-associated metabolic effects of WBC in healthy subjects and, although the very limited amount, in subjects with dysmetabolic conditions, it is licit to support an effect of cryostimulation on the systemic metabolic profile [51, 53, 54] by inducing homeostatic responses in tissues involved in energy use and storage (skeletal muscle [55], adipose tissue [50, 55], bone [56]). However, besides these evidences, reports in this field are still quantitatively and qualitatively limited and, therefore, it is hard to draw definitive conclusions.

Lipids are the main energy source, at rest and during exercise, and thermogenic substrate and cold stress primarily affect lipid metabolism [40]. A first confirmation of this hypothesis came from the observation that increasing the amount of WBC sessions from 5 to 10 and 20, there were increasing effects. Indeed, while 5 sessions resulted ineffective in healthy young males, 10 sessions 10 sessions reduced triglycerides (TG) by a third. Twenty sessions decreased, not only TG, from 108.0 ± 50.0 to 69.4 ± 27.2 mg/dL, but also total cholesterol (TC, from 172.6 ± 44.5 to 151.8 ± 53.8 mg/dL) and LDL cholesterol (from 97.7 ± 48.3 to 72.8 ± 52.0 mg/dL) and increased HDL cholesterol (from 53.2 ± 16.5 to 63.1 ± 27.4 mg/dL) and non-esterified fatty acids (NEFA, from 0.64 ± 0.4 to 0.79 ± 0.3 mmol/L) and their relative ratios. No effects were recorded for glycaemia [54]. The effects on TG, LDL and HDL were confirmed in obese adults who underwent a combined 20 WBC sessions and aerobic training, for 6 months [51]. Further, in young physically active males, recovery with WBC (two sessions per day, for 5 days) from 30-min step-up/ step-down associated with decrease in TC (43%) and LDL (52%) while passive recovery associated with their increase [53]. Pilch et al. although reported no significant changes in lipid profile, following WBC, they described a positive trend in metabolic balance of adipose tissue in class I obese [57]. Importantly, according to Ziemann and colleagues, the effectiveness of WBC depended on the cardiorespiratory fitness (CF): the lower was CF the greater were the improvement in CF [50]. Finally, again the Lubkowska's group described that, in 45 healthy male military academy students, 20 consecutive exposures to WBC, and even more 30 exposures, induced the already mentioned positive changes in TC, LDL and HDL, associated with a decreased ApoB:ApoA-I ratio, that represent constituents of LDL and HDL, respectively [58].

As cold affects lipid metabolism, it is expected to affect directly or indirectly the function of both WAT and BAT [45, 59]. Evidences support this hypothesis and researches demonstrate that they are both activated during cold exposure; however, BAT is particularly 'consumed' under cold stress, thus contributing to energy homeostasis [40].

Effects on Metabolic Inflammation

Chronic metabolic inflammation, also known as LGI, is a chronic inflammatory states associated with the toxic effects of lipids accumulated in WAT and liver and driven by the chronically, but even slightly, elevated circulating IL-6. A positive energy balance (i.e. high-energy intake and low-energy expenditure) causes accumulation of lipids into WAT. Adipocytes' dimensions increase until they reach a critical size that makes them too distant from the oxygen source (i.e. capillaries). The consequent hypoxia causes the death of adipocytes and necrosis of WAT. The released mediators attract and activate macrophages that release cytokines. The net result is that the entire WAT shifts towards a pro-inflammatory phenotype characterised by increased secretion of pro-inflammatory mediators (IL-6, TNFα, plasminogen activator inhibitor 1 (PAI1), leptin, macrophage chemoattractant protein 1 (MCP1), IL-18, resistin, visfatin) and the inhibition of the anti-inflammatory species (adiponectin) [60, 61]. Activation of the innate branch of immunity together with the often coexisting hyperglycaemia, hyperinsulinemia and hypercortisolism initiate a vicious cycle that further pushes inflammation and amplifies its deleterious effects. Chronically elevated IL-6, contrarily temporarily defined increases, fails in stimulating the translocation to the plasma membrane of the insulin-dependent glucose transporter (GLUT4), expressed by the skeletal muscle and the adipose tissue. This is further impaired by TNFα that inhibits insulin action. LGI is associated with metabolic syndrome (insulin resistance, type 2 diabetes, cardiovascular disease, atherosclerosis and fatty liver disease) and ageing and lifestyle factors (smoking, obesity, dietary patterns, cognitive decline and cachexia), and it is a relevant independent predictor of all-cause mortality [62].

WBC improves the circulating profile associated with metabolic inflammation and, in obese subjects, 10 sessions, increased the anti-inflammatory IL-10 and decreased the pro-inflammatory IL-6, TNFα and adipokines (resistin, visfatin) with a greater effects in those subjects with worse metabolic phenotype [50]. The same author described in a similar cohort of middle-aged obese men, the decrease in the systemic inflammatory marker C-reactive protein (CRP) and the increase of the thermogenic muscle-derived mediator irisin, after 10 sessions of WBC, in a CF-dependent manner [55]. Accordingly, CWI induced irisin and inhibited fibroblast growth factor 21 (FGF21) suggestive of non-shivering thermogenesis [63], and WBC has been reported to decrease the circulating level of FGF21 in female volleyball players [64].

The unbalanced production of radical species is associated with inflammation and is a key pathogenic factor in metabolic inflammation [62]. WBC effectively counteracts the production of pro-oxidant species and stimulates the expression of components of the antioxidant system, such as uric acid, superoxide dismutase (SOD) and total antioxidants [65]. These effects could be relevant in contrasting the onset and progression of metabolic dysfunctions.

Effects on the Endocrine Function of Adipose Tissue

Another way to counteract the deleterious effects of adiposity is to inhibit the expression of the endocrine mediators (i.e. adipokines) produced by inflamed adipocytes. Resistin and visfatin, two main WAT-derived inflammatory mediators, were induced in low CF while reduced in high CF class 1 and 2 obese subjects, while adiponectin and leptin resulted to be unaffected [50]. On the contrary, possibly due to the heterogeneity of the study cohort, no changes were recorded by Lubkowska and co-workers in adiponectin, resistin and leptin after 6 months of WBC [51]. Similar results were reported, for adiponectin, by Pilch et al. in obese subjects after 10 and 20 WBC sessions, although leptin decreased [57]. This latter effect may be due to the partial restoration of β-3 adrenergic receptors expression that is impaired in obesity [66].

The baseline adiposity could be the key for the explanation of the heterogeneity in the effects of WBC on adipokines since most of their expression is strikingly associated with fat mass.

Effects of WBC on Endocrine Axis

As a stressful stimulation, importantly affecting the homeostasis, extreme cold exposure, during cryostimulation, activates the awareness response. Importantly, the beneficial effects of WBC are only partially related to the acute response, but they rely on the recovery phase when a new homeostasis is reached. This 'secondary' set of responses becomes evident when exposure is repeated. Most of the knowledge in this field comes from studies made on athletes that use WBC for recovery purposes, and patients affected by autoimmune inflammatory diseases [40].

Even in this case, the information available is not definitive and mostly incomplete. The aim of this section is to give a short overview of the current knowledge on the demonstrated effects of WBC on the main studied hormone axes. Noteworthy, studies on sex hormones and thyroid function are lacking.

Neurohumoral Axis

Part of the neurohumoral response has been already described above. The activation of the SNS represents, perhaps, the key response which underlies all the other responses (i.e. insulative and thermogenic) and effects (analgesic, anti-inflammatory, activating the metabolism). Briefly, cold activates the thermal receptors of the nerves afferent to CNS; sympathetic efferent nerve terminals release NA and acetylcholine (ACh) that act, respectively, on β2-adrenergic receptors and α7nAChR and induce several intracellular responses all converging on nuclear factor κB (NF-κB) [67–70]. This is a main effect that presupposes to the anti-inflammatory effect of cold application since the inhibition of NF-κB, that is, the molecular hub of inflammation, affects the expression of several downstream effectors involved in inflammation and oxidative stress, such as IL-1β [71, 72], IL-6 [73], TNFα [72], IL-10 [74], inducible nitric oxide synthase (iNOS) and myeloperoxidase (MPO) [72, 75], SOD, glutathione peroxidase (GPx) [65] and intracellular adhesion molecule 1 (ICAM-1) [76]. Inhibition of NF-κB limits the M1 differentiation macrophages while supporting the maintenance of M0 phenotype or the shift through the M2 regulatory phenotype [32]. Further, cold directly limits enzymatic activities and expression of pain mediators and more relevantly those that result hyper-activated at the time of the stimulus, for example, collagenases [77] and matrix metalloproteinases (MMPs) [78, 79], prostaglandin E2 (PGE2) [74, 80] and histamine. In this latter case, painful stimuli cause the release of neuropeptides from sensory nerves that activate mast cells and induce the release of histamine. Throughout a positive feedback, histamine further stimulates the release of neuropeptides from sensory fibres. Therefore, cold stimulation limits painful sensation through this pathway, too [81].

Cold-induced analgesia is also associated with direct activation of gate control, increased nociceptor excitability threshold, reduced nerve conduction rate and decreased muscle spasm rate and strength. Circulating NA also reaches the spinal cord via the posterior spinal arteries supplying, where pain afferent neurons from skin end [82].

As described above, NA also activates α-adrenoreceptors expressed by smooth muscle cells of the vasculature and induces vasoconstriction [83]. Other than being an insulative response, vasoconstriction decreases vascular permeability, therefore limiting oedema and bleeding [33]. Moreover, the inhibition of NF-κB downregulates the expression of vascular endothelial growth factor (VEGF), with consequent inhibition of angiogenesis further supporting the limitation of peripheral blood flow, although in the case of chronic exposure [84].

Taken together, the overall neurohumoral response to cold stimulus accounts for most of the analgesic, anti-inflammatory, anti-oedema and anti-bleeding effects of WBC.

Hypothalamus-Pituitary-Adrenal Gland Axis

In their seminal paper, Leppäluoto and colleagues described that in healthy females, exposed to either CWI (0–2 °C) or WBC (−110 °C) three times per week over 12 weeks, adrenocorticotropic hormone (ACTH) was decreased starting from week 4 as a potential mechanism of adaptation to the chronic stimulation [47]. Therefore, according to this observation, WBC and more general cold-exposure, might not affect the function of the HPA axis. This was confirmed in different settings, where athletes from different disciplines underwent WBC or CWI in the course of specific training programmes. For instance, WBC did not affect cortisol level in elite synchronised swimmers after a normal training week, although the control group (i.e. those subject not undergone to WBC) experienced a decline in the hormone levels

[85]. Similarly, a single WBC exposure did not affect cortisol level in professional soccer players after repeated-sprint exercise [86] and after severe intermittent running [87].

Contrarily, Minett et al. described a decrease in cortisol, together with CK levels, in subjects who underwent to CWI after intermittent-sprint exercise [88] and in professional rugby players during a training camp [89], while it was increased in professional tennis players submitted to a moderate-intensity training programme and 10 WBC sessions over 5 days [90].

Conclusions

WBC and extreme cold exposure have established beneficial effects on well-being and, as emerging, on metabolism. Most of them are related to the activation of the SNS and the consequent neurohumoral response that drives all the physiological responses (insulative and metabolic). Although there are evidences about the potential application of cryostimulatory protocols in the treatment of dysmetabolic conditions, the knowledge about the molecular mechanisms of action of cold is still very limited. Improved knowledge, coming from well-designed case-control studies and randomised clinical trials, would surely represent a milestone on which to build appropriate and effective cold-based therapeutic strategies.

References

1. Ocobock C, Lacy S, Niclou A. Between a rock and a cold place: Neanderthal biocultural cold adaptations. Evol Anthropol. 2021;30(4):262–79.
2. Makinen TM. Different types of cold adaptation in humans. Front Biosci (Schol Ed). 2010;2(3):1047–67.
3. Steegmann AT Jr. Human cold adaptation: an unfinished agenda. Am J Hum Biol. 2007;19(2):218–27.
4. Stocks JM, et al. Human physiological responses to cold exposure. Aviat Space Environ Med. 2004;75(5):444–57.
5. Castellani JW, Young AJ. Human physiological responses to cold exposure: acute responses and acclimatization to prolonged exposure. Auton Neurosci. 2016;196:63–74.
6. Young AJ, et al. Human thermoregulatory responses to cold air are altered by repeated cold water immersion. J Appl Physiol (1985). 1986;60(5):1542–8.
7. Hingley E, et al. Physiology of cold water immersion: a comparison of cold water acclimatised and no-cold water acclimatised participants during static and dynamic immersions. Br J Sports Med. 2011;45:e1.
8. Bird F, et al. The physiological and subjective responses to repeated cold water immersion in a group of 10–12 year olds. J Sport Sci Med. 2012;11:779.
9. Parsons K. Human thermal environments. 2nd ed. London: CRC Press; 2002. p. 560.
10. Frank SM, et al. Relative contribution of core and cutaneous temperatures to thermal comfort and autonomic responses in humans. J Appl Physiol (1985). 1999;86(5):1588–93.
11. Castellani JW, et al. Thermoregulation during cold exposure after several days of exhaustive exercise. J Appl Physiol (1985). 2001;90(3):939–46.
12. Bell DG, Tikuisis P, Jacobs I. Relative intensity of muscular contraction during shivering. J Appl Physiol (1985). 1992;72(6):2336–42.

13. Sell H, Deshaies Y, Richard D. The brown adipocyte: update on its metabolic role. Int J Biochem Cell Biol. 2004;36(11):2098–104.
14. Saito M, et al. High incidence of metabolically active brown adipose tissue in healthy adult humans: effects of cold exposure and adiposity. Diabetes. 2009;58(7):1526–31.
15. van Marken Lichtenbelt WD, et al. Cold-activated brown adipose tissue in healthy men. N Engl J Med. 2009;360(15):1500–8.
16. Virtanen KA, et al. Functional brown adipose tissue in healthy adults. N Engl J Med. 2009;360(15):1518–25.
17. Levy SB, et al. Brown adipose tissue, energy expenditure, and biomarkers of cardio-metabolic health among the Yakut (Sakha) of northeastern Siberia. Am J Hum Biol. 2018;30(6):e23175.
18. Ocobock C, et al. Elevated resting metabolic rates among female, but not male, reindeer herders from subarctic Finland. Am J Hum Biol. 2020;32(6):e23432.
19. Cypess AM, et al. Identification and importance of brown adipose tissue in adult humans. N Engl J Med. 2009;360(15):1509–17.
20. Levy SB. Field and laboratory methods for quantifying brown adipose tissue thermogenesis. Am J Hum Biol. 2019;31(4):e23261.
21. Bostrom P, et al. A PGC1-alpha-dependent myokine that drives brown-fat-like development of white fat and thermogenesis. Nature. 2012;481(7382):463–8.
22. Lombardi G, et al. Implications of exercise-induced adipo-myokines in bone metabolism. Endocrine. 2016;54(2):284–305.
23. Young AJ. Homeostatic responses to prolonged cold exposure: human cold acclimatization. In: Fregly MJ, Blatteis CM, editors. Handbook of physiology: environmental physiology. Bethesda, MD: American Physiological Society; 1996. p. 419–38.
24. Leonard WR, et al. Climatic influences on basal metabolic rates among circumpolar populations. Am J Hum Biol. 2002;14(5):609–20.
25. Snodgrass JJ, et al. Basal metabolic rate in the Yakut (Sakha) of Siberia. Am J Hum Biol. 2005;17(2):155–72.
26. Leonard WR, et al. Seasonal variation in basal metabolic rates among the Yakut (Sakha) of northeastern Siberia. Am J Hum Biol. 2014;26(4):437–45.
27. Kang BS, et al. Changes in body temperature and basal metabolic rate of the ama. J Appl Physiol (1985). 1963;18(3):483–8.
28. Davis TR. Chamber cold acclimatization in man. J Appl Physiol. 1961;16:1011–5.
29. Nishimura T, et al. Relationship between seasonal cold acclimatization and mtDNA haplogroup in Japanese. J Physiol Anthropol. 2012;31(1):22.
30. van der Lans AA, et al. Cold acclimation recruits human brown fat and increases nonshivering thermogenesis. J Clin Invest. 2013;123(8):3395–403.
31. White GE, Wells GD. Cold-water immersion and other forms of cryotherapy: physiological changes potentially affecting recovery from high-intensity exercise. Extrem Physiol Med. 2013;2(1):26.
32. Guillot X, et al. Cryotherapy in inflammatory rheumatic diseases: a systematic review. Expert Rev Clin Immunol. 2014;10(2):281–94.
33. Demoulin C, Vanderthommen M. Cryotherapy in rheumatic diseases. Joint Bone Spine. 2012;79(2):117–8.
34. Zalewski P, et al. Whole-body cryostimulation increases parasympathetic outflow and decreases core body temperature. J Therm Biol. 2014;45:75–80.
35. Douzi W, et al. 3-min whole body cryotherapy/cryostimulation after training in the evening improves sleep quality in physically active men. Eur J Sport Sci. 2019;19(6):860–7.
36. Louis J, et al. The use of whole-body cryotherapy: time- and dose-response investigation on circulating blood catecholamines and heart rate variability. Eur J Appl Physiol. 2020;120(8):1733–43.
37. Costello JT, et al. Muscle, skin and core temperature after −110 degrees c cold air and 8 degrees c water treatment. PLoS One. 2012;7(11):e48190.
38. Savic M, Fonda B, Sarabon N. Actual temperature during and thermal response after whole-body cryotherapy in cryo-cabin. J Therm Biol. 2013;38:186–91.

39. Costello JT, et al. Whole-body cryotherapy (extreme cold air exposure) for preventing and treating muscle soreness after exercise in adults. Cochrane Database Syst Rev. 2015;9:CD010789.
40. Lombardi G, Ziemann E, Banfi G. Whole-body cryotherapy in athletes: from therapy to stimulation. An updated review of the literature. Front Physiol. 2017;8:258.
41. Fontana JM, et al. Whole-body cryostimulation in obesity. A scoping review. J Therm Biol. 2022;106:103250.
42. Gordon CJ. The therapeutic potential of regulated hypothermia. Emerg Med J. 2001;18(2):81–9.
43. Gordon CJ, et al. Direct and indirect methods for determining plasma volume during thermo-neutral and cold-water immersion. Eur J Appl Physiol. 2003;89(5):471–4.
44. Pilch W, et al. Blood pro-oxidant/antioxidant balance in young men with class II obesity after 20 sessions of whole body cryostimulation: a preliminary study. Redox Rep. 2021;26(1):10–7.
45. Hanssen MJ, et al. Short-term cold acclimation recruits Brown adipose tissue in obese humans. Diabetes. 2016;65(5):1179–89.
46. Wiecek M, et al. Whole-body cryotherapy is an effective method of reducing abdominal obesity in menopausal women with metabolic syndrome. J Clin Med. 2020;9(9):2797.
47. Leppaluoto J, et al. Effects of long-term whole-body cold exposures on plasma concentrations of ACTH, beta-endorphin, cortisol, catecholamines and cytokines in healthy females. Scand J Clin Lab Invest. 2008;68(2):145–53.
48. Lombardi G, Ziemann E, Banfi G. Whole-body cryotherapy: possible application in obesity and diabesity. In: Capodaglio P, editor. Rehabilitation interventions in the patient with obesity. Cham, Switzerland: Springer Nature Switzerland AG; 2020. p. 173–88.
49. Pilch W, et al. The effect of whole-body cryostimulation on body composition and leukocyte expression of HSPA1A, HSPB1, and CRP in obese men. Cryobiology. 2020;94:100–6.
50. Ziemann E, et al. Whole-body cryostimulation as an effective method of reducing low-grade inflammation in obese men. J Physiol Sci. 2013;63(5):333–43.
51. Lubkowska A, et al. Body composition, lipid profile, Adipokine concentration, and antioxidant capacity changes during interventions to treat overweight with exercise Programme and whole-body Cryostimulation. Oxidative Med Cell Longev. 2015;2015:803197.
52. Speakman JR. Obesity and thermoregulation. Handb Clin Neurol. 2018;156:431–43.
53. Ziemann E, et al. Whole-body cryostimulation as an effective way of reducing exercise-induced inflammation and blood cholesterol in young men. Eur Cytokine Netw. 2014;25(1):14–23.
54. Lubkowska A, et al. Changes in lipid profile in response to three different protocols of whole-body cryostimulation treatments. Cryobiology. 2010;61(1):22–6.
55. Dulian K, et al. The whole body cryostimulation modifies irisin concentration and reduces inflammation in middle aged, obese men. Cryobiology. 2015;71(3):398–404.
56. Galliera E, et al. Bone remodelling biomarkers after whole body cryotherapy (WBC) in elite rugby players. Injury. 2012;44(8):1117–21.
57. Pilch W, et al. Different changes in Adipokines, lipid profile, and TNF-alpha levels between 10 and 20 whole body Cryostimulation sessions in individuals with I and II degrees of obesity. Biomedicines. 2022;10(2):269.
58. Lubkowska A, et al. The effect of repeated whole-body cryostimulation on the HSP-70 and lipid metabolisms in healthy subjects. Physiol Res. 2019;68(3):419–29.
59. Cheng L, et al. Brown and beige adipose tissue: a novel therapeutic strategy for obesity and type 2 diabetes mellitus. Adipocytes. 2021;10(1):48–65.
60. Lombardi G. Exercise-dependent modulation of bone metabolism and bone endocrine function: new findings and therapeutic perspectives. J Sci Sport Exercise. 2019;1:20–8.
61. Lombardi G, Ziemann E, Banfi G. Physical activity and bone health: what is the role of immune system? A narrative review of the third way. Front Endocrinol (Lausanne). 2019;10:60.
62. Khandekar MJ, Cohen P, Spiegelman BM. Molecular mechanisms of cancer development in obesity. Nat Rev Cancer. 2011;11(12):886–95.
63. Lee P, et al. Irisin and FGF21 are cold-induced endocrine activators of brown fat function in humans. Cell Metab. 2014;19(2):302–9.

64. Jaworska J, et al. A 2-week specific volleyball training supported by the whole body Cryostimulation protocol induced an increase of growth factors and counteracted deterioration of physical performance. Front Physiol. 2018;9:1711.
65. Miller E, et al. Effect of short-term cryostimulation on antioxidative status and its clinical applications in humans. Eur J Appl Physiol. 2012;112(5):1645–52.
66. Collins S, et al. Impaired expression and functional activity of the beta 3- and beta 1-adrenergic receptors in adipose tissue of congenitally obese (C57BL/6J Ob/Ob) mice. Mol Endocrinol. 1994;8(4):518–27.
67. Pournot H, et al. Time-course of changes in inflammatory response after whole-body cryotherapy multi exposures following severe exercise. PLoS One. 2011;6(7):e22748.
68. Mourot L, Cluzeau C, Regnard J. Hyperbaric gaseous cryotherapy: effects on skin temperature and systemic vasoconstriction. Arch Phys Med Rehabil. 2007;88(10):1339–43.
69. Pavlov VA, Tracey KJ. The cholinergic anti-inflammatory pathway. Brain Behav Immun. 2005;19(6):493–9.
70. Tracey KJ. Reflex control of immunity. Nat Rev Immunol. 2009;9(6):418–28.
71. Hildebrand F, et al. Effects of hypothermia and re-warming on the inflammatory response in a murine multiple hit model of trauma. Cytokine. 2005;31(5):382–93.
72. Zhang H, et al. Therapeutic effect of post-ischemic hypothermia duration on cerebral ischemic injury. Neurol Res. 2008;30(4):332–6.
73. Straub RH, et al. Acute cold stress in rheumatoid arthritis inadequately activates stress responses and induces an increase of interleukin 6. Ann Rheum Dis. 2009;68(4):572–8.
74. Banfi G, et al. Effects of whole-body cryotherapy on serum mediators of inflammation and serum muscle enzymes in athletes. J Therm Biol. 2009;34(2):55–9.
75. Kang J, et al. The effects of systemic hypothermia on a murine model of thoracic aortic ischemia reperfusion. J Vasc Surg. 2010;52(2):435–43.
76. Cao J, et al. Influence of selective brain cooling on the expression of ICAM-1 mRNA and infiltration of PMNLs and monocytes/macrophages in rats suffering from global brain ischemia/reperfusion injury. Biosci Trends. 2008;2(6):241–4.
77. Harris ED Jr, McCroskery PA. The influence of temperature and fibril stability on degradation of cartilage collagen by rheumatoid synovial collagenase. N Engl J Med. 1974;290(1):1–6.
78. Suehiro E, et al. Increased matrix metalloproteinase-9 in blood in association with activation of interleukin-6 after traumatic brain injury: influence of hypothermic therapy. J Neurotrauma. 2004;21(12):1706–11.
79. Truettner JS, Alonso OF, Dietrich WD. Influence of therapeutic hypothermia on matrix metalloproteinase activity after traumatic brain injury in rats. J Cereb Blood Flow Metab. 2005;25(11):1505–16.
80. Stalman A, et al. Temperature-sensitive release of prostaglandin E(2) and diminished energy requirements in synovial tissue with postoperative cryotherapy: a prospective randomized study after knee arthroscopy. J Bone Joint Surg Am. 2011;93(21):1961–8.
81. Wojtecka-Lukasik E, et al. Cryotherapy decreases histamine levels in the blood of patients with rheumatoid arthritis. Inflamm Res. 2010;59(Suppl 2):S253–5.
82. Pertovaara A, Kalmari J. Comparison of the visceral antinociceptive effects of spinally administered MPV-2426 (fadolmidine) and clonidine in the rat. Anesthesiology. 2003;98(1):189–94.
83. Shepherd JT, Rusch NJ, Vanhoutte PM. Effect of cold on the blood vessel wall. Gen Pharmacol. 1983;14(1):61–4.
84. Coassin M, et al. Hypothermia reduces secretion of vascular endothelial growth factor by cultured retinal pigment epithelial cells. Br J Ophthalmol. 2010;94(12):1678–83.
85. Schaal K, et al. Whole-body Cryostimulation limits overreaching in elite synchronized swimmers. Med Sci Sports Exerc. 2015;47(7):1416–25.
86. Russell M, et al. The effects of a single whole-body cryotherapy exposure on physiological, performance, and perceptual responses of professional academy soccer players after repeated Sprint exercise. J Strength Cond Res. 2017;31(2):415–21.

87. Krueger M, et al. Whole-body cryotherapy (−110 °C) following high-intensity intermittent exercise does not alter hormonal, inflammatory or muscle damage biomarkers in trained males. Cytokine. 2019;113:277–84.
88. Minett GM, et al. Cold-water immersion decreases cerebral oxygenation but improves recovery after intermittent-sprint exercise in the heat. Scand J Med Sci Sports. 2014;24(4):656–66.
89. Grasso D, et al. Salivary steroid hormones response to whole-body cryotherapy in elite rugby players. J Biol Regul Homeost Agents. 2014;28(2):291–300.
90. Ziemann E, et al. Five-day whole-body cryostimulation, blood inflammatory markers, and performance in high-ranking professional tennis players. J Athl Train. 2012;47(6):664–72.

Cellular Cold Perception

3

Raffaella Cancello

Temperature sensitivity is a crucial aspect of our somatosensory system, finely tuned to help us perceive potentially harmful thermal conditions in nature and seek out the optimal temperature range for survival. At the systemic level, temperature perception relies on the detection by afferent sensory neurons located in either the dorsal root ganglia (DRG) or trigeminal ganglia (TG) [1–3]. These neurons include specific afferent populations, primarily small C-fibers and medium Aδ-fibers, which are activated at distinct temperature thresholds [1]. For instance, a significant group of sensory afferents associated with perceiving noxious heat exhibit a thermal activation threshold of approximately 45 °C in vitro, corresponding to the temperature at which noxious heat is physically perceived [4]. Similarly, there are afferents signals that respond to thermal thresholds in the warm range (30–40 °C), innocuous cool range (<30–15 °C), and noxious cold range (<15 °C) [5, 6]. These coordinated signals contribute to our overall perception of any given environmental temperature.

In addition to the thermal perception of sensory neurons, a family of receptors directly involved in signal transduction induced by thermal variations were discovered in the 1990s: the transient receptor potential channel family (TRP) [7]. The transient receptor potential (TRP) channels are a family of ion potential channels that are involved in various sensory processes, including sensory perception (*e.g.*, temperature, taste, pain), cellular signaling, and ion homeostasis, and are involved in numerous disease conditions. These channels have been extensively studied and are associated with specific sensory modalities [7].

R. Cancello (✉)
Obesity Unit and Laboratory of Nutrition and Obesity Research, Department of Endocrine and Metabolic Diseases, IRCCS Istituto Auxologico Italiano, Milan, Italy
e-mail: r.cancello@auxologico.it

© The Author(s), under exclusive license to Springer Nature Switzerland AG 2024

P. Capodaglio (ed.), *Whole-Body Cryostimulation*,
https://doi.org/10.1007/978-3-031-18545-8_3

The discovery of TRP channels is an ongoing process that spans several decades. The first hypotheses on the existence of thermal receptors date back to the 1990s. The TRP channel studies began in 1969 when Cosens and Manning discovered a mutant blind phenotype in Drosophila in the presence of constant bright light [8]. This mutant, named transient receptor potential (*trp*), was then cloned and mutations in the *trp* gene identified [8]. Montell and Rubin in 1989 recognized TRP as a transmembrane protein, but they also concluded that it did not encode the light-sensitive channels [9]. In the late 1990s, three independent research groups identified and characterized the TRP channels in Drosophila and mammals [10–12]. These channels were named canonical TRP channels due to their structural similarity to TRPL and their involvement in store-operated calcium entry [13]. In the early 2000s, extensive efforts led to the identification of additional members of the TRP channel family. These discoveries included the characterization of TRPV channels (*e.g.*, TRPV1, known as the capsaicin receptor), TRPM channels (*e.g.*, TRPM8, known as the cold and menthol receptor), TRPA channels (*e.g.*, TRPA1, known as the mustard oil and environmental irritant receptor), and others [13]. Until 2002, little was known about how temperature drops activate the subpopulation of somatosensory fibers responsible for cold detection. In that year, David Julius and Ardem Patapoutian independently published two seminal studies describing the molecular machine that allows mammals to detect cold [5]. Using two different strategies, they found the answer in the TRP channel TRPM8, the 80 members of the transient receptor potential melastatin family, providing a new and exciting candidate to understand the molecular mechanism of cold sensing. They also showed that this Ca^{2+}-permeable nonselective cation channel, expressed in trigeminal ganglia (TG) and dorsal root ganglia (DRG) neurons, was activated by natural and artificial cooling compounds [5], explaining Hensel and Zotterman's foundational observations that menthol sensitizes and potentiates the cold-evoked electrical responses of cold thermoreceptor fibers [6]. In 2004, two independent groups reported that TRPM8 is a voltage-dependent channel activated by membrane depolarization [7, 8, 14, 15]. However, evidence demonstrating TRPM8 activation by cold and its expression in cold thermoreceptor neurons was insufficient to unequivocally establish its contribution to cold sensing in mammals. The generation of three different TRPM8 knockout mice (TRPM8$^{-/-}$) revealed that animals lacking functional expression of the TRPM8 channel display an evident impairment in their ability to avoid cold temperatures in a temperature preference chamber and an attenuated response to evaporative cooling, highlighting its relevance as a crucial molecular cold transducer [16–18].

In 2021, David Julius and Ardem Patapoutian were jointly awarded the Nobel Prize in Physiology or Medicine for their discoveries related to the identification and functional characterization of TRP channels. David Julius was recognized for his work on the capsaicin receptor TRPV1 [19], while Ardem Patapoutian was honored for his contributions to the identification of various TRP channels involved in sensory perception [20].

Actually, mammalian TRP channels have been grouped into six subfamilies: TRPC (canonical or classical), TRPV (vanilloid), TRPML (mucolipin), TRPP (polycystin), TRPA (ankyrin-like), and TRPM (melastatin) [21]. A seventh subfamily, TRPN, has members in lower vertebrates and invertebrates only [21]. All seven members of this subfamily are structurally similar having six transmembrane helices, a putative hydrophobic pore forming loop, three to four ankyrin repeats, coiled-coil domains in the N- and C-terminus, a C-terminal proline-rich region, a calmodulin/IP3 binding region, and what is known as the TRP motif. The TRPC channels have been shown to form both heterotetramers and homotetramers within the TRP channel superfamily, with different members having certain preferences; for example, TRPC1 forms physiologically relevant functional channels with several TRPC channels, including TRPC4, TRPV1, and TRPP2 [7, 21].

Over the years, researchers have focused on characterizing the functional properties, activation mechanisms, and physiological roles of different TRP channels. TRP channels have been found to participate in various physiological processes, including sensory perception (e.g., temperature, taste, pain), cellular signaling, ion homeostasis, and numerous disease conditions. The TRP channel family consists of several subfamilies, each with distinct properties and activation mechanisms. Some well-known TRP channels include TRPV1, TRPV2, TRPA1, TRPM8, and TRPC channels. These channels have been extensively studied and are associated with specific sensory modalities. For example, TRPV1 is activated by capsaicin, the compound responsible for the hot and spicy sensation of chili peppers. It is involved in nociception, the perception of pain.

Cooling is selectively sensed by two members of the TRP family, namely, the TRPM8 and TRPA1 (ANKTM1) receptors that are activated by a temperature between 15 and 28 °C and lower than 18 °C, respectively (Fig. 3.1) [22]. In addition

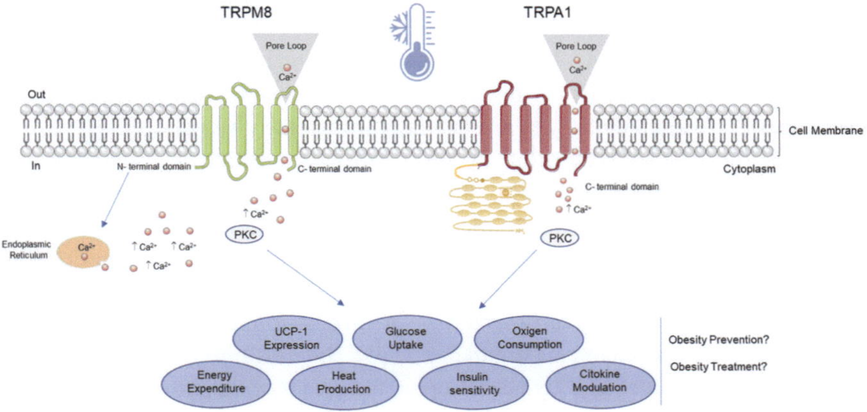

Fig. 3.1 Schematic signaling pathways involved in TRPM8 and TRPA1 channel cellular activation by cold temperatures and potential effects relevant to obesity prevention and treatment

to activation by mild cooling, TRPM8 can be activated also by natural and pharmacological compounds such as menthol, a cooling agent from the mint plant that is responsible for the fresh sensation after its administration, and icilin, a TRPM8 agonist chemically unrelated to menthol [23, 24] and various other substances, such as the recently found selective agonists WS-12 and CPS-369 [25].

TRMP8

One of the most studied members of the TRPM subfamily is the TRPM8, which is best known for its cold-sensing ability. The TRPM8 is a cold-activated ion channel that plays an essential role in the detection of environmental temperatures and is also a target for natural and synthetic cooling agents such as menthol. The TRPM8 variant was first recognized as a receptor transducing cold stimuli in the somatosensory system and is mainly expressed in sensory neurons [5] but it is also expressed in different nonneuronal cell types, such as mast cells, macrophages, bladder, prostate, sperm [26–28], as well as in other cancer cells (melanoma and breast cancer cells) [29, 30]. The role of the TRPM8 receptor in nonneuronal tissues and cancer cells has not been clearly established and studies are still ongoing. TRPM8 is a nonselective, Ca^{2+} permeable cation channel [31, 32]. Of the TRPM subfamily, TRPM8 is the most selective for Ca^{2+} with a selectivity ratio (PCa/PNa) of 3.3 [33]. Upon activation, TRPM8 allows the intracellular influx of calcium ions, leading to depolarization of cell membrane (in sensory neurons) and generation of electrical signals that are transmitted to the central nervous system for further processing. In nonneuronal cells, the phosphatidylinositol 4,5-bisphosphate, commonly referred to as PIP2(4,5), is a well-established intracellular regulator of TRPM8. The enzyme phospholipase C (PLC) hydrolyzes PIP2(4,5) to form the two classical second messengers: inositol 1,4,5 trisphosphate (IP3) and diacylglycerol (DAG). IP3 binds to its receptor in the endoplasmic reticulum and releases Ca^{2+}, whereas DAG is an activator of protein kinase C (PKC) enzymes. Activation of PLC is expected to lead not only to reduction of PIP2 levels but also to the activation of PKC both via the formation of DAG and directly by Ca^{2+} influx through the channel.

Besides the TRPM8 activation by mild to moderate cold temperatures, this receptor is also activated by "cold mimicking" compounds such as menthol [34]. Almost all the analgesic potency of menthol comes from the activation of TRPM8. The activation of TRPM8 by menthol has been extensively studied. Proudfoot et al. [35] demonstrated that peripherally (4 mM) or centrally (200 nM) menthol infusion in a model of neuropathic pain marked reverse behavioral reflex sensitization to noxious heat and mechanical stimulation [35]. Interestingly, the activation of TRPM8 can be regulated also by neurotrophic factors [36, 37], phosphatidylinositol bisphosphate (PIP2) [38, 39], Ca^{2+}-independent phospholipase A2 (iPLA2), and polyunsaturated fatty acids [40], forming a complex network. The TRPM8 desensitization occurs when the channel becomes refractory to an activating stimulus by adopting a conformational state where the passage of ions is not allowed. In the context of the nociceptive system, the desensitization functions as a protective mechanism in which hyperexcitation (or cell death) by ion-dependent signaling pathways is avoided [41]. The activity of the cold- and menthol-activated TRPM8 diminishes over time in the presence of extracellular Ca^{2+} [42, 43]. Both agonists and antagonists of TRPM8 have sensorial and therapeutic applications, with antagonists being explored for management of cold hypersensitivity associated with neuropathic pain [44].

The downstream effects of TRPM8 activation are still under investigation but this receptor possesses a central role in inflammatory regulation, macrophage differentiation, colitis protection, prostate cancer, and CGRP release in sensory neurons [45, 46]. In Trpm8$^{-/-}$ mice, a knockout model of TRPM8, heightened susceptibility to DSS-induced colitis compared to wild-type (WT) mice was reported [18, 47]. Notably, the analysis of splenic samples from Trpm8$^{-/-}$ mice revealed elevated levels of IL-6 and IL-1β, which are both potent pro-inflammatory cytokines [45, 47]. These findings provide valuable insights into the involvement of the Trpm8 protein in modulating the inflammatory response associated with colitis [48]. Recently, thanks to genome-wide expression analysis of human osteoarthritic chondrocytes, the expression of 19 different TRP genes was identified [49].

Ma et al. demonstrated that mouse brown adipocytes express TRPM8 which, when activated with menthol, induced an increase in UCP1 expression, independently of the adrenergic system [50]. Menthol significantly increases the core temperatures and prevents diet-induced obesity and related glucose abnormalities in wild-type mice but not in TRPM8$^{-/-}$ and UCP1$^{-/-}$ mice [50].

TRPM8 is present also in human white adipocytes and its activation by natural (menthol) and synthetic (icilin) agonists induces a dose-dependent rise in intracellular Ca^{2+} along with the induction of UCP1 expression, an increase of mitochondria membrane potential, glucose uptake, and heat production [51]. These effects resemble those observed in BAT during in vivo cold exposure mediated by adrenergic stimulation [52–54]. Thus, stimulation of the cold-sensitive TRPM8 receptor expressed in human white adipocytes mimics the effects induced by cold exposure in stimulating these cells to behave as brown-like adipocytes or by activating "beige" adipocytes as recently described [55]. TRPM8 agonist icilin and menthol stimulation increased insulin-induced glucose uptake in human white adipocytes after treatment [51]. The white adipocytes stimulated by menthol are characterized by changes in mitochondria morphology and localization with a preferential distribution very close around lipid droplets, all features mimicking what is commonly observed in activated brown adipocytes undergoing active lipolysis [52] suggesting that TRPM8 receptor stimulation in white adipocytes induces the appearance of morphological characteristics that are typical of thermogenically active adipocytes [51]. Hence, the TRPM8 receptor activation may play a role in the "browning/ beiging" of white adipocytes or in the recruitment of a beige adipocyte population within WAT. In adipocytes, different TRPM channels have been implicated in adipose physiological processes, including adipogenesis (the formation and differentiation of fat cells), lipid metabolism, adipokine secretion, energy metabolism regulation, and inflammation of adipose tissues, suggesting the potential role of TRP channels in human obesity treatment and prevention [56–60]. Targeting the TRPM8 channel could be a promising strategy for clinical treatment and prevention of human obesity and related metabolic diseases.

TRPA1

The transient receptor potential ankyrin 1 (TRPA1) is a second TRP channel variant involved in cold perception, especially in response to extreme cold temperatures. The TRPA1 name is based on the presence of 14 ankyrin repeats located in the NH_2 terminus of the channel, an unusual structural feature that may be relevant to its interactions with intracellular components [61]. It was first cloned in 1999 by Jacquemar et al. from lung fibroblasts [62]. TRPA1 gene consists of 73.635 bases and 29 exons and is present on the eighth chromosome in humans. Homologous genes of TRPA1 have been identified in both mammalian species like dogs, non-human primates, cattle, pigs and non-mammalian species including birds, fishes, and nematodes [63]. Initially, it was believed that the TRPA1 channel was expressed in the sensory neurons of dorsal root ganglia (DRG), trigeminal ganglia (TG), and nodose ganglia, [16, 64]; however, growing evidence from different studies suggested nonneuronal expression of TRPA1 in various organs including the heart, lungs, brain, pancreas, gastrointestinal tract, and urinary bladder [65–67]. Enterochromaffin cells and myenteric nerves present in the small and large intestines express TRPA1 [68]. In the stomach, the pyloric region showed the expression of TRPA1 [69]. In the gastrointestinal tract, TRPA1 acts as a chemo-sensor for various stimuli from the luminal environment and modulates the function in the intestine along with intestinal odorant receptors [70]. High TRPA1 expression has been detected in rat pancreatic beta islets [71], lung cells [72, 73], mouse inner ear [74, 75], keratinocytes, fibroblasts [76], enterochromaffin cells of human and rat colon [68], melanocytes [77], and human dental pulp fibroblast [78].

TRPA1 is primarily involved in the detection of an extremely wide variety of exogenous stimuli that may produce cellular damage. TRPA1 has been reported to be activated by cold, heat, and mechanical stimuli, and its function is modulated by multiple factors, including Ca^{2+}, metals (in trace), pH, reactive oxygen, nitrogen, and carbonyl species [61–63]. TRPA1 is involved in acute and chronic pain, as well as inflammation regulation. The TRPA1 is also known as the "mustard oil receptor" due to its activation by compounds found in mustard oil and other irritants [16, 63]. For several years the intrinsic sensitivity to cold of TRPA1 was debated, until recent studies that unequivocally showed that human TRPA1 was effectively activated by cold temperatures [63, 79–81]. In vivo, cold-induced activation of mouse TRPA1 was shown to occur in a Ca^{2+} independent manner and at the single-channel level in cell-attached and inside-out patches [16, 63]. As for TRPM8, the TRPA1 stimulation initiates thanks to intracellular signaling cascades involving calcium influx, activation of protein kinases, modulation of ion channels, and neurotransmitter release. Activation leads to the opening of the channel pore, allowing the influx of calcium ions (Ca^{2+}) and sodium ions (Na^+) into the cell. This influx of ions depolarizes the cell membrane, leading to the generation of an electrical signal. The increase in intracellular calcium levels plays a crucial role in TRPM8-mediated signaling. Calcium ions bind to various intracellular proteins and enzymes, initiating downstream signaling pathways. The expression of TRPA1 is limited in a subset of nociceptive neurons of the trigeminal ganglion and DRG and is a sensor for a wide variety of environmental stimuli, such as intense cold activation temperature of <18 °C (close to 8 °C, the reported threshold of noxious cold), reactive chemicals, and endogenous signals associated with cell injury to elicit protective responses [63]. TRPA1 is activated by some irritating compounds that directly activate TRPA1 such as cinnamaldehyde, allyl isothiocyanate, allicin, formalin, and bradykinin as inflammatory mediators [82]. TRPA1 has been implicated in several painful and inflammatory conditions and is considered a promising potential target for the development of analgesic, antipruritic, and anti-inflammatory pharmacotherapeutics [82]. Karashima et al. [82] showed the bell-shaped dose-response curve of menthol to channels by whole-cell and single-channel recordings of heterologous TRPA1, demonstrate a bimodal sensitivity of TRPA1 to menthol, further proved that menthol acts as an effective agonist of TRPA1 at relatively low concentrations (100–300 µM), but acts as an antagonist at higher concentrations of ≥300 mM by causing reversible channel blocking, although this high-concentration blocking effect was only found in rodent models, not human models [82, 83]. Despite the extensive knowledge about TRPA1 physiology, the molecular players and mechanisms underlying its trafficking remain largely unknown. Recent evidence suggests that TRPA1 trafficking, following activation, depends at least partially on SNAP receptor protein (SNARE)-mediated vesicle transport [63]. Since the effect of TRPA1 activation on trafficking is dependent on the localized influx of Ca^{2+}, it will be crucial to identify the Ca^{2+}-dependent mediators involved in this process and hopefully identify new potential drug targets.

TRPA1 regulates energy metabolism and thermogenesis in adipocytes and in high-fat diet (HFD) obese mice the oral administration of allyl-isothiocyanate reduces body weight, accumulation of lipid droplets in the liver, and white adipocyte mean size [83]. Cinnamaldehyde activates TRPA1 in mouse gastric epithelial cells and upregulates fatty acid oxidation-related genes in adipose tissue [69]. Oleuropein aglycone, as an agonist of TRPA1 and TRPV1, enhances the expression of UCP1 in BAT and promotes fat thermogenesis by promoting the secretion of norepinephrine [84–86]. It has been hypothesized that menthol-induced thermogenesis in adipocytes probably also involved the TRPA1 receptor as well but the mechanisms remain to be elucidated. Activation of TRPA1 induces the release of the 5-hydroxytryptamine receptor (5-HT) from EC cells, leading to delayed gastric emptying. TRPA1-mediated secretion of 5-HT and potentially other gut hormones could therefore influence gastric motility and food intake. Tamura et al. [86] found that dietary supplementation with the TRPA1 agonist, cinnamaldehyde, reduced adiposity in mice fed a high-fat, high-sugar diet. However, cinnamaldehyde did not alter food intake but instead led to increased energy expenditure [86], reflected by increased expression of UCP1 in BAT. The allyl isothiocyanate (AITC), a specific

TRPA1 agonist, has been extensively studied for the treatment of diabetes. AITC has been reported to improve insulin secretion in diabetic rats [87]. In vivo study on HFD-fed mice showed preventive effects of AITC on the development of insulin resistance and stimulation of insulin secretion from the pancreas and blood glucose levels were found to be lowered along with the inhibition of lipid peroxidation [87, 88]. TRPA1 agonist AITC has been reported to have anti-diabetic, anti-inflammatory, and antioxidant properties. Therefore, TRPA1 may contribute to regulating metabolic complications of people living with obesity.

TRP Channel and Energy Homeostasis

Several studies have demonstrated that TRP channels are involved in the regulation of energy homeostasis, adipose tissue function, gut hormone release, glucose metabolism, and thermogenesis of brown adipose tissue and that TRP channels play a role in regulating body weight. Studies of genetic linkage demonstrated a role for TRPC4, TRPM8, TRPML, and TRPP2 genes in obesity. [89–92]. In a Turkish population, the rs12472151 polymorphism of the TRPM8 gene was associated with metabolic syndrome [93]. Mice with a deficiency of TRPM8 are obese and cold intolerant [94] and chronic administration of the TRPM8 agonist icilin decreases body weight in diet-induced obesity (DIO) mice boosting energy expenditure [95]. There is no expression of TRPM8 in the endocrine pancreas; however, mice lacking TRPM8 have an increased insulin sensitivity, which results from a compensatory mechanism following enhanced insulin clearance in TRPM8$^{-/-}$ mice. TRPM8 has recently been indicated in association with pancreatic adenocarcinoma, where it might serve as a potential biomarker [96].

The combination of sub-effective doses of TRP channel agonists has lipid preventing, glucose utilizing, and browning effects on the 3T3-L1 adipose cell line, reduces weight gain, WAT hypertrophy, insulin resistance, and hepatic steatosis, and improves glucose homeostasis, promoting browning and BAT activation in HFD-obese mice. In vitro, in primary cultures of human adipocytes, menthol and icilin significantly increased UCP1 mRNA and protein levels, thermogenesis, glucose uptake, mitochondrial membrane potential, and mitochondrial elongation and clustering around lipid droplets independent of genes involved in mitochondrial biogenesis through TRPM8 activation and consequent Ca^{2+} influx [51].

Few studies are available for humans. In 20 healthy adult individuals, topical menthol significantly increased metabolic rate (+18%), cutaneous vasoconstriction, body heat storage, and rectal temperature compared to control and oral menthol administration [97]. A single oral L-menthol administration generated minor effects on enhancing thermogenesis and metabolic rate in humans compared to a single skin L-menthol administration [81]. However, L-menthol absorption in the body was very high following the oral administration. Thus, it is logical to hypothesize that human metabolism and WAT thermogenic activity may increase following a long-term L-menthol oral administration [81]. Further studies are then required to confirm whether daily menthol oral administration is a promising candidate treatment for browning induction.

Our understanding of the relationship between TRP channels and energy homeostasis is still evolving, and more research is needed to fully elucidate the mechanisms involved. Nonetheless, these studies suggest that TRP channels (in particular TRPM8 and TRPa1) may serve as potential therapeutic targets for metabolic disorders and weight management in the future.

Conclusion

TRP channels are polymodal channels that can be activated by a multitude of stimuli, including cold exposure. While they were initially recognized for their role in sensory physiology, recent studies have revealed that TRP channels are also crucial players in various other physiological and pathological conditions, such as renal physiology, cardiac health, cancer, and energy homeostasis. In particular, their involvement in energy homeostasis has garnered significant interest due to the urgent need for developing novel and safe therapeutic strategies to address the global obesity pandemic. One area of interest is the impact of TRPM8 and TRPA1 activation in response to cold stimuli, such as through whole-body cryotherapy (WBC), on white adipose tissue (WAT) thermogenic phenotype and metabolism in individuals living with obesity. While research in this specific context is limited, investigating the effects of TRPM8 and TRPA1 activation in response to cold stimuli in people living with obesity could provide valuable insights into potential therapeutic approaches for controlling and reducing obesity. Further research is then needed to fully elucidate these relationships and to develop targeted interventions that leverage TRP channels for managing obesity and related metabolic disorders.

References

1. Hensel H. Thermoreception and temperature regulation. Monogr Physiol Soc. 1981;38:1–321.
2. Scott SA. Sensory neurons: diversity, development, and plasticity. New York: Oxford University Press; 1992.
3. Schlader ZJ, Simmons SE, Stannard SR, Mundel T. The independent roles of temperature and thermal perception in the control of human thermoregulatory behavior. Physiol Behav. 2011;103:217–24.
4. Jessen C. Temperature regulation in humans and other mammals. Berlin: Springer-Verlag; 2001.
5. McKemy DD. The molecular and cellular basis of cold sensation. ACS Chem Neurosci. 2013;4(2):238–47. https://doi.org/10.1021/cn300193h.
6. Hensel H, Zotterman Y. The response of the cold receptors to constant cooling. Acta Physiol Scand. 1951;22(2–3):96–105. https://doi.org/10.1111/j.1748-1716.1951.tb00758.x.
7. Patapoutian A, Peier A, Story G, et al. ThermoTRP channels and beyond: mechanisms of temperature sensation. Nat Rev Neurosci. 2003;4:529–39. https://doi.org/10.1038/nrn1141.
8. Cosens DJ, Manning A. Abnormal electroretinogram from a drosophila mutant. Nature. 1969;224:285–7.

9. Montell C, Rubin GM. Molecular characterization of drosophila trp locus, a putative integral membrane protein required for phototransduction. Neuron. 1989;2:1313–23.
10. Minke B, Selinger Z. Inositol lipid pathway in fly photoreceptors: excitation, calcium mobilization and retinal degeneration. Prog Retinal Res. 1991;11:99–124.
11. Hardie RC, Raghu P. Visual transduction in Drosophila. Nature. 2001;413:186–93.
12. Clapham DE. TRP channels as cellular sensors. Nature. 2003;426:517–24.
13. Pedersen SF, Owsianik G, Nilius B. TRP channels: an overview. Cell Calcium. 2005;38(3–4):233–52. https://doi.org/10.1016/j.ceca.2005.06.028.
14. Brauchi S, Orio P, Latorre R. Clues to understanding cold sensation: thermodynamics and electrophysiological analysis of the cold receptor TRPM8. Proc Natl Acad Sci USA. 2004;101:15494–9.
15. Voets T, Droogmans G, Wissenbach U, Janssens A, Flockerzi V, Nilius B. The principle of temperature-dependent gating in cold- and heat-sensitive TRP channels. Nature. 2004;430:748–54.
16. Bautista DM, Jordt SE, Nikai T, et al. TRPA1 mediates the inflammatory actions of environmental irritants and proalgesic agents. Cell. 2006;124(6):1269–82. https://doi.org/10.1016/j.cell.2006.02.023.
17. Colburn RW, Lubin ML, Stone DJ Jr, et al. Attenuated cold sensitivity in TRPM8 null mice. Neuron. 2007;54(3):379–86. https://doi.org/10.1016/j.neuron.2007.04.017.
18. Dhaka A, Viswanath V, Patapoutian A. Trp ion channels and temperature sensation. Annu Rev Neurosci. 2006;29:135–61. https://doi.org/10.1146/annurev.neuro.29.051605.112958.
19. Caterina MJ, Rosen TA, Tominaga M, Brake AJ, Julius D. A capsaicin-receptor homologue with a high threshold for noxious heat. Nature. 1999;398(6726):436–41. https://doi.org/10.1038/18906.
20. Patapoutian A, Peier AM, Story GM, Viswanath V. ThermoTRP channels and beyond: mechanisms oftemperature sensation. Nat Rev Neurosci. 2003;4:529–39.
21. Li H. TRP Channel classification. Adv Exp Med Biol. 2017;976:1–8. https://doi.org/10.1007/978-94-024-1088-4_1.
22. Pan Y, Thapa D, Baldissera L Jr, Argunhan F, Aubdool AA, Brain SD. Relevance of TRPA1 and TRPM8 channels as vascular sensors of cold in the cutaneous microvasculature. Pflugers Arch. 2018;470(5):779–86. https://doi.org/10.1007/s00424-017-2085-9.
23. Bharate SS, Bharate SB. Modulation of thermoreceptor TRPM8 by cooling compounds. ACS Chem Neurosci. 2012;3(4):248–67. https://doi.org/10.1021/cn300006u.
24. Andersson DA, Chase HW, Bevan S. TRPM8 activation by menthol, icilin, and cold is differentially modulated by intracellular pH. J Neurosci. 2004;24(23):5364–9. https://doi.org/10.1523/JNEUROSCI.0890-04.2004.
25. Sherkheli MA, Vogt-Eisele AK, Bura D, Beltran Marques LR, Gisselmann G, Hatt H. Characterization of selective TRPM8 ligands and their structure activity response (S.A.R) relationship. J Pharm Pharm Sci. 2010;13:242–53.
26. Cho Y, Jang Y, Yang YD, Lee CH, Lee Y, Oh U. TRPM8 mediates cold and menthol allergies associated with mast cell activation. Cell Calcium. 2010;48(4):202–8. https://doi.org/10.1016/j.ceca.2010.09.001.
27. De Blas GA, Darszon A, Ocampo AY, et al. TRPM8, a versatile channel in human sperm. PLoS One. 2009;4(6):e6095. https://doi.org/10.1371/journal.pone.0006095.
28. Tyagi P. Pathophysiology of the urothelium and detrusor. Can Urol Assoc J. 2011;5(5 Suppl 2):S128–30. https://doi.org/10.5489/cuaj.11181.
29. Valero M, Morenilla-Palao C, Belmonte C, Viana F. Pharmacological and functional properties of TRPM8 channels in prostate tumor cells. Pflugers Arch. 2011;461(1):99–114. https://doi.org/10.1007/s00424-010-0895-0.
30. Van Haute C, De Ridder D, Nilius B. TRP channels in human prostate. ScientificWorldJournal. 2010;10:1597–611. https://doi.org/10.1100/tsw.2010.149.
31. McKemy DD. TRPM8: the cold and menthol receptor. In: Liedtke WB, Heller S, editors. TRP Ion Channel function in sensory transduction and cellular signaling cascades. Boca Raton (FL): CRC Press/Taylor & Francis; 2007.

32. Liu Z, Wu H, Wei Z, et al. TRPM8: a potential target for cancer treatment. J Cancer Res Clin Oncol. 2016;142(9):1871–81. https://doi.org/10.1007/s00432-015-2112-1.
33. Zholos A, Johnson C, Burdyga T, Melanaphy D. TRPM channels in the vasculature. Adv Exp Med Biol. 2011;704:707–29. https://doi.org/10.1007/978-94-007-0265-3_37.
34. Pertusa M, Solorza J, Madrid R. Molecular determinants of TRPM8 function: key clues for a cool modulation. Front Pharmacol. 2023;14:1213337. https://doi.org/10.3389/fphar.2023.1213337.
35. Proudfoot CJ, Garry EM, Cottrell DF, et al. Analgesia mediated by the TRPM8 cold receptor in chronic neuropathic pain. Curr Biol. 2006;16(16):1591–605. https://doi.org/10.1016/j.cub.2006.07.061.
36. Lippoldt EK, Elmes RR, McCoy DD, Knowlton WM, McKemy DD. Artemin, a glial cell line-derived neurotrophic factor family member, induces TRPM8-dependent cold pain. J Neurosci. 2013;33(30):12543–52. https://doi.org/10.1523/JNEUROSCI.5765-12.2013.
37. Knowlton WM, Palkar R, Lippoldt EK, et al. A sensory-labeled line for cold: TRPM8-expressing sensory neurons define the cellular basis for cold, cold pain, and cooling-mediated analgesia. J Neurosci. 2013;33(7):2837–48. https://doi.org/10.1523/JNEUROSCI.1943-12.2013.
38. Premkumar LS, Raisinghani M, Pingle SC, Long C, Pimentel F. Downregulation of transient receptor potential melastatin 8 by protein kinase C-mediated dephosphorylation. J Neurosci. 2005;25:11322–9.
39. Rohacs T, Lopes CMB, Michailidis I, Logothetis DE. PI(4,5)2 regulates the activation and desensitization of TRPM8 channels through the TRP domain. Nat Neurosci. 2005;8:626–34.
40. Andersson DA, Nash M, Bevan S. Modulation of the cold-activated channel TRPM8 by lyso-phospholipids and polyunsaturated fatty acids. J Neurosci. 2007;27:3347–55.
41. Rosenbaum T, Morales-Lázaro SL, Islas LD. TRP channels: a journey towards a molecular understanding of pain. Nat Rev Neurosci. 2022;23(10):596–610. https://doi.org/10.1038/s41583-022-00611-7.
42. Yudin Y, Rohacs T. Regulation of TRPM8 channel activity. Mol Cell Endocrinol. 2012;353(1–2):68–74. https://doi.org/10.1016/j.mce.2011.10.023.
43. Diver MM, Cheng Y, Julius D. Structural insights into TRPM8 inhibition and desensitization. Science. 2019;365(6460):1434–40. https://doi.org/10.1126/science.aax6672.
44. Liu Y, Mikrani R, He Y, et al. TRPM8 channels: a review of distribution and clinical role. Eur J Pharmacol. 2020;882:173312. https://doi.org/10.1016/j.ejphar.2020.173312.
45. Trusiano B, Tupik JD, Allen IC. Cold sensor, hot topic: TRPM8 plays a role in monocyte function and differentiation. J Leukoc Biol. 2022;112(3):361–3. https://doi.org/10.1002/JLB.3CE0222-099R.
46. Hornsby E, King HW, Peiris M, et al. The cation channel TRPM8 influences the differentiation and function of human monocytes. J Leukoc Biol. 2022;112:365–81. https://doi.org/10.1002/JLB.1HI0421-181R.
47. Dhaka A, Murray AN, Mathur J, Earley TJ, Petrus MJ, Patapoutian A. TRPM8 is required for cold sensation in mice. Neuron. 2007;54(3):371–8. https://doi.org/10.1016/j.neuron.2007.02.024.
48. Khalil M, Babes A, Lakra R, et al. Transient receptor potential melastatin 8 ion channel in macrophages modulates colitis through a balance-shift in TNF-alpha and interleukin-10 production. Mucosal Immunol. 2016;9:1500–13. https://doi.org/10.1038/mi.2016.11.
49. Halonen L, Pemmari A, Nummenmaa E, et al. Human osteoarthritic chondrocytes express nineteen different TRP-genes-TRPA1 and TRPM8 as potential drug targets. Int J Mol Sci. 2023;24(12):10057. https://doi.org/10.3390/ijms241210057.
50. Ma S, Yu H, Zhao Z, et al. Activation of the cold-sensing TRPM8 channel triggers UCP1-dependent thermogenesis and prevents obesity. J Mol Cell Biol. 2012;4(2):88–96. https://doi.org/10.1093/jmcb/mjs001.
51. Rossato M, Granzotto M, Macchi V, et al. Human white adipocytes express the cold receptor TRPM8 which activation induces UCP1 expression, mitochondrial activation and heat production. Mol Cell Endocrinol. 2014;383(1–2):137–46. https://doi.org/10.1016/j.mce.2013.12.005.

52. Cinti S. Transdifferentiation properties of adipocytes in the adipose organ. Am J Physiol Endocrinol Metab. 2009;297(5):E977–86. https://doi.org/10.1152/ajpendo.00183.2009.
53. Cancello R, Zingaretti MC, Sarzani R, Ricquier D, Cinti S. Leptin and UCP1 genes are reciprocally regulated in brown adipose tissue. Endocrinology. 1998;139(11):4747–50. https://doi.org/10.1210/endo.139.11.6434.
54. Cinti S, Cancello R, Zingaretti MC, et al. CL316,243 and cold stress induce heterogeneous expression of UCP1 mRNA and protein in rodent brown adipocytes. J Histochem Cytochem. 2002;50(1):21–31. https://doi.org/10.1177/002215540205000103.
55. Boström P, Wu J, Jedrychowski MP, et al. A PGC1-α-dependent myokine that drives brown-fat-like development of white fat and thermogenesis. Nature. 2012;481(7382):463–8. https://doi.org/10.1038/nature10777.
56. Bishnoi M, Khare P, Brown L, Panchal SK. Transient receptor potential (TRP) channels: a metabolic TR(i)P to obesity prevention and therapy. Obes Rev. 2018;19:1269–92. https://doi.org/10.1111/obr.12703.
57. Bishnoi M, Kondepudi KK, Gupta A, Karmase A, Boparai RK. Expression of multiple transient receptor potential channel genes in murine 3T3-L1 cell lines and adipose tissue. Pharmacol Rep. 2013;65:751–5. https://doi.org/10.1016/s1734-1140(13)71055-7.
58. Uchida K, Sun W, Yamazaki J, Tominaga M. Role of Thermo-sensitive transient receptor potential channels in Brown adipose tissue. Biol Pharm Bull. 2018;41:1135–44. https://doi.org/10.1248/bpb.b18-00063.
59. Gao P, Yan Z, Zhu Z. The role of adipose TRP channels in the pathogenesis of obesity. J Cell Physiol. 2019;234:12483–97.
60. Zhai M, Yang D, Yi W, Sun W. Involvement of calcium channels in the regulation of adipogenesis. Adipocytes. 2020;9:132–41. https://doi.org/10.1080/21623945.2020.1738792.
61. Zhang H, Wang C, Zhang K, et al. The role of TRPA1 channels in thermosensation. Cell Insight. 2022;1(6):100059. https://doi.org/10.1016/j.cellin.2022.100059.
62. Jaquemar D, Schenker T, Trueb B. An ankyrin-like protein with transmembrane domains is specifically lost after oncogenic transformation of human fibroblasts. J Biol Chem. 1999;274(11):7325–33. https://doi.org/10.1074/jbc.274.11.7325.
63. Talavera K, Startek JB, Alvarez-Collazo J, et al. Mammalian transient receptor potential TRPA1 channels: from structure to disease. Physiol Rev. 2020;100(2):725–803. https://doi.org/10.1152/physrev.00005.2019.
64. Story GM, Peier AM, Reeve AJ, et al. ANKTM1, a TRP-like channel expressed in nociceptive neurons, is activated by cold temperatures. Cell. 2003;112(6):819–29. https://doi.org/10.1016/s0092-8674(03)00158-2.
65. De Logu F, De Siena G, Landini L, et al. Non-neuronal TRPA1 encodes mechanical allodynia associated with neurogenic inflammation and partial nerve injury in rats. Br J Pharmacol. 2023;180(9):1232–46. https://doi.org/10.1111/bph.16005.
66. Kannler M, Lüling R, Yildirim AÖ, Gudermann T, Steinritz D, Dietrich A. TRPA1 channels: expression in non-neuronal murine lung tissues and dispensability for hyperoxia-induced alveolar epithelial hyperplasia. Pflugers Arch. 2018;470(8):1231–41. https://doi.org/10.1007/s00424-018-2148-6.
67. Wang Z, Ye D, Ye J, et al. The TRPA1 channel in the cardiovascular system: promising features and challenges. Front Pharmacol. 2019;10:1253. Published 2019 Oct 18. https://doi.org/10.3389/fphar.2019.01253.
68. Nozawa K, Kawabata-Shoda E, Doihara H, et al. TRPA1 regulates gastrointestinal motility through serotonin release from enterochromaffin cells. Proc Natl Acad Sci USA. 2009;106(9):3408–13. https://doi.org/10.1073/pnas.0805323106.
69. Camacho S, Michlig S, de Senarclens-Bezençon C, et al. Anti-obesity and anti-hyperglycemic effects of cinnamaldehyde via altered ghrelin secretion and functional impact on food intake and gastric emptying. Sci Rep. 2015;5:7919. https://doi.org/10.1038/srep07919.
70. Kaji I, Yasuoka Y, Karaki S, Kuwahara A. Activation of TRPA1 by luminal stimuli induces EP4-mediated anion secretion in human and rat colon. Am J Physiol Gastrointest Liver Physiol. 2012;302(7):G690–701. https://doi.org/10.1152/ajpgi.00289.2011.

71. Cao DS, Zhong L, Hsieh TH, et al. Expression of transient receptor potential ankyrin 1 (TRPA1) and its role in insulin release from rat pancreatic beta cells. PLoS One. 2012;7(5):e38005. https://doi.org/10.1371/journal.pone.0038005.
72. Caceres AI, Brackmann M, Elia MD, Bessac BF, del Camino D, D'Amours M, Witek JS, Fanger CM, Chong JA, Hayward NJ, Homer RJ, Cohn L, Huang X, Moran MM, Jordt SE. A sensory neuronal ion channel essential for airway inflammation and hyperreactivity in asthma. Proc Natl Acad Sci USA. 2009;106(22):9099–104. https://doi.org/10.1073/pnas.0900591106.
73. Nassini R, Pedretti P, Moretto N, Fusi C, Carnini C, Facchinetti F, Viscomi AR, Pisano AR, Stokesberry S, Brunmark C, Svitacheva N, McGarvey L, Patacchini R, Damholt AB, Geppetti P, Materazzi S. Transient receptor potential ankyrin 1 channel localized to non-neuronal airway cells promotes non-neurogenic inflammation. PLoS One. 2012;7(8):e42454. https://doi.org/10.1371/journal.pone.0042454.
74. Corey DP, García-Añoveros J, Holt JR, Kwan KY, Lin SY, Vollrath MA, Amalfitano A, Cheung EL, Derfler BH, Duggan A, Géléoc GS, Gray PA, Hoffman MP, Rehm HL, Tamasauskas D, Zhang DS. TRPA1 is a candidate for the mechanosensitive transduction channel of vertebrate hair cells. Nature. 2004;432(7018):723–30. https://doi.org/10.1038/nature03066.
75. Stepanyan RS, Indzhykulian AA, Vélez-Ortega AC, Boger ET, Steyger PS, Friedman TB, Frolenkov GI. TRPA1-mediated accumulation of aminoglycosides in mouse cochlear outer hair cells. J Assoc Res Otolaryngol. 2011;12(6):729–40. https://doi.org/10.1007/s10162-011-0288-x.
76. Jain A, Brönneke S, Kolbe L, Stäb F, Wenck H, Neufang G. TRP-channel-specific cutaneous eicosanoid release patterns. Pain. 2011;152(12):2765–72. https://doi.org/10.1016/j.pain.2011.08.025.
77. Atoyan R, Shander D, Botchkareva NV. Non-neuronal expression of transient receptor potential type A1 (TRPA1) in human skin. J Invest Dermatol. 2009;129(9):2312–5. https://doi.org/10.1038/jid.2009.58.
78. El Karim IA, Linden GJ, Curtis TM, About I, McGahon MK, Irwin CR, Killough SA, Lundy FT. Human dental pulp fibroblasts express the "cold-sensing" transient receptor potential channels TRPA1 and TRPM8. J Endod. 2011;37(4):473–8. https://doi.org/10.1016/j.joen.2010.12.017.
79. Caspani O, Heppenstall PA. TRPA1 and cold transduction: an unresolved issue? J Gen Physiol. 2009;133:245–9. https://doi.org/10.1085/jgp.200810136.
80. Chen J, Hackos DH. TRPA1 as a drug target--promise and challenges. Naunyn Schmiedeberg's Arch Pharmacol. 2015;388(4):451–63. https://doi.org/10.1007/s00210-015-1088-3.
81. Kwan KY, Corey DP. Burning cold: involvement of TRPA1 in noxious cold sensation. J Gen Physiol. 2009;133:251–6. https://doi.org/10.1085/jgp.200810146.
82. Karashima Y, Damann N, Prenen J, et al. Bimodal action of menthol on the transient receptor potential channel TRPA1. J Neurosci. 2007;27(37):9874–84. https://doi.org/10.1523/JNEUROSCI.2221-07.2007.
83. Lo CW, Chen CS, Chen YC, et al. Allyl Isothiocyanate ameliorates obesity by inhibiting Galectin-12. Mol Nutr Food Res. 2018;62(6):e1700616. https://doi.org/10.1002/mnfr.201700616.
84. Oi-Kano Y, Iwasaki Y, Nakamura T, et al. Oleuropein aglycone enhances UCP1 expression in brown adipose tissue in high-fat-diet-induced obese rats by activating β-adrenergic signaling. J Nutr Biochem. 2017;40:209–18. https://doi.org/10.1016/j.jnutbio.2016.11.009.
85. Tamura Y, Iwasaki Y, Narukawa M, Watanabe T. Ingestion of cinnamaldehyde, a TRPA1 agonist, reduces visceral fats in mice fed a high-fat and high-sucrose diet. J Nutr Sci Vitaminol (Tokyo). 2012;58(1):9–13. https://doi.org/10.3177/jnsv.58.9.
86. Sahin N, Orhan C, Erten F, et al. Effects of allyl isothiocyanate on insulin resistance, oxidative stress status, and transcription factors in high-fat diet/streptozotocin-induced type 2 diabetes mellitus in rats. J Biochem Mol Toxicol. 2019;33(7):e22328. https://doi.org/10.1002/jbt.22328.

87. Ahn J, Lee H, Im SW, Jung CH, Ha TY. Allyl isothiocyanate ameliorates insulin resistance through the regulation of mitochondrial function. J Nutr Biochem. 2014;25(10):1026–34. https://doi.org/10.1016/j.jnutbio.2014.05.006.

88. Bishnoi M, Khare P, Brown L, S.K. Panchal transient receptor potential (TRP) channels: a metabolic TR(i)P to obesity prevention and therapy. Obes Rev. 2018;19(9):1269–92. https://doi.org/10.1111/OBR.12703.

89. Zhu Z, Luo Z, Ma S, D. Liu TRP channels and their implications in metabolic diseases Pflueg arch Eur. J Physiol. 2011;461(2):211–23. https://doi.org/10.1007/S00424-010-0902-5.

90. Ahern GP. Ahern Transient receptor potential channels and energy homeostasis. Trends Endocrinol Metabol. 2013;24(11):554–60.

91. Uchida K, Dezaki K, Yoneshiro T, Watanabe T, Yamazaki J, Saito M, et al. Involvement of thermosensitive TRP channels in energy metabolism. J Physiol Sci. 2017;67(5):549–60.

92. Tabur S, Oztuzcu S, Duzen IV, Eraydin A, Eroglu S, Ozkaya M, et al. Role of the transient receptor potential (TRP) channel gene expressions and TRP melastatin (TRPM) channel gene polymorphisms in obesity-related metabolic syndrome. Eur Rev Med Pharmacol Sci. 2015;19:1388–97. https://doi.org/10.1530/endoabs.37.EP609.

93. Reimúndez A, Fernández-Peña C, García G, Fernández R, Ordás P, Gallego R, et al. Deletion of the cold thermoreceptor TRPM8 increases heat loss and food intake leading to reduced body temperature and obesity in mice. J Neurosci. 2018;38(15):3643–56.

94. Clemmensen C, Jall S, Kleinert M, et al. Coordinated targeting of cold and nicotinic receptors synergistically improves obesity and type 2 diabetes. [published correction appears in Nat Commun. 2018 Nov 20;9(1):4975]. Nat Commun. 2018;9(1):4304. https://doi.org/10.1038/s41467-018-06769-y.

95. Liskiewicz D, Zhang Q, Barthem CS, Jastroch M, Liskiewicz A, Khajavi N, Grandl G, Coupland C, Kleinert M, Garcia-Caceres C, Novikoff A, Maity G, Boehm U, Tschöp MH, Müller TD. Neuronal loss of TRPM8 leads to obesity and glucose intolerance in male mice. Mol Metab. 2023;72:101714. https://doi.org/10.1016/j.molmet.2023.101714.

96. Sanders OD, Rajagopal JA, Rajagopal L. Menthol to induce non-shivering thermogenesis via TRPM8/PKA signaling for treatment of obesity. J Obes Metab Syndr. 2021;30(1):4–11. https://doi.org/10.7570/jomes20038Cc.

97. Valente A, Carrillo AE, Tzatzarakis MN, et al. The absorption and metabolism of a single L-menthol oral versus skin administration: effects on thermogenesis and metabolic rate. Food Chem Toxicol. 2015;86:262–73. https://doi.org/10.1016/j.fct.2015.09.018.

Subjective Cold Perception

4

Romain Bouzigon

The beneficial effects of the whole-body cryostimulation (WBC) exposure are based on an external cold stimulus [1]. The cold perception felt by the exposed person leads to the stimulation of the hypothalamus which activates cold adaptations. This "feeling," named "cold perception," is then very important to induce the desired effect. The cold perception is a sensory perception. In cognitive psychology, a sensory perception is a subject's reaction to an external stimulation characterized by chemical and neuronal phenomena at the level of the organs and the central nervous system (CNS). This perception is provided by the senses. The central nervous system collects and processes sensory information. Then the resulting awareness depends on the past and the actual state of the subject. Cold perception is tactile because it comes from the skin thermoreceptors. It is then composed of two factors: (1) an objective afferent signal from the skin to the CNS, more precisely to the hypothalamus, and (2) the interpretation of this signal [2].

The objective afferent signal comes from the skin. The interaction between the human body and the external environment (in our case the cryocabin or cryochamber) occurs principally at the skin level, and skin temperature may reflect the balance between heat loss to the environment and heat produced by metabolically active tissues [3]. The skin is a sensory organ and belongs to the somatosensory system. It allows the perception of much information from the external environment like cognitive information (hot, cold, pain, etc.) [2]. This information is transmitted to the brain. The cold external stimuli (hot and cold) activate skin sensors called

R. Bouzigon (✉)
Laboratoire Axe Sport Performance, Université de Franche-Comté, UFR STAPS Besançon, Besançon, France

Sports Performance Optimization Complex, Society Inside the Athletes 3.0, Besançon, France

Society Aurore Concept, Noisiel, France

© The Author(s), under exclusive license to Springer Nature Switzerland AG 2024
P. Capodaglio (ed.), *Whole-Body Cryostimulation*,
https://doi.org/10.1007/978-3-031-18545-8_4

thermoreceptors. These receptors are free nerve endings. The cold receptors are nearer to the surface than the hot receptors. The best-known cold-sensitive nerve channels are those of transient receptor potential (TRP) M8 (vanilloid) and TRPA1 (ankyrin). The TRPA1 channel works principally in ice stimuli and for temperatures under 18 °C and the TRPM8 channel mostly in cold stimuli at 10–25 °C [4–6]. Internally the cold thermal stimulus is transmitted by thermal nerve cells to various hypothalamus areas like the preoptic area (POA), which plays a central role in thermoregulation. The thermoreceptors produce a constant electrical discharge rate when the temperature remains constant. When the temperature drops suddenly, the discharge rate increases considerably [7]. The rate is from about 10–20 impulses/s at a normal skin temperature to a maximum of 120–140 impulses/s. The cold sensors are endings of sensory nerve fibers. These fibers are group III fibers or Aδ fibers. They are myelinated, not bulky (1–5 μm), and less fast than the other sensory nerve fibers (5–30 m/s). The afferent message then goes into the spinal cord before joining the hypothalamus.

The hypothalamus is the human thermostat. It allows to know core and skin temperature and triggers thermogenesis or thermolysis in function of these temperatures. The thermogenesis consists mainly of (1) peripheral vasoconstriction to decrease heat exchange with the external environment and keep the internal temperature for the organs and (2) the triggering of shivering to create heat. The thermolysis is permitted by perspiration and its evaporation. This behavioral thermoregulation allows the prevention of thermal injuries from the external environment.

The important point for this part is the place of the perception inside this response. Today it is difficult to know if the intensity of the cold adaptation response triggered by the hypothalamus is linked to the objective afferent signal from the thermoreceptors or to our perceptual interpretation of this signal.

The perceptual interpretation of the signal depends on several factors: The initial skin temperature, the speed of temperature change and the size, the stimulated surface, the gender, the age, and the ethnic origin [8]. We know that Inuit or some Siberian populations have genetic variants on a single chromosome. Two genes, WARS2 and TBX15, allow them to have different body fat distribution, especially with differentiation on the brown fat cells that are involved in heat generation [9]. The cold perception could be different for these populations.

Thermal perception is composed of two basic elements: thermal sensation (discriminative component) and thermal comfort (hedonic component). The thermal sensation is the perception of the hot and cold stimuli, and the thermal comfort is the "pleasantness or unpleasantness" feeling linked [4, 10]. These two components of thermal perception would be independent. Indeed a study demonstrated that facial cooling induced a similar cold sensation in both hot and cold environments but the thermal pleasantness was evoked only in a hot environment [11]. Another study supports these findings by showing that the two components involved the activation of different parts of the CNS [10]. The discriminative component involved activation of the medial prefrontal cortex extending to the anterior cingulate cortex, insula, middle frontal cortex, and parietal lobes. The hedonic components involved activation of the medial prefrontal cortex, posterior cingulate cortex, and inferior parietal lobes.

Table 4.1 Studies that assessed the perception of cold, in particular thermal sensation and thermal comfort, during exposure to WBC

Study	Technology and protocol used	Perception scales used	Results
Bouzigon et al. (2017) [18] Validation of a new whole-body cryotherapy chamber based on forced convection	WBC Cryantal development (Noisiel, France). 30 s at −13.4 °C and 3″ at −34.5 °C Wind chill technology with an average of 2.4 m/s of win Healthy volunteers accustomed to WBC. This study was based on only one exposure.	**Thermal sensation:** "On average, how did you feel during the exposure?" Nine-point scale of "4—Very hot, 3—Hot, 2—Warm, 1—Slightly warm, 0—Neutral, −1—Slightly cool, −2—Cool, −3—Cold, −4—Very cold" [12] **Thermal comfort:** "On average, how did you feel during the exposure?" The scale graduated from "0—Excellent" to "10—Unbearable" [13]	**Thermal sensation:** The mean perceived temperature during a 3-min exposure was −3.0 ± 0.8, corresponding to "cold" **Thermal comfort:** Mean score = 6.0 ± 1.9, corresponding to "not very good" sensations
Smolander et al. (2004) [16] Thermal sensation and comfort in women exposed repeatedly to whole-body cryotherapy and winter swimming in ice-cold water	WBC Zimmer (Deutschland). Subjects pass through the first chamber (−10 °C) and the second chamber (−60 °C) before coming into the therapy chamber (−110 °C) Twenty healthy women (35–45 years and body mass index <28) were exposed to three 2-min exposures per week for 3 months	**Thermal sensation:** Nine-point scale "4—Very hot, 3—Hot, 2—Warm, 1—Slightly warm, 0—Neutral, −1—Slightly cool, −2—Cool, −3—Cold, −4—Very cold" [12] **Thermal comfort:** "Do you find this" Five-point scale "0 = comfortable, 1 = slightly uncomfortable, 2 = uncomfortable, 3 = very uncomfortable, 4 = extremely uncomfortable" [12]	**Thermal sensation:** Before exposure = "neutral" After exposure = between "cool" and "slightly cool" the first month; "slightly cool" and "neutral" the second and the third months **Thermal comfort:** Between "comfortable" and "slightly uncomfortable"

(continued)

Table 4.1 (continued)

Study	Technology and protocol used	Perception scales used	Results
Bouzigon et al. (2018) [21] Thermal sensations during a partial-body Cryostimulation exposure in elite basketball players	PBC Mecacel (Mouroux, France) 3 min at −130 °C Twenty-four international-level basketball players (13 females and 11 males, aged 25.7 ± 3.5 years) from the French national team participated in this study	**Thermal comfort:** "How cold do you feel right now?" Scale graduated from "0—Neutral" to "10—Unbearable" [13] Asked every 30 s during exposure	**Thermal sensation:** Seemed to increase every 30 s during PBC exposure in all athletes After 3 min: 5.7— "Cool" sensation In females, the BMI became significantly and negatively correlated with thermal sensation during the last minute
Costello et al. (2012) [19] Muscle, skin and Core temperature after −110 °C cold air and 8 °C water treatment	WBC Zimmer (Germany) 20 s at −60 °C and 3 min 40 at −110 °C Twenty healthy active males	Both thermal perceptions: Post and post 5′ after exposure **Thermal sensation:** "How are you feeling now?" Scale graduated from −4 to 4 [12] **Thermal comfort:** Scale graduated from 0 to 4, "0 = comfortable, 1 = slightly uncomfortable, 2 = uncomfortable, 3 = very uncomfortable, 4 = extremely uncomfortable" [12]	**Thermal sensation:** Post exp.: −1.8, between "slightly cool" and "cool" 5′ post exp.: −0.7, between "neutral" and "slightly cool" **Thermal comfort:** Subjects tended to find the WBC "uncomfortable"
Cuttel et al. (2017) [14] Individualizing the exposure of −110 °C whole body cryotherapy: The effects of sex and body composition	WBC Juka (Poland) 30 s at −60 °C and 2′ at −110 °C 18 untrained participants (10 males and 8 females)	**Thermal sensation:** A 9-point scale from 0 (considered as unbearably cold) to 8 (unbearably hot), with 4 (neutral) [25] **Thermal comfort:** A 9-point scale from 4 (very comfortable) to −4 (very uncomfortable) with 0 (neutral)	**Thermal sensation:** Males tended to find WBC "cool" immediately post treatment whereas females found WBC "slightly warm" (only significative difference between thermal sensation and sexes immmediatly post WBC) **Thermal comfort:** Male 1 and female 2.5 (NS)

Table 4.1 (continued)

Study	Technology and protocol used	Perception scales used	Results
Douzi et al. (2019) [20] Partial body cryostimulation after training improves sleep quality in professional soccer players	PBC Krion (Saint Petersburg, Russia) −180 °C during 1′30, or 2 × 1′30 or 3′ Nine male football professional players from the Niort football club	**Thermal comfort:** "How cold do you feel right now?" A 10-point scale from 0 ("neutral") to 10 ("unbearably cold") [13]	The perception of cold was significantly higher ($p < 0.001$) after the 180-s exposure (8.0 ± 1.2) than after the 90-s and the 2 × 90-s exposures (4.6 ± 1.8 and 5.3 ± 1.2, respectively)
Selfe et al. (2014) [15] The effect of three different (−135 °C) whole body cryotherapy exposure durations on elite Rugby league players	WBC Juka (Poland) 30 s at −60 °C and 1, 2, or 3 min at −135 °C Fourteen (24 years; mean weight 77.6 kg; mean height 183.2 cm) professional rugby league players from Wigan warriors RLFC	**Thermal sensation:** "How are you feeling now?" A scale from −4 to 4 [12] **Thermal comfort:** "Do you find this" 0 = comfortable; 1 = slightly comfortable; 2 = uncomfortable; 3 = very uncomfortable; 4 = extremely uncomfortable [12]	**Thermal sensation:** NS between 2- and 3′; however between 1- and 2′ exposures, there was a significant reduction: – post 1′: "Slightly cool" – post 2′: "Cold" or "very cold" – post 3′: "Very cold"
Theurot et al. (2021) [22] Impact of acute partial body cryostimulation on cognitive performance, cerebral oxygenation, and cardiac autonomic activity	PBC—Unknown technology 3′ at −150 °C Eighteen healthy active participants	**Thermal comfort:** 0 = neutral, 2 = slightly cool, 4 = cool, 6 = cold, 8 = very cold, 10 = unbearable cold [13]	After exposure: "8—Very cold"
Westerlund et al. (2003) [17] Thermal responses during and after whole-body cryotherapy (−110 °C)	WBC Zimmer −10 °C, −60 °C, and 2′ at −110 °C Nine sedentary and healthy females and one male	**Thermal sensation** How do you feel at this precise moment Scale graduated from −4 to 4 [12]	The subjects' thermal sensations immediately after WBC varied from "cold" (−3) to "slightly cool" (−1)

(continued)

Table 4.1 (continued)

Study	Technology and protocol used	Perception scales used	Results
Fonda et al. (2014) [23] Effects of whole-body cryotherapy duration on thermal and cardio-vascular response	PBC Criomed (Kherson, Ukraine) 90, 120, 150 and 180″ at −140 °C Twelve healthy young participants	**Thermal comfort** Every 15 s during the session, participants were asked to grade a level of thermal discomfort on a 10 cm visual–analog scale 0 = no thermal discomfort and 10 = unbearable thermal discomfort	4 at 30″ and 7 at 180″

Fig. 4.1 Thermal sensation scale of ISO 10051

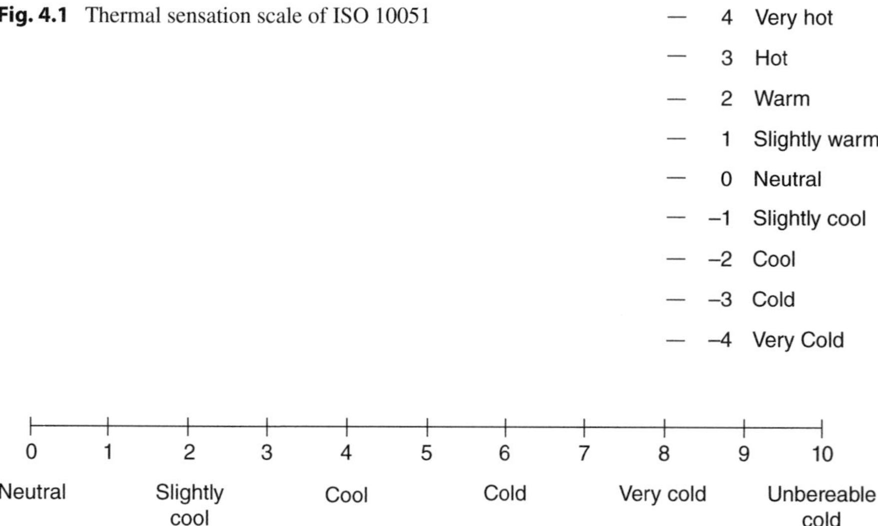

Fig. 4.2 Thermal comfort scale of Lundgren et al. [13]

Cold Perception during Whole-Body Cryotherapy

Several studies assessed cold perception, especially thermal sensation and thermal comfort, during a WBC exposure (Table 4.1). Most of them used the same scales. The thermal sensation is most of the time the ISO 10051 scale [12]. It is a nine-point scale "4—Very hot, 3—Hot, 2—Warm, 1—Slightly warm, 0—Neutral, −1—Slightly cool, −2—Cool, −3—Cold, −4—Very cold" and the question asked for people is usually "How are you feeling now?" (Fig. 4.1). For thermal comfort, several studies used the scale of the ISO 10051 and others scale of Lundgren et al. [13]. The Lundgren scale is graduated from "0—Excellent" to "10—Unbearable" (Fig. 4.2). The question is "How cold do you feel right now?"

It may be interesting to standardize two scales for these two components. The authors could already use the same scales. In the same way, it will be interesting to use the same question for each scale. In the literature some authors ask the question "How do you feel 'right now'?" and others, how do you feel 'on average during the exposure'?" The choice of the question is important because the answers may vary. For example, in the study of Cuttel et al. [14], the females feel "slightly warm" immediately after the exposure. So be careful if we want to know the cold feeling inside the chambers during exposure.

Generally, studies showed that people who practiced WBC and PBC did not suffer too much from the exposure. For 1′ exposure, the thermal sensation was "slightly cool" [15]; for 2′ exposure from "cool" to "very cold" [15–17]; and for 3′ from "cool" to "very cold" [15, 18, 19].

For the thermal comfort, a 1′30 exposure was between "average" and "not very cool" [20]; for 2′ between "neutral" and "slightly cool" [16]; and for 3′ between "not very good" and "bad" [18, 20–23].

Even if some authors demonstrated a greater skin temperature variation after WBC exposure in females than in males [14, 24], only one study found a difference in thermal sensation between both [14]. In this study, the difference was found for the thermal sensation immediately after exposure and not inside the chamber during exposure. Females felt "slightly warm" and males "cool". The other studies found no difference in thermal sensation or comfort between sexes [18, 21, 22]. Interestingly, Bouzigon et al. [21] showed that the body mass index was significantly and negatively correlated with the thermal comfort value after 2 min 30 s, and 3 min of exposure in PBC in females.

To our knowledge, no study assessed the difference in thermal sensation and comfort in function of the morphological characteristics of the participants.

References

1. Bouzigon R, Grappe F, Ravier G, Dugue B. Whole- and partial-body cryostimulation/cryotherapy: current technologies and practical applications. J Thermal Biol. 2016;61:67–81.
2. Boulais N, Misery L. The epidermis: a sensory tissue. Eur J Dermatol. 2008;18(2):119–27.
3. Cholewka A, Drzazga Z, Sieron A. Monitoring of whole body cryotherapy effects by thermal imaging: preliminary report. Phys Med. 2006;22(2):57–62.
4. Ntoumani M, Dugue B, Rivas E, Gongaki K. Thermoregulation and thermal sensation during whole-body water immersion at different water temperatures in healthy individuals: a scoping review. J Thermal Biol. 2023;112:103430.
5. Romanovsky AA. Thermoregulation: some concepts have changed. Functional architecture of the thermoregulatory system. Am J Physiol Regul Integr Comp Physiol. 2007;292(1):R37–46.
6. Wang H, Siemens J. TRP ion channels in thermosensation, thermoregulation and metabolism. Temperature (Austin). 2015;2(2):178–87.
7. Papenfuss W. Power from the cold, whole body cryotherapy at −110 degrees, a short-lasting physical therapy with a long-lasting effect. Edition; 2012. 143 p.

8. Karjalainen S. Thermal comfort and gender: a literature review. Indoor Air. 2012;22(2):96–109.
9. Racimo F, Gokhman D, Fumagalli M, Ko A, Hansen T, Moltke I, et al. Archaic adaptive introgression in TBX15/WARS2. Mol Biol Evol. 2017;34(3):509–24.
10. Aizawa Y, Harada T, Nakata H, Tsunakawa M, Sadato N, Nagashima K. Assessment of brain mechanisms involved in the processes of thermal sensation, pleasantness/unpleasantness, and evaluation. IBRO Rep. 2019;6:54–63.
11. Nakamura M, Yoda T, Crawshaw LI, Yasuhara S, Saito Y, Kasuga M, et al. Regional differences in temperature sensation and thermal comfort in humans. J Appl Physiol (1985). 2008;105(6):1897–906.
12. Standardisation IOf. ISO 10051 FS. Ergonomics of the thermal environment-assessment of the influence of the thermal environment using subjective judgment scales. Geneva; 1995.
13. Lundgren P, Henriksson O, Kuklane K, Holmer I, Naredi P, Bjornstig U. Validity and reliability of the cold discomfort scale: a subjective judgement scale for the assessment of patient thermal state in a cold environment. J Clin Monit Comput. 2014;28(3):287–91.
14. Cuttell S, Hammond L, Langdon D, Costello J. Individualising the exposure of −110 °C whole body cryotherapy: the effects of sex and body composition. J Thermal Biol. 2017;65:41–7.
15. Selfe J, Alexander J, Costello JT, May K, Garratt N, Atkins S, et al. The effect of three different (−135 °C) whole body cryotherapy exposure durations on elite rugby league players. PLoS One. 2014;9(1):e86420.
16. Smolander J, Mikkelsson M, Oksa J, Westerlund T, Leppaluoto J, Huttunen P. Thermal sensation and comfort in women exposed repeatedly to whole-body cryotherapy and winter swimming in ice-cold water. Physiol Behav. 2004;82(4):691–5.
17. Westerlund T, Oksa J, Smolander J, Mikkelsson M. Thermal responses during and after whole-body cryotherapy (−110 °C). J Thermal Biol. 2003;28(8):601–8.
18. Bouzigon R, Arfaoui A, Grappe F, Ravier G, Jarlot B, Dugue B. Validation of a new whole-body cryotherapy chamber based on forced convection. J Thermal Biol. 2017;65:138–44.
19. Costello JT, Culligan K, Selfe J, Donnelly AE. Muscle, skin and Core temperature after −110°C cold air and 8°C water treatment. PLoS One. 2012;7(11):e48190.
20. Douzi W, Dupuy O, Theurot D, Boucard G, Dugue B. Partial-body cryostimulation after training improves sleep quality in professional soccer players. BMC Res Notes. 2019;12(1):141.
21. Bouzigon R, Ravier G, Dugue B, Grappe F. Thermal sensations during a partial-body Cryostimulation exposure in elite basketball players. J Hum Kinet. 2018;62:55–63.
22. Theurot D, Dugue B, Douzi W, Guitet P, Louis J, Dupuy O. Impact of acute partial-body cryostimulation on cognitive performance, cerebral oxygenation, and cardiac autonomic activity. Sci Rep. 2021;11(1):7793.
23. Fonda B, De Nardi M, Sarabon N. Effects of whole-body cryotherapy duration on thermal and cardio-vascular response. J Thermal Biol. 2014;42:52–5.
24. Hammond LE, Cuttell S, Nunley P, Meyler J. Anthropometric characteristics and sex influence magnitude of skin cooling following exposure to whole body cryotherapy. Biomed Res Int. 2014;7:1.
25. Gagge AP, Stolwijk JA, Hardy JD. Comfort and thermal sensations and associated physiological responses at various ambient temperatures. Environ Res. 1967;1(1):1–20.

Muscular and Cerebral Tissue Oxygenation and Blood Flow

5

Dimitri Theurot, Benoit Dugué, and Olivier Dupuy

Introduction

For many years, cryostimulation has been proposed as a recovery technique that can improve and accelerate recovery processes in order to improve athlete performance, reduce the risks of injury and reduce the risk of negative adaptation to training, such as overtraining [1]. Several meta-analyses have reported a positive effect on muscular performance [2] and also on reducing pain and inflammation [3]. One of the proposed mechanisms to rationalise the utilisation of cryostimulation in post-exercise recovery processes centres around the observed vascular responses following cold exposure. At the muscular level, the literature suggests that the reduction in blood flow resulting from tissue cooling could lead to a decrease in inflammatory processes and post-exercise oedema [4–6]. Consequently, the drop in muscular blood flow and cellular metabolism due to cold exposure might curtail secondary muscle damage caused by inflammation [7–9], thus promoting recovery.

However, the literature often focuses on the peripheral effects of recovery techniques, often overlooking aspects of the central nervous system. At the brain level, there has been a limited number of studies that have specifically examined the effects of cold-water immersion or cold-air cryotherapy on the modulation of cerebral blood flow and cerebral oxygenation. Also, most of these studies were focused on cerebral haemodynamic recovery after a physical exercise associated

D. Theurot · B. Dugué
Laboratory MOVE, Faculty of Sport Sciences (STAPS), University of Poitiers, Poitiers, France

O. Dupuy (✉)
Laboratory MOVE, Faculty of Sport Sciences (STAPS), University of Poitiers, Poitiers, France

School of Kinesiology and Physical Activity Sciences (EKSAP), Faculty of Medicine, Université de Montreal, Montreal, Canada
e-mail: olivier.dupuy@univ-poitiers.fr

P. Capodaglio (ed.), *Whole-Body Cryostimulation*,
https://doi.org/10.1007/978-3-031-18545-8_5

with heat stress [10] or during a cold shock [11, 12] which is not representative of cold-water immersion protocol used in post-exercise recovery. However, inadequate cerebral oxygenation can occur during intense exercise, leading to the development of central fatigue [13, 14]. Therefore, investigating the effect of cooling strategies such as cryostimulation and cold-water immersion on cerebral oxygenation is a step forward in the understanding of the beneficial effect of these strategies on post-exercise recovery. Finally, it is important to note that vascular responses and tissue oxygenation variation triggered by cold exposure have primarily been studied in the context of cold-water immersion, and fewer studies exist regarding cryostimulation exposure.

Muscular Oxygenation and Blood Flow

Cold-Water Immersion

The scientific literature regarding the effect of cold-water immersion tends to corroborate the reduction in muscular oxygenation and muscular blood flow following exposure. As an illustration, cold water immersion has been evidenced to lower microvascular perfusion in the cooled muscle after a physical exercise involving continuous moderate-intensity exercise and high-intensity interval training (HIIT), potentially heightening muscular recovery [15]. These observations were also previously noted in a study aiming to determine the effects of cold-water immersion on the repetition of a maximal 15-min cycling performance. The performance remained consistent following cold-water immersion, whereas active recovery led to a performance decline during the second exercise session. This sustained performance was also linked to a reduction in blood flow to the lower and upper limbs after the cold-water immersion [16]. Recently, Jones also observed that in cold water immersion there is a reduced muscle oxygen consumption at rest [17]. These observations also seem to apply to exercise. Cold-water immersion prior to physical exercise appears to affect muscle oxygenation responses. In fact, Stanley observed that cold water immersion, prior to physical exercise, was accompanied by a reduction in muscular oxygen consumption during intermittent exercise, probably due to vasoconstriction [18]. It also seems that immersion in cold water is accompanied by a reduction in the aerobic system activity [18].

Interestingly, the influence of water temperature was explored in two separate investigations. The initial study investigated femoral artery blood flow before and after a 10-min session of cold-water immersion at 8 °C or cool-water immersion at 22 °C among a cohort of nine male participants. This immersion was administered after a 30-min rest period. The outcomes of this study unveiled a substantial decline in femoral artery blood flow, with a comparable magnitude observed for both water temperatures [19]. A subsequent work continued to investigate these water temperatures on femoral artery blood flow. However, in this study, the cold-water immersions were conducted following a session of resistance exercise. The findings indicated a comparable reduction in femoral artery blood flow under both temperature conditions [20].

These results imply that the hydrostatic pressure exerted during immersion induces vascular adaptations that induce a similar reduction in muscular blood flow, whether in cool water at 22 °C or cold water at 8 °C.

In summary, the collective findings of these studies demonstrate that cold water immersion leads to a reduction in both blood flow and muscular oxygenation. Nonetheless, it is challenging to conclude whether these physiological responses are induced by water temperature, hydrostatic pressure or a combination of these two factors.

Whole- and Partial-Body Cryostimulation

The scientific literature offers a limited number of studies that investigate the impact of whole and partial-body cryostimulation on muscular blood flow and oxygenation. The limited availability of research concerning whole and partial-body cryostimulation could potentially be attributed to the greater accessibility and more widespread utilisation of cold-water immersion within the realm of sport recovery. Furthermore, the few studies addressing this subject tend to yield more divergent outcomes in comparison to the relatively more consistent results obtained from cold-water immersion.

A study conducted by Selfe et al. [21] marked the initial exploration into the effects of cryostimulation on muscular oxygenation. This research was centred on investigating how capillary blood flow in the gastrocnemius muscles responded to three different durations of exposure to −135 °C whole-body cryostimulation, as assessed through near-infrared spectroscopy (NIRS). During the first 5 min following exposure, there was a noticeable decrease in concentrations of oxyhaemoglobin ($[HbO_2]$) and deoxyhaemoglobin ([HHb]) across all cryostimulation conditions. However, between 5 and 20 min after exposure, both $[HbO_2]$ and [HHb] concentrations increased, surpassing the values observed before the exposure. The authors argue that this pattern suggests a widening of blood volume within the venous compartment due to vasodilation induced by exposure of cryostimulation [21]. Three studies conducted more recently explored the impact of whole-body cryostimulation [22, 23] and partial-body cryostimulation [24] on femoral artery blood flow [22, 23] and vastus lateralis oxygenation [24]. In these three studies, the effect of cryostimulation was compared to cold-water immersion. The results showed a significant reduction of the femoral artery blood flow [23] and a significant reduction of the vastus lateralis oxygenation [24]. However, contrasting results were found by Haq et al. [22]. In this study, femoral artery blood flow measured after whole-body cryostimulation was similar to pre-exposure values which was not the case after immersion in cold water (10 min, 15 °C). The authors argued that this feature could explain the decrease in muscle strength observed after the regular use of cold bathing after strength exercise training. A reduction in blow flow could in fact reduced the arrival of free amino acids needed for muscle recovery and possible ergogenic effects. Using a near infrared imaging technique (fNIRS) at microvascular level, it has recently been shown that cryostimulation induced a reduction in oxygen consumption at rest [25]. These results may directly derive from a reduction in muscle or arterial blood flow observed in the above-mentioned studies or a reduction in oxidative metabolism.

In summary, the available data regarding the impact of cryostimulation on muscular blood flow and oxygenation are extremely limited. These data are incongruent and do not unequivocally confirm the muscular vascular responses to cryostimulation. Nevertheless, it is noteworthy to observe that certain studies directly compare the effects of these two cooling techniques.

Cold-Water Immersion vs. Whole- and Partial-Body Cryostimulation

Comparing the effects of cold-water immersion and cryostimulation is not a straightforward endeavour. Indeed, the diversity of protocols encompassing exercise types, environmental conditions and the range of studied populations prevents direct comparison of results across different studies. Nonetheless, scattered throughout the literature, are a few studies that directly compare the effects of these two cooling techniques.

In the first study, a comparative analysis was conducted concerning the muscular vascular responses from whole-body cryostimulation and cold-water immersion. Following a period of continuous moderate-intensity exercise, ten male participants were subjected to either a 2-min whole-body cryostimulation session at $-110\,°C$ or a cold-water immersion session up to the waist for 10 min at 8 °C. The outcomes revealed a significant decline in muscular blood flow discerned between the 'pre-cooling' measurements and those taken post-recovery. Moreover, the attenuation of blood flow was notably more pronounced after the cold-water immersion as compared to whole-body cryostimulation [23]. Similarly, Hohenauer et al. [24] conducted a study comparing the impact of cold-water immersion and cryostimulation on the oxygenation status of the vastus lateralis muscle of 19 male participants. Following a muscle-damaging protocol, participants undertook either a 10-min cold-water immersion at 10 °C up to the waist or 2 min at $-135\,°C$ during a partial-body cryostimulation session. The outcomes of this study unveiled notably diminished levels of muscular oxygenation among the cohort subjected to cold-water immersion compared to whole-body cryostimulation. This difference was significant from 10 to 40 min post-exposure [24]. More recently, the same researchers reproduced this protocol on a cohort of 28 females. Both cooling techniques induced the same decrease in muscular oxygenation compared to the control group [26].

These findings indicate that both cold water immersion and cryostimulation elicit a decrease in muscular blood flow and muscular oxygenation. Moreover, the magnitude of the decrease seems more important with cold-water immersion. Nevertheless, this greater reduction is not associated with enhanced recovery, suggesting that the degree of muscular oxygenation decline does not necessarily correspond to the extent of recovery.

Cerebral Oxygenation

Cold-Water Immersion

Recovery processes also depend to a large extent on the recovery of neurophysiological processes in the central nervous system. Despite the potential effect of cerebral oxygenation on post-exercise recovery, only one study investigated the effect of cold-water immersion on this physiological parameter. Indeed, in a study proposed by Minett et al., 9 participants underwent 3 experimental sessions consisting of 2 bouts of a 35-min intermittent exercise interspersed by a 15-min of passive recovery. Following this exercise, participants were submitted to either a 20-min cold-water immersion at 10 °C, a passive recovery at room temperature (32 °C), or a MIX condition consisting of using a cold wet towel over the head, and a cooling jacket for 20 min. Compared to the other conditions, the cold-water immersion significantly reduced cerebral oxygenation until 1-h post-intervention [10]. However, cold-water immersion hastened the recovery of maximal voluntary contraction. These observations suggest that the potential means by which CWI could mitigate central fatigue are distinct from alterations in cerebral perfusion and oxygenation [5].

Whole- and Partial-Body Cryostimulation

To this date, only one study investigated the effect of partial-body cryostimulation on cerebral oxygenation. Cerebral oxygenation was measured before, during, and after a 3-min partial-body cryostimulation at -150 °C in a cohort of 9 male and 9 female participants [27]. During the cryostimulation exposure, the results unveiled a significant reduction in tHb and HbO_2 levels both in male and female subjects, accompanied by a marked elevation in HHb. Moreover, this elevated HHb level remained significantly higher than the control group solely in male participants following the cryostimulation session whereas all other parameters returned to baseline values. Cerebral oxygenation was also measured during a Stroop task conducted before and after the cold exposure. The results indicate a greater cerebral oxygenation after the partial-body cryostimulation mainly marked by higher HHb values in the PBC group compared to the control group in male participants only. These results were also associated with faster reaction time at the Stroop task in male participants following the cold exposure [27].

As this study is the only one investigating the effect of cryostimulation on cerebral oxygenation, it is presently impossible to assert the effect of cryostimulation on this physiological mechanism. More studies are required to understand cerebrovascular responses to cryostimulation and their potential implication in post-exercise recovery.

Conclusion

To conclude, this brief review highlighted the potential effect of cold-water immersion and cryostimulation on muscular and cerebral oxygenation and blood flow. Although it seems rather clear that cold-water immersion induces a reduction of muscular tissue oxygenation and perfusion, these results are more equivocal concerning the effect of cryostimulation. This physiological response to cold exposure is also proposed as one of the key mechanisms explaining the beneficial effects of these two cooling techniques. Concerning brain oxygenation, the scare literature does not allow a clear conclusion. The first studies focused on these physiological responses indicate a reduction of cerebral oxygenation during the exposure that might be followed by greater cerebral oxygenation only following cryostimulation. More studies will be needed to better understand haemodynamic responses to cold exposure and elucidate its effect on post-exercise recovery.

References

1. Bouzigon R, Dupuy O, Tiemessen I, De Nardi M, Bernard JP, Mihailovic T, Theurot D, Miller ED, Lombardi G, Dugué BM. Cryostimulation for post-exercise recovery in athletes: a consensus and position paper. Front Sports Act Living. 2021;3:688828. https://doi.org/10.3389/fspor.2021.688828.
2. Moore E, Fuller JT, Bellenger CR, Saunders S, Halson SL, Broatch JR, Buckley JD. Effects of cold-water immersion compared with other recovery modalities on athletic performance following acute strenuous exercise in physically active participants: a systematic review, meta-analysis, and meta-regression. Sports Med. 2023;53:687–705. https://doi.org/10.1007/s40279-022-01800-1.
3. Dupuy O, Douzi W, Theurot D, Bosquet L, Dugué B. An evidence-based approach for choosing post-exercise recovery techniques to reduce markers of muscle damage, soreness, fatigue, and inflammation: a systematic review with meta-analysis. Front Physiol. 2018;9:403. https://doi.org/10.3389/fphys.2018.00403.
4. Banfi G, Melegati G, Barassi A, Dogliotti G, Melzi d'Eril G, Dugué B, et al. Effects of whole-body cryotherapy on serum mediators of inflammation and serum muscle enzymes in athletes. J Thermal Biol. 2009;34:55–9. https://doi.org/10.1016/j.jtherbio.2008.10.003.
5. Ihsan M, Watson G, Abbiss CR. What are the physiological mechanisms for post-exercise cold water immersion in the recovery from prolonged endurance and intermittent exercise? Sports Med. 2016;46:1095–109. https://doi.org/10.1007/s40279-016-0483-3.
6. Leeder J, Gissane C, van Someren K, Gregson W, Howatson G. Cold water immersion and recovery from strenuous exercise: a meta-analysis. Br J Sports Med. 2012;46:233–40. https://doi.org/10.1136/bjsports-2011-090061.
7. Bouzigon R, Grappe F, Ravier G, Dugué B. Whole- and partial-body cryostimulation/cryotherapy: current technologies and practical applications. J Thermal Biol. 2016;61:67–81. https://doi.org/10.1016/j.jtherbio.2016.08.009.
8. Merrick MA. Secondary injury after musculoskeletal trauma: a review and update. J Athl Train. 2002;37:209–17.
9. Swenson C, Swärd L, Karlsson J. Cryotherapy in sports medicine. Scand J Med Sci Sports. 2007;6:193–200. https://doi.org/10.1111/j.1600-0838.1996.tb00090.x.
10. Minett GM, Duffield R, Billaut F, Cannon J, Portus MR, Marino FE. Cold-water immersion decreases cerebral oxygenation but improves recovery after intermittent-sprint exercise in the

heat: cooling for recovery in the heat. Scand J Med Sci Sports. 2014;24:656–66. https://doi.org/10.1111/sms.12060.

11. Mantoni T, Belhage B, Pedersen LM, Pott FC. Reduced cerebral perfusion on sudden immersion in ice water: a possible cause of drowning. Aviat Space Environ Med. 2007;78:374–6.

12. Mantoni T, Rasmussen JH, Belhage B, Pott FC. Voluntary respiratory control and cerebral blood flow velocity upon ice-water immersion. Aviat Space Environ Med. 2008;79:765–8. https://doi.org/10.3357/ASEM.2216.2008.

13. Nybo L, Møller K, Volianitis S, Nielsen B, Secher NH. Effects of hyperthermia on cerebral blood flow and metabolism during prolonged exercise in humans. J Appl Physiol. 2002;93:58–64. https://doi.org/10.1152/japplphysiol.00049.2002.

14. Nybo L, Rasmussen P. Inadequate cerebral oxygen delivery and central fatigue during strenuous exercise. Exerc Sport Sci Rev. 2007;35:110. https://doi.org/10.1097/jes.0b013e3180a031ec.

15. Ihsan M, Watson G, Lipski M, Abbiss CR. Influence of postexercise cooling on muscle oxygenation and blood volume changes. Med Sci Sports Exerc. 2013;45:876–82. https://doi.org/10.1249/MSS.0b013e31827e13a2.

16. Vaile J, O'Hagan C, Stefanovic B, Walker M, Gill N, Askew CD. Effect of cold water immersion on repeated cycling performance and limb blood flow. Bri J Sports Med. 2011;45:825–9. https://doi.org/10.1136/bjsm.2009.067272.

17. Jones B, Waterworth S, Tallent J, Rogerson M, Morton C, Moran J, Southall-Edwards R, Cooper CE, McManus C. Influence of cold-water immersion on lower limb muscle oxygen consumption, as measured by near-infrared spectroscopy. J Athl Train. 2023; https://doi.org/10.4085/1062-6050-0532.22. (in press)

18. Stanley J, Peake JM, Coombes JS, Buchheit M. Central and peripheral adjustments during high-intensity exercise following cold water immersion. Eur J Appl Physiol. 2014;114:147–63. https://doi.org/10.1007/s00421-013-2755-z.

19. Gregson W, Black MA, Jones H, Milson J, Morton J, Dawson B, et al. Influence of cold water immersion on limb and cutaneous blood flow at rest. Am J Sports Med. 2011;39:1316–23. https://doi.org/10.1177/0363546510395497.

20. Mawhinney C, Jones H, Low DA, Green DJ, Howatson G, Gregson W. Influence of cold-water immersion on limb blood flow after resistance exercise. Eur J Sport Sci. 2017a;17:519–29.

21. Selfe J, Alexander J, Costello JT, May K, Garratt N, Atkins S, et al. The effect of three different (−135 °C) whole body cryotherapy exposure durations on elite rugby league players. PLoS ONE. 2014;9:e86420. https://doi.org/10.1371/journal.pone.0086420.

22. Haq A, Ribbans WJ, Hohenauer E, Baross AW. The comparative effect of different timings of whole body cryotherapy treatment with cold water immersion for post-exercise recovery. Front Sports Act Living. 2022;4:940516. https://doi.org/10.3389/fspor.2022.940516.

23. Mawhinney C, Low DA, Jones H, Green DJ, Costello JT, Gregson W. Cold water mediates greater reductions in limb blood flow than whole body cryotherapy. Med Sci Sports Exerc. 2017b;49:1252–60. https://doi.org/10.1249/MSS.0000000000001223.

24. Hohenauer E, Costello JT, Stoop R, Küng UM, Clarys P, Deliens T, et al. Cold-water or partial-body cryotherapy? Comparison of physiological responses and recovery following muscle damage. Scand J Med Sci Sports. 2018;28:1252–62. https://doi.org/10.1111/sms.13014.

25. Theurot D, Dupuy O, Louis J, Douzi W, Morin R, Arc-Chagnaud C, Dugué B. Partial-body cryostimulation does not impact peripheral microvascular responsiveness but reduces muscular metabolic O_2 consumption ($mV\dot{O}_2$) at rest. Cryobiology. 2023;112:104561. https://doi.org/10.1016/j.cryobiol.2023.104561.

26. Hohenauer E, Costello JT, Deliens T, Clarys P, Stoop R, Clijsen R. Partial-body cryotherapy (−135 °C) and cold-water immersion (10 °C) after muscle damage in females. Scand J Med Sci Sports. 2020;30:485–95. https://doi.org/10.1111/sms.13593.

27. Theurot D, Dugué B, Douzi W, Guitet P, Louis J, Dupuy O. Impact of acute partial-body cryostimulation on cognitive performance, cerebral oxygenation, and cardiac autonomic activity. Sci Rep. 2021;11:1–11. https://doi.org/10.1038/s41598-021-87089-y.

Muscle Exercise

6

Ewa Ziemann

Whole-body cryostimulation (WBC) is a very popular treatment among both recreational and professional athletes. In winter, during lockdown caused by COVID-19, cold exposure has become a very popular, available form of physical activity, due to the fact that there is a widespread belief of its regenerative and an anti-inflammatory effect [1]. Based on current literature, a number of factors are required to describe the effects of WBC on skeletal muscle function including: time of its application (before or post-exercise), amount of WBC sessions, the type of contraction that predominates during exercise (dynamic, static, plyometric or eccentric), adaptation to exercise (participants status unaccustomed, beginners or well trained), age and gender, body composition of participants or finally physical fitness and type of exercise (endurance, resistance or interval), which type of effort the application was associated with. All those factors have a significant impact on muscle functions in response to WBC. Although muscle recovery has been the most claimed and, possibly, the most debated effect of WBC it is also necessary to emphasise that muscle functions are not limited to the generation of power, improvement of locomotion, posture or breathing, which could enhance performance. Cold conditions might have reduced metabolism, which is generally important due to the fact that skeletal muscle is one of the largest energy stores with substantial amounts of triglycerides and glycogen. It is worth to note that skeletal muscle contractions during cold exposure [2, 3] are stimulated by muscle shivering and enhance the endocrine function by releasing certain muscle-derived peptides: myokines [4] and exerkines [5], which may prevent or even reverse negative effects of many health problems [6]. At the same time shivering skeletal muscle induced by low exposure is the most important

E. Ziemann (✉)
Department of Athletics, Strength and Conditioning, Poznan University of Physical
Education, Poznan, Poland

P. Capodaglio (ed.), *Whole-Body Cryostimulation*,
https://doi.org/10.1007/978-3-031-18545-8_6

way for the maintenance of body temperature [7]. The lack of unequivocal conclusions related to the effects on musculoskeletal conditions of WBC results from the variety of protocols used, both in single and repeated sessions with varying frequency, and combinations with different exercise protocols or regular training.

Muscle Damage

One of the most common circumstances of using the WBC is its use after an eccentric effort. Various cryotherapy protocols as well as damage induction tests and measurements of markers monitoring the extent of damage make it difficult to define precise recommendations. WBC can be applied directly post-eccentric exercise and in the following days after inducing delayed-onset muscle soreness (DOMS). The main aim of this cold-treatment is to reduce pain and stimulate an anti-inflammatory response. DOMS, or exercise-induced muscle damage (EIMD), is caused by performing unaccustomed exercise with eccentric muscle contraction or exhaustive exercise by well-adapted-to-exercise subjects. This leads to muscle damage, an inflammation, an efflux of muscle proteins into the circulation and soreness on several days post-exercise. It has particularly meaning that fewer leukocytes are mobilised to the injured tissue. Sarcomere disruptions and muscle membrane damage leading to a reduced pro-inflammatory response and consequently less secondary muscle damage [8].

Among the many procedures that induce EIMD and at the same time are combined with WBC, we can mention: downhill runs, sessions on an eccentric cycle ergometer (Cyclus2 Eccentric Trainer), step up/down exercise and plyometric exercise. Some of them involve only partially eccentric work of muscle fibres (step up/down exercise), others rely only on eccentric contractions (an eccentric cycle ergometer). Not only different methods of inducing muscle damage are presented in scientific papers, but also various tests carried out before and after application of WBC were used in order to assess the effects of coldness. Among the many, the most common are isometric and isokinetic assessment using the Biodex System, ramp test, specific eccentric or training test, for example a preliminary 400-m freestyle swimming time trial or specific judo/tennis tests. In addition, together with perceived sensations of muscle pain and tiredness, different blood indicators were measured to assess muscle damage such as creatine kinase (CK), lactate dehydrogenase (LDH) activity, myoglobin and the concentration of pro- and anti-inflammatory cytokines. Some of them directly correlate with muscle damage, while others play a signalling role in the anti-inflammatory response and, consequently, in the induction of adaptive changes. For example, following cell damage (sarcomeres disruption) leukocytes are also mobilized to the injured tissue by soluble intercellular adhesion molecule-1 (sICAM-1), producing reactive oxygen species and pro-inflammatory cytokines in the injured tissue by neutrophils, lymphocytes and monocytes resulting in intramuscular degradation and an amplification of muscle damage [8, 9]. This can be observed by an increase in muscle proteins in systemic circulation 24–48 h following the initial bout of exercise. Carrying out the same effort will again reduce muscle damage, but very often the magnitude of the secondary response to muscle damage may depend on the balance between pro- and anti-inflammatory cytokines [10].

Ferreira-Junior et al. [11] observed the WBC-induced attenuation in sICAM-1 immediately after EIMD and suggested that the reduced acute inflammatory response is responsible for muscle damage. WBC reduces muscle temperature and causes vasoconstriction, which leads to decreased permeability of blood vessels to immune cells. These processes, vasoconstriction and reduced number of leukocytes can be just obtained by reaching the muscles through the inhibition of sICAM-1 [11]. The drop of sICAM-1 was also noted in rugby players post-five consecutive daily sessions of WBC and this decrease was accompanied by 40% decrease in creatine kinase (CK) and LDH activity [12]. The same tendency accompanied by 30% reduction of CK activity after single and 34% post-six sessions in kayakers was registered by Wozniak and co-workers [13]. In professional rugby players, after a 7-day training camp with two daily WBC sessions, lactate dehydrogenase (LDH) and aspartate aminotransferase (AST) activities were increased, as consequent to high workload, whilst CK was slightly but significantly decreased. Moreover, the kidney function (estimated glomerular filtration rate, eGFR), which could be impaired following muscle damages, was unaffected by the treatment [14]. The drop of CK activity in response to training camp among high professional tennis players was noted also after 10 sessions of WBC but applied twice a day for 5 days ($-120\,°C$, 3 min) [15].

Another report published by Hausswirth et al. investigated the effect of three recovery modalities, including WBC in the nine runners who performed three identical repetitions of a damaging simulated trail run. WBC was randomly applied within the first hour (post), 24 h (post 24 h) and 48 h (post 48 h), after each strenuous running exercise. Maximal muscle strength and perceived sensations were recovered and significantly differ in comparison to other recovery methods after the first WBC session (post 1 h). The possible decrease in maximal isometric force, after 3 isometric voluntary contractions of knee extensor muscles, was used for judging muscle damage due to strenuous exercise. The best results were observed after WBC at 1 h, 24 h and 48 h post-exercise [16]. WBC-enhanced psychological recovery within days after exercise included a decreased perception of muscular fatigue and pain, as early as after the first session of WBC, while pain sensation was lowered only at 48 h after by FIR, and it did not change at all as a result of passive recovery after the end of exercise. Well-being, evaluated through a standardized questionnaire as for tiredness and pain, was improved after 24 h by WBC and after 48 h by FIR. However, the increase in serum activity of CK, typical of strenuous exercise, was not improved by 3 WBC sessions [16]. Ziemann et al. noted a reduction of physiological cost (measured via indirect calorimetry using breath-by-breath pulmonary gas exchange MetaMax 3B, Cortex Biophysik) of eccentric exercise up/down step repeated post-10 sessions of WBC within young men. Along with lower physiological cost of second bout of eccentric work, lower CK was registered in response to exercise among those subjects who underwent WBC. In addition, an increase in the anti-inflammatory cytokine interleukin 10 (IL-10) and a decrease in the pro-inflammatory cytokine IL-1β was observed after the second workout following cold treatment. These beneficial changes in blood indicators were accompanied by a significant improvement in pain perception [10]. Reduction in another indicator of muscle damage, myoglobin, was registered in response to second eccentric exercise after 1 month of resistance training supported three times a week by WBC in young, inactive subjects unaccustomed to exercise [17].

The diminishing of inflammation is very often recorded in WBC experiments, even after a single session of WBC. Pournot et al. recently reported that a single exposure to WBC significantly alleviated inflammation after a strenuous exercise run mainly composed of eccentric contractions [18]. Positive effects after 96 h were registered among physically active subjects, who performed a single maximal eccentric contraction of the left knee extensors, through two WBC sessions (-110 °C) 24 h and 48 h after exercise. The effects were negative at 24 h and 48 h post-exercise [19]. On the other hand, opposite results are also available. Kruger et al. did not observe beneficial changes on hormonal, inflammatory and muscle damage biomarkers after a single WBC-session following intermittent high-intensity running exercise (HIR). Eleven endurance athletes were tested twice in a randomized crossover design with 5×5 min of HIR followed by 1 h of passive recovery, including either WBC (-110 °C, 3 min) or a 3-min walking. Time-to-exhaustion difference between a ramp-test protocol before running and 1 h post-recovery was lower in WBC-treated subjects. Authors also noted that performing HIR induced significant increases in all biomarkers except sICAM-1 in two applied recovery conditions and increased levels of cortisol following exercise were negatively correlated with subsequent running performance in both conditions. WBC improves acute recovery during high-intensity intermittent exercise in thermoneutral conditions. This could be induced by enhanced oxygenation of the working muscles, as well as by reduction of cardiovascular strain and increased work economy at submaximal intensities [20].

Physical Efficiency

Data regarding the impact of WBC on aerobic or anaerobic capacity are limited and not always unambiguous. The beneficial effects of WBC are much more often observed in the post-exercise regeneration of endurance training than in the unequivocal effect on physical performance. In turn, the level of physical fitness itself is indicated as a factor modifying the effects of WBC. In people with higher levels of cardiorespiratory fitness level (CFL), the effects of WBC are less pronounced than in inactive, poorly adapted and with low levels of CFL. Nonetheless, some reports also presented that WBC augments training-induced aerobic adaptations and performance [21]. In recreational and professional sports training, it is important not only to directly increase physical performance, but also to prevent overreaching or overtraining, especially in periods of intensified training. A particularly interesting study on this topic is the one written by Schaal et al. In a randomized controlled trial, they investigated the effect of the aspect of the 10 top level female synchronized swimmers' recovery by preserving sleep quantity during intensified training supported by daily WBC treatment. Authors noted that WBC limited the appearance of physiological signs associated with functional overreaching during maximal exercise, such as reduced sympathetic activation and lactate accumulation. They evaluated the effects of 10 sessions of WBC applied post the whole day training workload. Additionally, the results of specific swimming test 200-m intervals or 400 m test trial suggested improved fitness, with reduced physical effort and perceived difficulty for a fixed workload [22]. Ziemann et al. investigated the effect of 10 sessions of WBC (twice a day) but applied during 5 days, also combined with training among high-ranking professional tennis players [15]. In order to assess the impact of WBC on rate of recovery, they used the specific tennis test before and post intervention. Low levels of lactate and higher effectiveness of tennis strokes were registered among WBC tennis players, unlike the control group. Furthermore, this WBC protocol ameliorated the cytokine profile, resulting in a decrease of the tumour necrosis factor alpha (TNFα) and an increase in interleukin 6 (IL-6) [15]. In addition, athletes' performance remained unchanged after 10 sessions of WBC in professional judokas, who used to train for 2 weeks and combined high intensity training with cold exposure. However, the subjects perceived the positive changes induced by the intervention in response to the specific training workload and the specific judo test. The increase of growth factor concentrations (BDNF: brain-derived neurotrophic factor; IGF-1: insulin-like growth factor) and the improvement of amino acid profile (proline and leucine) contributed to maintaining a high level of muscle function (low level of lactate after judo test and better scores in judo test, maintained muscle strength) [23]. Similar growth factor sequelae (BDNF and IGF-1 concentrations) was obtained also by Jaworska et al. in other experiments involving academic volleyball players. Authors suggested that the shifts of BDNF and IGF-1 offset a decline of physical performance, which was recorded after 2 weeks intervention. However, the extent of the drop was smaller in the WBC group. In the same report, motor abilities tested pre- and post-commencing the training programme revealed that women from WBC group achieved better results in the serve accuracy and concentration tests compared to men. This alternation was explained by a drop of tryptophan concentration suggesting its faster uptake. Such observation has special significance because among the different effects of WBC, the most investigated domain was improvement in mental health [24]. Despite the fact that in this study cognitive functions were assessed selectively, the authors tried to explain the observed changes by blood shifts tryptophan. In contrast to the above four reports, Klimek et al. have shown an improvement in tolerance to pain, highlighted by an increase in blood lactate concentration, which ultimately caused an improvement in anaerobic capacity after 10 sessions of WBC in 30 healthy young subjects [25]. In summary, we conclude that physical fitness is a factor that strongly modifies the WBC response and that there is a lack of information on whether this treatment directly improves human capacity but prevents its decline.

Training

One of the issues related to the use of WBC is the impact on the potential improvement in exercise capacity, the other being the effect on adaptive changes. While there are many data regarding the changes or lack of WBC on exercise capacity, data on the combination of WBC and regular exercise training are limited. Recently, numerous reports, including cold water immersion (CWI), have revealed that repeated cryotherapy can blunt training adaptations. These studies have advanced the concept that especially resistance training combined with cold treatment may impair muscle strength and inhibit muscle hypertrophy [26, 27]. Data on how to use different cold procedures interchangeably are inconsistent. Costello and co-workers compared effects of a single CWI (4-min at 8 °C) and CRY session (3.40-min at −110 °C), and found that their impacts on muscle and core temperatures were similar, differing only in the aspect of skin cooling [28]. However, regarding above mentioned papers with the use of CWI, potential associated mechanisms include blunted arterial diameter gains and expression of anabolic signals. Instead, the limited papers include descriptions of the effects of short training cycles combined with WBC: recovery training in tennis [15], 2 weeks of specific training in volleyball [29] and judo [23]; both applied among top professional athletes, and 2 weeks of high interval intensity training supported or not by WBC [1]. In these studies, WBC was applied daily, twice or once daily, and always after training, respectively. The results of applying WBC not every day but a few times a week (two or three) in conjunction with diverse training protocols were recently described by Jaworska (resistance training and three times a week) [17] and Haq (endurance and strength training and two times a week) [30]. The physical workload was described in detail, and final conclusions revealed that the effects were quite beneficial. Jaworska et al. noted improvement in mean power and isokinetic muscle strength in extension after the 4-week intervention. The induced changes were accompanied by shifts in exerkines' concentrations: a drop in myostatin and an elevation in IL-15 concentration in participants undergoing both resistance training and cold treatment [17]. In contrast to Roberts et al., who observed attenuated muscle adaptation to long-term resistance training supported by CWI (12 weeks, 24 sessions, workload 8, 10 and 12 1-RM respectively); Jaworska and colleagues enhanced the physical workload to 80% of 1-RM load in last week of 4 weeks of total period of training [26]. Haq also indicated that the 6-week concurrent and progressive training programme was effective in improving lower body strength, jump power and body composition, regardless of whether it was supported by a 2-day WBC. Repeated WBC did not appear to have a detrimental impact on these fitness attributes but it could hinder improvements in countermovement jumping power [30]. Young and healthy subjects were involved in these two reports, and authors did not present the duration of the induced changes. Kozlowska noted that among middle-aged people the changes induced by HIIT applied in conjunction with WBC alternation were temporary. Thus, Haq rightly points out that further research should focus more on clarifying the potential mechanisms by which repetitive WBC can affect physiological adaptations to sports training programmes, especially regarding muscle power. In addition, further investigations should evaluate parameters such as electromyography and muscle hypertrophy markers (e.g. protein synthesis rates and muscle fibre cross-sectional areas) to elucidate how repetitive WBC may mediate potential mechanisms of strength and power development [30].

Myokines/Exerkines

Changes in musculoskeletal conditions may be strongly related to alternations in proteins realising during shivering or in response to exercise when applied together with WBC. In experimental work including WBC, only a few myokines have been extensively studied for their effects on skeletal muscle, such as IL-6, IL-15, BDNF, FGF21, irisin, myostatin and insulin-like growth factor (IGF). Both exercise and cold exposure could activate the same pathways [31]. Irisin is considered a hormone-like myokine produced in abundance by skeletal muscle in response to exercise or cold [32]. In 2012, it was shown to elicit the browning response in white fat (WAT), causing its transdifferentiation into brown fat [33]. This action of irisin is combined with the promotion of uncoupling protein 1 (UCP1) expression in WAT, probably through p38 mitogen-activated protein kinase (MAPK) signalling, which consequently causes increased energy expenditure and improved metabolic profile [33, 34]. Further studies revealed that irisin is one of the metabolic regulators with anti-diabetic properties, able to stimulate glucose uptake in adipocytes and myofibres and to improve glucose homeostasis [35]. Fitness level has been observed to impact irisin secretion in response to WBC [36]. The 10 consecutive sessions of WBC lead to an increase in serum irisin in non-active men with obesity, while it has no effect in active men with obesity. Furthermore, values recorded 24 h after the last cryo-session were significantly correlated with adipose tissue but inversely with skeletal muscle mass. This observation suggested that the subcutaneous adipose tissue could be the main source of irisin in response to cold exposures, and thus this protein could be considered a thermogenic adipo-myokine. The broad spectrum of effects of irisin leads to the question of whether this myokine has an effect on muscle function and adaptive changes in response to short, and long, lasting training. Fatourous, in his extensive review containing analysis of 74 exercise studies concerning this topic, cannot endorse a specific role for irisin in human metabolism at rest or in response to acute or chronic exercise [37]. However, some data might suggest that exposure to extreme cold may stimulate pathways responsible not so much for a direct impact on physical performance, but for improving communication between the muscles and the nervous system. For example, it was shown that FNDC5/irisin together with other myokine cathepsin B (CATB) contribute to the modification of BDNF concentration [38] and in that way are involved in improving brain function [39]. Although Jaworksa and co-workers did not observe changes in irisin concentration in response to a training programme combined with WBC, they registered the increase of other exerkine: BDNF and at the same time the increase of volleyball task effectiveness, especially among female athletes. Another work published by Kozlowska-Flis and co-workers revealed an effect on irisin in response to WBC combined with other exercise protocols: six sessions of HIIT [1]. The question of the beneficial effect of WBC connected with exercise may depend on baseline physical capacity of subjects and these results are very often more pronounced among non-active subjects, characterised by low fitness level. Kozlowska-Flis et al. did not observe changes in serum irisin but in their report recorded that 6 units of HIIT training were enough to cause a significant increase of other cold-induced myokine FGF21 (fibroblast growth factor 21) in inactive individuals with obesity. This increase was associated with an elevation in the circulating level of adiponectin and the improvement of metabolic profile, i.e. a reduction in TG and an improvement in HOMA-B. Interestingly, WBC-supported HIIT did not induce similar changes [1]. FGF21 acts in the control of glucose and lipid homeostasis. It regulates the expression of genes involved in gluconeogenesis, lipogenesis, lipolysis and fatty acid oxidation. FGF21 has been shown to improve pancreatic β-cell survival and function [40]. Thus, FGF21 can support the action of irisin. Taking into consideration that recent reports emphasise the physiological role of irisin, alteration of its levels in heart failure and the possible existing mechanisms of irisin in metabolic remodelling and cardiac hypertrophy [41, 42]; it is necessary to establish in further research the factors that modify the effect of WBC on irisin, and the role of WBC on irisin cannot be completely ruled out. It is also known that irisin may have functions in the musculoskeletal system, and there is evidence for possible effects on the skeleton. Data obtained on mice indicate that this molecule can have a role in the control of bone mass, with positive effects on cortical mineral density and geometry. Thus, irisin is an additional link in bone–muscle crosstalk. Despite numerous studies, the question of how irisin communicates with other organs, there is no clear answer. The search for the irisin receptor is still ongoing. Research by Kim and co-authors partially explains the mechanism of action of irisin. The researchers identified a protein from the integrin family in osteocytes that is responsible for the exchange of nutrients and metabolites through direct contact with blood vessels. Therefore, they participate in the maintaining bone tissue homeostasis through direct control of cytoskeleton shaping. Osteocytes regulate osteoclast function in two ways: by direct secretion of RANKL, the most potent osteoclastogenesis-inducing factor and through secretion of the protein sclerostin (Sost), a local modulator of bone remodelling, which also suppresses osteoprotegerin acting on the RANKL factor. Kim discovered that irisin binds to proteins of αV integrins, and biophysical studies have confirmed the interaction between irisin and αV/β5 integrin. Chemical inhibition of αV integrins blocks irisin signalling and function in osteocytes and fat cells. Irisin increases both osteocyte survival and sclerostin production [43]. Straburzynska-Lupa et al. investigated the effects of single and repeated exposures to WBC (10 consecutive sessions, $-110\ ^\circ$C) among young active, male subjects on biomarkers of bone remodelling and osteo-immune crosstalk: sclerostin, osteocalcin (OC), C-terminal cross-linked telopeptide of type I collagen (CTx-I), osteoprotegerin (OPG) and free soluble receptor activator for nuclear factor κ B ligand (sRANKL). RANKL and its decoy receptor osteoprotegerin constitute a fundamental cytokine system connecting the immune system and bone metabolism in order to link the pro- and anti-inflammatory balance to the calcium stores. RANKL is released from osteoblasts and lymphocytes and activates osteoclasts inducing bone resorption [3]. Osteoclasts express RANK, the specific receptor of RANKL, which induces an intracellular signal to reabsorb bone. The effects of RANKL on RANK are blocked by OPG (Banfi et al. 2010a). Results obtained by Straburzyunska-Lupa's group showed that changes in the sRANKL factor depend on the level of physical fitness and sclerostin could be a sensitive marker in the first contact with cold exposure. In addition, in Galliera's report, WBC applied to ten professional rugby players belonging to Italian National Team who were subjected to single daily sessions of WBC for 5 consecutive days ($-110\ °C$, 2 min) did not affect plasma RANK and RANKL concentrations, while it increased OPG and, thus, the OPG/RANKL ratio, an index of resorption-to-formation balance [44]. It is necessary to emphasise that bone health is essential in whole-body health but also in determining and sustaining athletes' performance [3, 45]. Due to high energy expenses associated with high-level physical activity [46], the risk of osteopenia and stress fractures, which is the inability of the skeleton to modify its own microarchitecture depending on applied loads, is always present. Muscles and bone tissue are a two-way connection. They interact with each other to maintain their structure and function. Research shows that the load that skeletal muscles overcome in response to resistance exercise is transferred to bone tissue, which not only initiates muscle protein synthesis, but also signals the need for energy to facilitate bone formation, thus providing evidence of a biomechanical interaction. Biochemical signals with a bidirectional action are coordinated by myokines/exerkines released by myocytes and by osteokines produced by osteocytes. WBC is considered as a significant medical tool which can modify this interaction [3]. Furthermore, not only re-modelling of bone mass is of special significance, but also the improvement of the quality of life of patients with ankylosing spondylitis (AS) due to the analgesic effect and reduction of morning stiffness. Report including 92 patients with AS indicated that adding cryotherapy at $-110\ °C$ to exercise therapy led to significantly reduced disease activity compared with exercise therapy alone [47]. Although most of the available studies do not indicate any real effect of WBC on muscle mass, it is interesting to note that exposure to the WBC can change myostatin concentration. It has particular meaning not only for athletes' efficiency but also for their health. It is known that the elevated level of myostatin corelates with low level of physical activity, some injuries or even with sarcopenia. Myostatin, known as GDF-8 growth differentiation factor 8 (MSTN) belongs to the cytokine family of transforming growth factor βeta (TGFβ) [48]. Because MSTN negatively regulates muscle stem cell proliferation and differentiation, it may act on muscle cells in an autocrine manner leading to inhibition of muscle myogenesis [49]. When released from the muscles, MSTN may act locally or systemically through activin type IIA receptors. Connecting MSTN with the receptor activates the Smad family transcription factors (Smad2 and Smad3), and these activate other transcription factors FOXO (1, 2 and 3), which leads to inhibition of the AKT/mTOR pathway. Muscle myostatin expression and its plasma concentration are downregulated after acute and long-term physical exercise thus allowing muscle hypertrophy. Most evidence suggests that regular aerobic training lowers myostatin levels, but there is also evidence that resistance training may have a similar effect. Jaworska noted that after a 4-week period of strength training combined with WBC (3 times a week, 3 minutes, $-110\,°C$ in cryo-chamber, the next day post-training). The statistically decline in serum myostatin was visible both after the entire training period and after the eccentric test exercise performed before and after the intervention in the group of people not adapted to resistance training [17]. Although the authors registered no changes in muscle mass, they did record a significant increase in maximal average power in the isokinetic knee extension strength test among subjects who combined training with WBC, while in the control group the strength level remained stable. A recently published paper indicated that a 3-h exposure to $7\,°C$ did not affect the expression of myostatin genes [50]. The reason for such a varied response may be related to the training used, differences in load and duration, which are likely to determine changes in myostatin levels. The decrease in myostatin concentration in response to training combined with cryo-therapy can be explained by the finding of Kong and co-authors that skeletal muscle and brown adipose tissue (BAT) are functionally related. They described the intriguing role of the transcription factor regulating interferon 4 (IRF4) in BAT, which mediates via myostatin in BAT communication with muscle tissue. They found that thermoneutrality or loss of IRF4 led to elevated serum myostatin levels and decreased exercise capacity [51]. Observed by Kong changes in myostatin concentration might explain results obtained by Kozlowska et al. who also noted the drop of MSTN among middle aged men who underwent 10 sessions of WBC. The decrease of myostatin was accompanied by the improvement of amino acid profile and glucose homeostasis. It has been mentioned that the molecular mechanisms by which myostatin acts as a negative regulator of muscle growth involves the inhibition of activation of satellite cells and myoblast proliferation through the decrease of muscle protein synthesis. Thus, Kozlowska's results are very promising for the improvement of muscle metabolism (lowered valine and asparagine concentrations post-WBC treatment). However, muscle parameters were assessed in this experiment, but based on the previously published study, the subjects participating in WBC had a similar level of fitness, expressed by maximal oxygen uptake (VO_2max) for WBC group 46.5 ± 5.1 mL kg^{-1} min^{-1} and for control 47.4 ± 4.6 mL kg^{-1} min^{-1}. Although the next report published by the same research group confirmed these results, the question of the persistence of changes in myokine concentration and their effects induced by WBCs remains open. One of these factors, which could have an impact on myokines, is subject's age. Sliwicka and co-workers noted that the shifts in myostatin induced by cold treatment and/or physical exercise were temporary in young men and returned to the baseline level within 24 h after the triggering factor had been applied. Therefore, the effect of exposure to extremely low temperature combined with training gives such good results in the form of lowering the level of myostatin. It is worth to note that together with the decrease in myostatin concentration, Jaworska observed significant changes in IL-15 concentration among subjects who underwent resistance training supported by WBC [17]. IL-15 is considered an important factor regulating muscle metabolism and hypertrophy [6]. Perez-Lopez et al. demonstrated that a single session of 4 sets of leg press and leg extension at 75% 1RM stimulated the IL-15/IL-15Rα signalling pathway together with an elevated serum concentration of IL-15, and such activation supported myofibrillar protein synthesis [52]. The increase of IL-15 was recorded both after a 2-week training cycle among professional volleyball players and daily cryostimulation (WBC every day) [29], as well as after a monthly period of resistance training combined with WBC (three times a week) for beginners. Thus, the results of these two studies may indicate that cold treatment did not attenuate IL-15 synthesis. Based on the current literature, it appears that WBC may be a practical tool to support the effects of single exercise sessions and regular workouts, especially among subjects who are beginning to be active. It is obvious that this is not a stimulus that significantly modified physical performance or body composition, but by improving muscle regeneration and flexibility and endocrine function it may have a beneficial effects on health.

References

1. Kozlowska-Flis M, Rodziewicz-Flis E, Micielska K, Kortas J, Jaworska J, Borkowska A, et al. Short and long-term effects of high-intensity interval training applied alone or with whole-body cryostimulation on glucose homeostasis and myokine levels in overweight to obese subjects. Front Biosci (Landmark Ed). 2021;26(11):1132–46.
2. Ziemann E, Olek RA, Grzywacz T, Antosiewicz J, Kujach S, Luszczyk M, et al. Whole-body cryostimulation as an effective method of reducing low-grade inflammation in obese men. J Physiol Sci. 2013;63(5):333–43.
3. Lombardi G, Ziemann E, Banfi G. Whole-body cryotherapy in athletes: from therapy to stimulation. an updated review of the literature. Front Physiol. 2017;8:258.
4. Giudice J, Taylor JM. Muscle as a paracrine and endocrine organ. Curr Opin Pharmacol. 2017;34:49–55.
5. Safdar A, Tarnopolsky MA. Exosomes as mediators of the systemic adaptations to endurance exercise. Cold Spring Harb Perspect Med. 2018;8(3)
6. Huh JY. The role of exercise-induced myokines in regulating metabolism. Arch Pharm Res. 2018;41(1):14–29.
7. Schnyder S, Handschin C. Skeletal muscle as an endocrine organ: PGC-1alpha, myokines and exercise. Bone. 2015;80:115–25.
8. Paulsen G, Mikkelsen UR, Raastad T, Peake JM. Leucocytes, cytokines and satellite cells: what role do they play in muscle damage and regeneration following eccentric exercise? Exerc Immunol Rev. 2012;18:42–97.
9. Peake J, Nosaka K, Suzuki K. Characterization of inflammatory responses to eccentric exercise in humans. Exerc Immunol Rev. 2005;11:64–85.
10. Ziemann E, Olek RA, Grzywacz T, Kaczor JJ, Antosiewicz J, Skrobot W, et al. Whole-body cryostimulation as an effective way of reducing exercise-induced inflammation and blood cholesterol in young men. Eur Cytokine Netw. 2014;25(1):14–23.
11. Ferreira-Junior JB, Bottaro M, Loenneke JP, Vieira A, Vieira CA, Bemben MG. Could whole-body cryotherapy (below −100 °C) improve muscle recovery from muscle damage? Front Physiol. 2014;5:247.
12. Banfi G, Melegati G, Barassi A, Dogliotti G, d'Eril GM, Dugué B, Corsi MM. Effects of whole-body cryotherapy on serum mediators of inflammation and serum muscle enzymes in athletes. J Therm Biol. 2009;34(2):55–9.
13. Wozniak A, Wozniak B, Drewa G, Mila-Kierzenkowska C, Rakowski A. The effect of whole-body cryostimulation on lysosomal enzyme activity in kayakers during training. Eur J Appl Physiol. 2007;100(2):137–42.

14. Lombardi G, Colombini A, Porcelli S, Mauri C, Zani V, Bonomi FG, Melegati G, Banfi G. Muscular damage and kidney function in rugby players after daily whole body cryostimulation. Physiology 2014;2014:1–7.

15. Ziemann E, Olek RA, Kujach S, Grzywacz T, Antosiewicz J, Garsztka T, et al. Five-day whole-body cryostimulation, blood inflammatory markers, and performance in high-ranking professional tennis players. J Athl Train. 2012;47(6):664–72.

16. Hausswirth C, Louis J, Bieuzen F, Pournot H, Fournier J, Filliard JR, et al. Effects of whole-body cryotherapy vs. far-infrared vs. passive modalities on recovery from exercise-induced muscle damage in highly-trained runners. PLoS One. 2011;6(12):e27749.

17. Jaworska J, Rodziewicz-Flis E, Kortas J, Kozlowska M, Micielska K, Babinska A, et al. Short-term resistance training supported by whole-body cryostimulation induced a decrease in myostatin concentration and an increase in isokinetic muscle strength. Int J Environ Res Public Health. 2020;17(15):5496.

18. Pournot H, Bieuzen F, Louis J, Mounier R, Fillard JR, Barbiche E, et al. Time-course of changes in inflammatory response after whole-body cryotherapy multi exposures following severe exercise. PLoS One. 2011;6(7):e22748.

19. Costello JT, Algar LA, Donnelly AE. Effects of whole-body cryotherapy (−110 °C) on proprioception and indices of muscle damage. Scand J Med Sci Sports. 2012;22(2):190–8.

20. Krueger M, Costello JT, Achtzehn S, Dittmar KH, Mester J. Whole-body cryotherapy (−110 °C) following high-intensity intermittent exercise does not alter hormonal, inflammatory or muscle damage biomarkers in trained males. Cytokine. 2019;113:277–84.

21. Kwiecien SY, McHugh MP. The cold truth: the role of cryotherapy in the treatment of injury and recovery from exercise. Eur J Appl Physiol. 2021;121(8):2125–42.

22. Schaal K, Le Meur Y, Louis J, Filliard JR, Hellard P, Casazza G, et al. Whole-body cryostimulation limits overreaching in elite synchronized swimmers. Med Sci Sports Exerc. 2015;47(7):1416–25.

23. Jaworska J, Laskowski R, Ziemann E, Zuczek K, Lombardi G, Antosiewicz J, et al. The specific Judo training program combined with the whole body cryostimulation induced an increase of serum concentrations of growth factors and changes in amino acid profile in professional Judokas. Front Physiol. 2021;12:627657.

24. Bouzigon R, Grappe F, Ravier G, Dugue B. Whole- and partial-body cryostimulation/cryotherapy: current technologies and practical applications. J Therm Biol. 2016;61:67–81.

25. Klimek AT, Lubkowska A, Szygula Z, Chudecka M, Fraczek B. Influence of the ten sessions of the whole body cryostimulation on aerobic and anaerobic capacity. Int J Occup Med Environ Health. 2010;23(2):181–9.

26. Roberts LA, Raastad T, Markworth JF, Figueiredo VC, Egner IM, Shield A, et al. Post-exercise cold water immersion attenuates acute anabolic signalling and long-term adaptations in muscle to strength training. J Physiol. 2015;593(18):4285–301.

27. Yamane M, Ohnishi N, Matsumoto T. Does regular post-exercise cold application attenuate trained muscle adaptation? Int J Sports Med. 2015;36(8):647–53.

28. Costello JT, Culligan K, Selfe J, Donnelly AE. Muscle, skin and core temperature after −110 °C cold air and 8 °C water treatment. PLoS One. 2012;7(11):e48190.

29. Jaworska J, Micielska K, Kozlowska M, Wnorowski K, Skrobecki J, Radziminski L, et al. A 2-week specific volleyball training supported by the whole body cryostimulation protocol induced an increase of growth factors and counteracted deterioration of physical performance. Front Physiol. 2018;9:1711.

30. Haq A, Ribbans WJ, Hohenauer E, Baross AW. The effect of repetitive whole body cryotherapy treatment on adaptations to a strength and endurance training programme in physically active males. Front Sports Act Living. 2022;4:834386.

31. Lee P, Linderman JD, Smith S, Brychta RJ, Wang J, Idelson C, et al. Irisin and FGF21 are cold-induced endocrine activators of brown fat function in humans. Cell Metab. 2014;19(2):302–9.

32. Xin C, Liu J, Zhang J, Zhu D, Wang H, Xiong L, et al. Irisin improves fatty acid oxidation and glucose utilization in type 2 diabetes by regulating the AMPK signaling pathway. Int J Obes. 2016;40(3):443–51.

33. Bostrom P, Wu J, Jedrychowski MP, Korde A, Ye L, Lo JC, et al. A PGC1-alpha-dependent myokine that drives brown-fat-like development of white fat and thermogenesis. Nature. 2012;481(7382):463–8.

34. Yang M, Wei D, Mo C, Zhang J, Wang X, Han X, et al. Saturated fatty acid palmitate-induced insulin resistance is accompanied with myotube loss and the impaired expression of health benefit myokine genes in C2C12 myotubes. Lipids Health Dis. 2013;12:104.

35. Perakakis N, Triantafyllou GA, Fernandez-Real JM, Huh JY, Park KH, Seufert J, et al. Physiology and role of irisin in glucose homeostasis. Nat Rev Endocrinol. 2017;13(6):324–37.

36. Dulian K, Laskowski R, Grzywacz T, Kujach S, Flis DJ, Smaruj M, et al. The whole body cryostimulation modifies irisin concentration and reduces inflammation in middle aged, obese men. Cryobiology. 2015;71(3):398–404.

37. Fatouros IG. Is irisin the new player in exercise-induced adaptations or not? A 2017 update. Clin Chem Lab Med. 2018;56(4):525–48.

38. Pedersen BK. Physical activity and muscle-brain crosstalk. Nat Rev Endocrinol. 2019;15(7):383–92.

39. Zhang J, Zhang W. Can irisin be a linker between physical activity and brain function? Biomol Concepts. 2016;7(4):253–8.

40. BonDurant LD, Ameka M, Naber MC, Markan KR, Idiga SO, Acevedo MR, et al. FGF21 regulates metabolism through adipose-dependent and -independent mechanisms. Cell Metab. 2017;25(4):935–44 e4.

41. Guo W, Zhang B, Wang X. Lower irisin levels in coronary artery disease: a meta-analysis. Minerva Endocrinol. 2020;45(1):61–9.

42. Li J, Xie S, Guo L, Jiang J, Chen H. Irisin: linking metabolism with heart failure. Am J Transl Res. 2020;12(10):6003–14.

43. Kim H, Wrann CD, Jedrychowski M, Vidoni S, Kitase Y, Nagano K, et al. Irisin mediates effects on bone and fat via alphaV integrin receptors. Cell. 2018;175(7):1756–68 e17.

44. Galliera E, Dogliotti G, Melegati G, Corsi Romanelli MM, Cabitza P, Banfi G. Bone remodelling biomarkers after whole body cryotherapy (WBC) in elite rugby players. Injury. 2013;44(8):1117–21.

45. Sansoni V, Vernillo G, Perego S, Barbuti A, Merati G, Schena F, et al. Bone turnover response is linked to both acute and established metabolic changes in ultra-marathon runners. Endocrine. 2017;56(1):196–204.

46. Lombardi G, Lanteri P, Graziani R, Colombini A, Banfi G, Corsetti R. Bone and energy metabolism parameters in professional cyclists during the Giro d'Italia 3-weeks stage race. PLoS One. 2012;7(7):e42077.

47. Romanowski MW, Straburzynska-Lupa A. Is the whole-body cryotherapy a beneficial supplement to exercise therapy for patients with ankylosing spondylitis? J Back Musculoskelet Rehabil. 2020;33(2):185–92.

48. Kirk B, Feehan J, Lombardi G, Duque G. Muscle, bone, and fat crosstalk: the biological role of myokines, osteokines, and adipokines. Curr Osteoporos Rep. 2020;18(4):388–400.

49. Elliott B, Renshaw D, Getting S, Mackenzie R. The central role of myostatin in skeletal muscle and whole body homeostasis. Acta Physiol (Oxf). 2012;205(3):324–40.

50. Zak RB, Shute RJ, Heesch MW, La Salle DT, Bubak MP, Dinan NE, et al. Impact of hot and cold exposure on human skeletal muscle gene expression. Appl Physiol Nutr Metab. 2017;42(3):319–25.

51. Kong X, Yao T, Zhou P, Kazak L, Tenen D, Lyubetskaya A, Dawes BA, Tsai L, Kahn BB, Spiegelman BM, Liu T, Rosen ED. Brown Adipose Tissue Controls Skeletal Muscle Function via the Secretion of Myostatin. Cell Metab. 2018;28(4):631–43.e3. https://doi.org/10.1016/j.cmet.2018.07.004. Epub 2018 Aug 2. PMID: 30078553; PMCID: PMC6170693.

52. Perez-Lopez A, McKendry J, Martin-Rincon M, Morales-Alamo D, Perez-Kohler B, Valades D, et al. Skeletal muscle IL-15/IL-15Ralpha and myofibrillar protein synthesis after resistance exercise. Scand J Med Sci Sports. 2018;28(1):116–25.

Metabolomics: Metabolite Changes in Response to Cold Stress with a Special Focus on Whole-body Cryostimulation

Wafa Douzi, Delphine Bon, and Benoit Dugué

Introduction

In order to investigate the impact of a specific stimulus or a series of stimuli exposures on a living system, one can have two approaches: a targeted one where the impact of a stimulus is studied on one variable (e.g. sICAM-1) [1, 2] or several variables (e.g. cytokines) [3] or a more holistic one where a global situation is evaluated with the determination of the variables that are sensitive to the stimulus (stimuli) [4, 5]. In this latter case, the quite recent developed OMICS technology has provided tools to obtain a deeper insight of the involved biological pathways and its various components after a specific stimulus.

OMICS refers to a set of technologies used to study various components of biological systems. These components include genomics (study of the entire genome), transcriptomics (study of all RNA transcripts), proteomics (study of all proteins), metabolomics (study of all metabolites) and others. By integrating data from these different "omics" fields, one can gain a comprehensive understanding of biological changes induced by different stimuli. OMICS techniques can, in fact, be used to study the effects of cold stresses and whole-body cryotherapy/cryostimulation on a variety of biological molecules, including genes, proteins, and metabolites, simultaneously. This holistic approach may enable the identification of complex molecular

W. Douzi(✉) · D. Bon · B. Dugué
Laboratory Mobilité, Vieillissement, Exercice (MOVE), Faculty of Sports Sciences,
University of Poitiers, Poitiers, France
e-mail: wafa.douzi01@univ-poitiers.fr; delphine.bon@univ-poitiers.fr
benoit.dugue@univ-poitiers.fr

P. Capodaglio (ed.), *Whole-Body Cryostimulation*,
https://doi.org/10.1007/978-3-031-18545-8_7

pathways and interactions that might not be apparent when studying individual components separately. Moreover, by analyzing changes in gene expression, protein levels or metabolite profiles one could discover potential biomarkers and regulatory mechanisms associated with the response to cold stress and whole-body cryotherapy/cryostimulation. In this chapter, we are going, in a first part, to present and described in a detailed way the **metabolomic approach**: how and in which circumstances such approach can be used, on which biological specimens it can provide valuable data, how to prepare the specimens, and how to analyze and interpret the obtained signals. In the second part, a summary of the knowledge that a metabolomic approach has been able to provide in the context of studying the effects of cold stresses and especially whole-body cryotherapy/cryostimulation will be presented. The aim of this review is to enlighten the reader about this specific approach, inform the researchers of the technical steps that have to be considered and encourage them to use such an approach to describe the effects of whole-body cryotherapy/cryostimulation on living organisms—especially in humans.

Metabolomic Approach

The objectives of a metabolomic study are always to provide better **diagnoses** (detection) and **prognoses** (prediction), to **monitor,** or to **better one's understanding** of an effect [6, 7]. The ultimate goal remaining to identify one unique disease **biomarker** with high sensitivity and high specificity allowing patient **stratification** or **classification**.

A metabolomic workflow can be separated into five main sequences [8]: (a) sample collection, (b) sample preparation, (c) analytical step, (d) data analysis and (e) pathway analysis. Each step requires certain considerations specific to the question asked, the chosen strategy, and the feasibility in a clinical protocol, which can already be cumbersome for the participant or the research or medical teams. Starting a metabolomics study remains quite difficult due to the variety of possible procedures, despite the efforts of many teams to propose standardized methods of reporting the experimental design of a study [9].

In this section, we present a short review on general elements and points of attention relating to the samples and to the analytical techniques used for metabolomic. We will introduce data analysis strategies and pathway analysis. Thus, the reader will have the necessary bibliography to be able to embark on a metabolomic analysis.

Biological Samples

Any type of biological samples can be the support of a metabolomic study.

The easiest matrix to access is **urine**. Its main advantages are the non-invasive collection procedure, its abundance, and the 4000 detected metabolites that are end products of metabolism and are consequently closely linked to the phenotype [7].

The collection, preservation, and preparation steps are straightforward. Contrariwise, urine reflects diet, hydration levels, time of day, age, gender, physical activity practiced and even intestinal flora. Some parameters can be monitored, such as diet or physical activity, and those that cannot be monitored must be considered in the study. Some recommendations do exist, even if there is still a lack of consensus [10]. For instance, a diet monitored over 24 h may be sufficient to mitigate dietary inter-individual effects; throughout the study, a single type of container from a single brand must be used; midstream urine morning collection is preferred. Regarding the preservation of urine, it could be necessary to add a preservative such as sodium azide [11] or borate [12], but there is no obligation [13, 14]. Moreover, a gentle centrifugation prior to storage is mandatory to remove cells without breaking them, and aliquots must be made to avoid too many freeze-thaw cycles [15].

Blood samples are also easy to access and represent more than 50% of the matrix used for metabolomic studies [6]. An advantage of blood is that it is obtained in a controlled environment, unlike urine, which can be collected at the participant's home. Procedures become a bit more complicated with blood [16]. Selection of the tube of collection is indeed essential. Serum is preferred to plasma because it does not require an anticoagulant additive, which can alter the spectra (such as citrate, EDTA or heparin). When serum is not accessible, opting for the right type of tube can become difficult depending on the chosen analytical technique. For some authors, lithium heparin seems to be the best choice, followed by EDTA, with citrated tubes being the worst choice [17]. For others, there is no real evidence that citrate must be excluded [15, 18].

In 2020, González-Domínguez et al. seem to have succeeded in making a synthesis of all these elements, and they proposed **best practices for blood and urine samples** [19].

While urine or blood can provide a final overview of a process, in response to disease or intervention, the other types of samples allow results to be interpreted more specifically. Thus, numerous metabolomic studies were performed using **tissue** from the brain [20], breast [21], lung [22], liver [23] or kidneys [24], for example. More rarely, **biofluids** such as saliva [25], seminal plasma [26], cerebrospinal fluid [27], bronchoalveolar fluid [28], synovial fluid [29], feces [30], amniotic fluid [31] or exhaled breath [32] have been used. It is also possible to carry out metabolomic analyses from **cell** cultures [33]. All those references allow us to obtain a panoramic view of different kinds of metabolomic studies that can be performed; no further details are provided here.

Sample Preparation

The large diversity of samples leads to an equally great diversity of pre-analytical sample processing protocols. Sometimes, it will be necessary to concentrate samples. **Freeze-drying** can be an option, and it is commonly used for plant analysis [34] or with fluids of which the metabolite concentration may be very low [35]. Furthermore, **precipitation** with methanol or acetonitrile makes it possible to reduce the complexity of the matrix by excluding proteins [36]. Given the complexity of the matrices, it is sometimes judicious to select the types of metabolites that one wishes to visualize. In this case, an **extraction** step, commonly used to reduce signal overlaps, can be performed before the analyses [37]. To explore polar metabolites, perchloric acid extraction is often used [38, 39]. To explore lipid metabolites (lipidomic), an MTBE extraction is appropriate [40]. If the experimenter wants to obtain information on the two types of metabolites, they should opt for a chloroform/methanol extraction [41, 42].

Analytical Techniques

When talking about metabolomics, the two main analytical techniques that come to mind are nuclear magnetic resonance (**NMR**) spectroscopy and mass spectrometry (**MS**). The choice depends on the quantity of the sample, the metabolite concentrations, and the type of sample [8]. Only a few works propose a combination of the two techniques to improve the quality of the studies [43].

Although very robust and unbiased, NMR is not preferred for low-concentration samples due to its low sensitivity. The increase in the power of the magnets and the development of cryoprobes reducing the electronic noise and thus enhancing the sensitivity and the resolution should allow the NMR to gain ground compared to the MS, which has the disadvantage of being less reproducible than NMR. On the other hand, NMR can allow analysis of slightly transformed samples, while MS requires a pre-analytical phase. Furthermore, since MS generates a much larger number of data, because of its higher sensitivity and spectral resolution, this analytical technique is almost always coupled with a separation step preceding the MS. Thus, we find metabolomic MS studies coupled with ion mobility [44], capillary electrophoresis [45] or, more often, liquid chromatography and gas chromatography [23] due to their widespread availability. The popularization of ultra-performance liquid chromatography (UPLC), which is more selective and more sensitive than high-performance liquid chromatography (HPLC), allows even more intense analysis throughputs. Other less common techniques have also proven interesting. This is the case of Raman or Fourier transform infrared (FTIR) spectroscopies [46].

Data Analysis

Once the samples have been analyzed, the spectra must be processed. This processing is generally well automated. It must be ensured that the baseline and the phasing of the spectra are correct. It is also necessary to check the alignment of the peaks or to choose between a direct integration or deconvolution. To transform processed spectrometric data into table data before the multivariate analysis, procedures are quite similar; only normalization and scaling steps can differ [47, 48].

Once the raw data have been transformed, the final step is chemometrics. At this point, there are two main ways of proceeding: a targeted or an untargeted analysis.

The objective of a **targeted analysis** is to search for a quantitative biomarker whose identity is known. A targeted analysis will focus on a defined group of metabolites in order to search for the metabolic pathways potentially involved in the phenomenon under consideration [49]. For an **untargeted analysis**, the strategy is holistic. We are looking for a profile, a signature characteristic for a pathology or a change in profile linked to a treatment or an intervention, without a priori [50]. Multivariate analysis will help us to visualize the difference between phenotypes. A principal component analysis (PCA) makes it possible to synthesize all the information contained in the spectra. Dots close together on a score plot means that the spectra are similar. If one dot is very far from all the others, it could be an outlier. This could also simply highlight a spectrum processing problem. When the PCA analysis reveals a tendency, it is reasonable to embark on a PLS-DA (partial least squares-discriminant analysis), which will help to define the peaks and therefore the metabolites involved in creating the differences between the spectra.

To be sure of the assignment of a metabolite to a peak, there are now many databases published in journals or online. Numerous initiatives are currently underway to optimize the **identification** of peaks, whether in NMR or in MS. Since 2008, Wishart's team have proposed valuable references: the human CSF metabolome [51], the human serum metabolome [52] and the human urine metabolome [53]. The Human Metabolome database, online, is now the most common reference used [54].

Pathway Analysis

Once a pattern change is determined, the **metabolic network** study is the final step. An online tool, Metaboanalyst, is a platform for the comprehensive analysis of metabolomic data [55]. One of the proposed options allows the highlighting of **metabolic pathways** of interest to propose new ideas for investigation.

From sample analysis to pathway analysis, it is necessary to have access to standardized procedures throughout the process of a metabolomics study [56, 57]. This was initiated in the Consortium for Metabonomic Toxicology (COMET) for rodents [58], but there is yet no equivalent for human research. However, in 2007, Summer et al. proposed minimum standards for reports that may help any researcher to published high values metabolomic studies [59]. In the same vein, data sharing projects are becoming more democratic with, in particular, Metabolomics Workbench [60], Metabolights [61] and COSMOS [62]. These projects will facilitate the transfer of experimental data between research teams [63] and easier access to metabolomics, including for the study of cryostimulation.

Metabolomics and Cold Stress

Exposure to cold elicits multiple molecular and cellular mechanisms. It was established that hypothermia reduces cellular metabolism to 50% at 30 °C and to 30% at 25 °C. For every 1 °C drop in body temperature, cellular metabolism decreases by

5–7% [64, 65]. Hypothermia has been used in organ preservation, surgical procedures and in treating brain injury to reduce metabolic rate and cellular requirement in oxygen and glucose [66]. Beneficial effects of therapeutic hypothermia have been explained by reducing levels of abnormal free radical production, excitatory amino acid, metabolic acidosis and enhancing cellular ion management and pH balance [67]. Indeed, hypothermia is often used as a therapeutic method which strengthens the cellular membrane and prevents the influx of deleterious ions after an ischemic event [66]. Such cellular changes could influence the energy metabolic pathways. It has been recognized that cold stress preserves cellular glucose reserves and ATP levels [67] and induces changes in lipid metabolism to heighten the energy expenditure by increasing lipolysis and free fatty acid turnover rate [68]. Exposure to cold induces also a change in electrolyte concentration through an increase in renal excretion leading to depletion of magnesium, potassium, and phosphate [69].

Knowing that practically all chemical reactions are impacted by temperature changes, hypothermia could differently regulate the fluxes and concentrations of various metabolites, leading therefore to metabolic and physiological changes [67]. Metabolic effects of mild hypothermia have been shown using nuclear magnetic resonance spectroscopy, which give an overview of the metabolic status of a cell, tissue or organism depending on genetic variations or external stimuli such as cold stress [70]. Metabolic responses of cells provide the final steps of cellular adaptation to stressors (thermal stress). It was demonstrated that a series of gene expression and biochemical adaptive responses are activated due to cold stress [71]. Exposure to low temperatures alters the lipid composition of cellular membranes and slows down the protein synthesis rate and cell proliferation and changes glucose homeostasis [72]. Kozłowska et al. [72] explored the impact of single and chronic cryotherapy on adipo-myokine profile, glucose homeostasis and amino acid profile; the authors observed that chronic whole-body cryostimulation (WBC) exposure had a positive effect on glucose homeostasis (reduction in blood glucose concentration and insulin level), adipo-myokine profile (increased irisin and adiponectin concentrations) and amino acid profile (reduced levels of valine and asparagine). These findings demonstrated that chronic WBC can effectively reduce the risk of the metabolic syndrome associated with hyperinsulinemia, increased levels of valine and asparagine, and muscle atrophy.

Animal [73] and human [29] metabolomic studies showed that the exposure to low temperature decrease marker of injury and inflammation by decreasing pro-inflammatory metabolites such as lactate, succinate, β-alanine, methionine, fumarate and acetate and increasing histidine, ornithine and glucose which might elicit anti-inflammatory and antioxidant effects [29, 73]. Furthermore, therapeutic hypothermia has been shown to increase ketone bodies and aromatic amino acids, especially tyrosine which may be related to enhanced immune activity [74]. In this line, we have previously [29] observed that exposure to local cryotherapy in knee arthritis patients led to a significant increase in the concentration of pyruvate, alanine, citrate and threonine in inflammatory synovial fluid. Our observations suggest that the increased level of metabolites involved in energy metabolism may explain the underlying molecular pathways that mediate the antioxidant and anti-inflammatory capacities of cryotherapy.

Metabolomic studies using different animal models [75, 76] showed that exposure to cold stress induces changes in endogenous amino acid concentration. Alanine and aspartate increased whilst glycine and serine levels decreased [75]. It has been reported that alanine preserves proteins from cold inactivation and may help to cold survival [75] by activating the antioxidant defence proteins (Heme oxygenase (HO)-1 and ferritin) [77]. The final amino acid upregulated due to freezing in the Antarctic midge is aspartate, and this increase could be a secondary response to a disruption in glycolysis, as demonstrated by increased levels of glycerol and alanine [75, 78]. Venero et al. [79] observed that rats exposed to cold stress had a higher urinary excretion of glutamate and aspartate, and a lower urinary excretion of glutamine and glycine. These findings are indicative of elevated glucocorticoid levels, which increase excitatory amino acids like aspartate and glutamate while decreasing inhibitory amino acids like gamma aminobutyric acid (GABA) and glycine. In response to cold stress, the levels of other amino acids increase such as tryptophan metabolites (nicotinate and 5-hydroxyindole-3-acetate). Urinary NMR analysis conducted on animal models [80] revealed that exposure to acute cold has a significant impact on metabolites involved in several pathways including the tricarboxylic acid (TCA) cycle (fumarate, citrate, pyruvate, succinate), muscle metabolism (creatinine) and gut microflora (hippurate). The urinary excretion of some metabolites (citrate, 2-oxoglutarate, succinate, fumarate and pyruvate) decreases, which may be attributed to the increased energy consumption and TCA cycle activity, which may be indicative of enhanced adrenergic nerve activity [81].

Gandhi et al. [75] reported changes in the relative concentration of various metabolites of urine samples obtained in mice exposed to cold, the authors observed a significant decrease in pyruvate, citrate, 2-oxoglutarate, succinate, fumarate, *N*-methylnicotinamide, creatinine, hippurate, phenylalanine, β-hydroxybutyrate, TMAO and acetoacetate following cold exposure. The decrease in phenylalanine levels could be explained by its increased conversion to catecholamines in response to cold stress [75]. Reduced creatinine levels may indicate a lower glomerular filtration rate and/or changes in the transport mechanism at the tubular level [75]. Hippurate levels also decrease in response to cold stress, which is indicative of marked up-regulation of gut microbiota activity [82]. The effects of chronic cold exposure have been investigated in rat serum and renal tissue samples [75, 76, 80]. NMR analysis revealed a significant continuous increase in metabolites such as lactate, alanine, and glucose following a prolonged cold exposure. Lactate concentration rise indicates activated anaerobic carbohydrate metabolism because of increased energy demands caused by cold exposure (the elevated lactate levels are consistent with incomplete glucose oxidation). Elevated glucose levels indicate increased glucose availability to muscles, implying that carbohydrate metabolism via glycolytic rather than oxidative pathways occur during prolonged cold exposure. An increase in alanine also indicates a metabolic shift towards energy conservation. In response to acute exposure to cold, creatinine levels rise and then fall indicating an altered glomerular filtration rate whereas during continuous exposure, the body adapts to the cold stress by maintaining homeostasis and creatinine levels begin to drop back to health-related reference values [76].

There is a growing body of literature examining the use of the metabolomic approach in investigating the impact of cold stress on metabolic pathways in animal models, whereas there is a paucity of human research in this area. The impact of cold-based therapeutic strategies such as cryotherapy on metabolic pathways need to be investigated to understand the underlying physiological mechanisms mediated by cold.

Conclusion

Chemical reactions are impacted by temperature changes. Exposure to cold could differently regulate the fluxes and concentrations of various metabolites, leading therefore to metabolic and physiological changes. Metabolomic studies combined with statistical analysis allow for non-invasive and simultaneous monitoring of multiple functional metabolites involved in various metabolic pathways within the body, leading to a better understanding of the systemic response to external stimuli such as cold stress.

References

1. Dugué B, Leppänen E, Gräsbeck R. Preanalytical factors (biological variation) and the measurement of serum soluble intercellular adhesion molecule-1 in humans: influence of the time of day, food intake, and physical and psychological stress. Clin Chem. 1999;45(9):1543–7.
2. Bieuzen F, Hausswirth C, Dugué B. Circulating soluble intercellular adhesion molecule-1 (sICAM-1) after exercise-induced muscular damage: does the use of whole-body cryostimulation influence its concentration in blood? Cryobiology. 2019;87:120–2.
3. Dugué B, Leppänen E. Adaptation related to cytokines in man: effects of regular swimming in ice-cold water: thermal stress and cytokines. Clin Physiol. 2000;20(2):114–21.
4. Douzi W, Bon D, Suikkanen S, Soukkio P, Boildieu N, Nenonen A, et al. ^{1}H NMR urinary metabolomic analysis in older adults after hip fracture surgery may provide valuable information for patient profiling—a preliminary investigation. Metabolites. 2022;12(8):744.
5. Enea C, Seguin F, Petitpas-Mulliez J, Boildieu N, Boisseau N, Delpech N, et al. ^{1}H NMR-based metabolomics approach for exploring urinary metabolome modifications after acute and chronic physical exercise. Anal Bioanal Chem. 2010;396(3):1167–76.
6. Bujak R, Struck-Lewicka W, Markuszewski MJ, Kaliszan R. Metabolomics for laboratory diagnostics. J Pharm Biomed Anal. 2015;113:108–20.
7. Zhang A, Sun H, Wu X, Wang X. Urine metabolomics. Clin Chim Acta. 2012;414:65–9.
8. Segers K, Declerck S, Mangelings D, Heyden YV, Eeckhaut AV. Analytical techniques for metabolomic studies: a review. Bioanalysis. 2019;11(24):2297–318.
9. The Standard Metabolic Reporting Structures Working Group. Summary recommendations for standardization and reporting of metabolic analyses. Nat Biotechnol. 2005;23(7):833–8.
10. Emwas AH, Luchinat C, Turano P, Tenori L, Roy R, Salek RM, et al. Standardizing the experimental conditions for using urine in NMR-based metabolomic studies with a particular focus on diagnostic studies: a review. Metabolomics. 2015;11(4):872–94.

11. Lauridsen M, Hansen SH, Jaroszewski JW, Cornett C. Human urine as test material in ^{1}H NMR-based metabonomics: recommendations for sample preparation and storage. Anal Chem. 2007;79(3):1181–6.

12. Smith LM, Maher AD, Want EJ, Elliott P, Stamler J, Hawkes GE, et al. Large-scale human metabolic phenotyping and molecular epidemiological studies via ^{1}H NMR spectroscopy of urine: investigation of borate preservation. Anal Chem. 2009;81(12):4847–56.

13. Maher AD, Zirah SFM, Holmes E, Nicholson JK. Experimental and analytical variation in human urine in ^{1}H NMR spectroscopy-based metabolic phenotyping studies. Anal Chem. 2007;79(14):5204–11.

14. Stevens VL, Hoover E, Wang Y, Zanetti KA. Pre-analytical factors that affect metabolite stability in human urine, plasma, and serum: a review. Metabolites. 2019;9(8):156.

15. Bernini P, Bertini I, Luchinat C, Nincheri P, Staderini S, Turano P. Standard operating procedures for pre-analytical handling of blood and urine for metabolomic studies and biobanks. J Biomol NMR. 2011;49(3–4):231–43.

16. Beckonert O, Keun HC, Ebbels TMD, Bundy J, Holmes E, Lindon JC, et al. Metabolic profiling, metabolomic and metabonomic procedures for NMR spectroscopy of urine, plasma, serum and tissue extracts. Nat Protoc. 2007;2(11):2692–703.

17. Sotelo-Orozco J, Chen SY, Hertz-Picciotto I, Slupsky CM. A comparison of serum and plasma blood collection tubes for the integration of epidemiological and metabolomics data. Front Mol Biosci. 2021;8:682134.

18. Paglia G, Del Greco FM, Sigurdsson BB, Rainer J, Volani C, Hicks AA, et al. Influence of collection tubes during quantitative targeted metabolomics studies in human blood samples. Clin Chim Acta. 2018;486:320–8.

19. González-Domínguez R, González-Domínguez Á, Sayago A, Fernández-Recamales Á. Recommendations and best practices for standardizing the pre-analytical processing of blood and urine samples in metabolomics. Metabolites. 2020;10(6):229.

20. Sjøbakk TE, Vettukattil R, Gulati M, Gulati S, Lundgren S, Gribbestad IS, et al. Metabolic profiles of brain metastases. Int J Mol Sci. 2013;14(1):2104–18.

21. Paul A, Kumar S, Raj A, Sonkar AA, Jain S, Singhai A, et al. Alteration in lipid composition differentiates breast cancer tissues: a ^{1}H HRMAS NMR metabolomic study. Metabolomics. 2018;14(9):119.

22. Benahmed MA, Elbayed K, Daubeuf F, Santelmo N, Frossard N, Namer IJ. NMR HRMAS spectroscopy of lung biopsy samples: comparison study between human, pig, rat, and mouse metabolomics. Magn Reson Med. 2014;71(1):35–43.

23. Ferrarini A, Poto CD, He S, Tu C, Varghese RS, Balla AK, et al. Metabolomic analysis of liver tissues for characterization of hepatocellular carcinoma. J Proteome Res. 2019;18(8):3067–76.

24. Nizioł J, Copié V, Tripet BP, Nogueira LB, Nogueira KOPC, Ossoliński K, et al. Metabolomic and elemental profiling of human tissue in kidney cancer. Metabolomics. 2021;17(3):30.

25. Saheb Sharif-Askari N, Soares NC, Mohamed HA, Saheb Sharif-Askari F, Alsayed HAH, Al-Hroub H, et al. Saliva metabolomic profile of COVID-19 patients associates with disease severity. Metabolomics. 2022;18(11):81.

26. Boguenet M, Bocca C, Bouet PE, Serri O, Chupin S, Tessier L, et al. Metabolomic signature of the seminal plasma in men with severe oligoasthenospermia. Andrology. 2020;8(6):1859–66.

27. Del Mar AM, Colsch B, Lamari F, Jardel C, Ichou F, Rastetter A, et al. Targeted versus untargeted omics—the CAFSA story. J Inherit Metab Dis. 2018;41(3):447–56.

28. Surowiec I, Karimpour M, Gouveia-Figueira S, Wu J, Unosson J, Bosson JA, et al. Multiplatform metabolomics assays for human lung lavage fluids in an air pollution exposure study. Anal Bioanal Chem. 2016;408(17):4751–64.

29. Douzi W, Guillot X, Bon D, Seguin F, Boildieu N, Wendling D, et al. ^{1}H-NMR-Based analysis for exploring knee synovial fluid metabolite changes after local cryotherapy in knee arthritis patients. Metabolites. 2020;10(11):E460.

30. Kim M, Vogtmann E, Ahlquist DA, Devens ME, Kisiel JB, Taylor WR, et al. Fecal metabolomic signatures in colorectal adenoma patients are associated with gut microbiota and early events of colorectal cancer pathogenesis. MBio. 2020;11(1):e03186–19.

31. Graca G, Duarte IF, Goodfellow BJ, Barros AS, Carreira IM, Couceiro AB, et al. Potential of NMR spectroscopy for the study of human amniotic fluid. Anal Chem. 2007;79(21):8367–75.
32. Peralbo-Molina A, Calderón-Santiago M, Priego-Capote F, Jurado-Gámez B, Luque de Castro MD. Identification of metabolomics panels for potential lung cancer screening by analysis of exhaled breath condensate. J Breath Res. 2016;10(2):026002.
33. Balcerczyk A, Damblon C, Elena-Herrmann B, Panthu B, Rautureau GJP. Metabolomic approaches to study chemical exposure-related metabolism alterations in mammalian cell cultures. Int J Mol Sci. 2020;21(18):6843.
34. Oikawa A, Otsuka T, Jikumaru Y, Yamaguchi S, Matsuda F, Nakabayashi R, et al. Effects of freeze-drying of samples on metabolite levels in metabolome analyses. J Sep Sci. 2011;34(24):3561–7.
35. Fernández-Peralbo MA, Calderón Santiago M, Priego-Capote F, Luque de Castro MD. Study of exhaled breath condensate sample preparation for metabolomics analysis by LC–MS/MS in high resolution mode. Talanta. 2015;144:1360–9.
36. Martineau E, Tea I, Loaec G, Giraudeau P, Akoka S. Strategy for choosing extraction procedures for NMR-based metabolomic analysis of mammalian cells. Anal Bioanal Chem. 2011;401(7):2133–42.
37. Mushtaq MY, Choi YH, Verpoorte R, Wilson EG. Extraction for metabolomics: access to the metabolome. Phytochem Anal. 2014;25(4):291–306.
38. Salek R, Cheng KK, Griffin J. Chapter seventeen—the study of mammalian metabolism through NMR-based metabolomics. In: Methods in enzymology. Academic Press; 2011. p. 337–51.
39. Kruger NJ, Troncoso-Ponce MA, Ratcliffe RG. ^{1}H NMR metabolite fingerprinting and metabolomic analysis of perchloric acid extracts from plant tissues. Nat Protoc. 2008;3(6):1001–12.
40. Matyash V, Liebisch G, Kurzchalia TV, Shevchenko A, Schwudke D. Lipid extraction by methyl-tert-butyl ether for high-throughput lipidomics. J Lipid Res. 2008;49(5):1137–46.
41. Belle JEL, Harris NG, Williams SR, Bhakoo KK. A comparison of cell and tissue extraction techniques using high-resolution ^{1}H-NMR spectroscopy. NMR Biomed. 2002;15(1):37–44.
42. Wu H, Southam AD, Hines A, Viant MR. High-throughput tissue extraction protocol for NMR- and MS-based metabolomics. Anal Biochem. 2008;372(2):204–12.
43. Marshall DD, Powers R. Beyond the paradigm: combining mass spectrometry and nuclear magnetic resonance for metabolomics. Prog Nucl Magn Reson Spectrosc. 2017;100:1–16.
44. Dwivedi P, Schultz AJ, Hill HH. Metabolic profiling of human blood by high resolution ion mobility mass spectrometry (IM-MS). Int J Mass Spectrom. 2010;298(1-3):78–90.
45. Zhang W, Ramautar R. CE-MS for metabolomics: developments and applications in the period 2018–2020. Electrophoresis. 2021;42(4):381–401.
46. Lopes J, Correia M, Martins I, Henriques AG, Delgadillo I, da Cruz e Silva O, et al. FTIR and Raman spectroscopy applied to dementia diagnosis through analysis of biological fluids. J Alzheimers Dis. 2016;52(3):801–12.
47. Ren S, Hinzman AA, Kang EL, Szczesniak RD, Lu LJ. Computational and statistical analysis of metabolomics data. Metabolomics. 2015;11(6):1492–513.
48. Khakimov B, Mobaraki N, Trimigno A, Aru V, Engelsen SB. Signature Mapping (SigMa): an efficient approach for processing complex human urine ^{1}H NMR metabolomics data. Anal Chim Acta. 2020;1108:142–51.
49. Roberts LD, Souza AL, Gerszten RE, Clish CB. Targeted metabolomics. Curr Protoc Mol Biol. 2012;98(1):30–2.
50. Schrimpe-Rutledge AC, Codreanu SG, Sherrod SD, McLean JA. Untargeted metabolomics strategies—challenges and emerging directions. J Am Soc Mass Spectrom. 2016;27(12):1897–905.
51. Wishart DS, Lewis MJ, Morrissey JA, Flegel MD, Jeroncic K, Xiong Y, et al. The human cerebrospinal fluid metabolome. J Chromatogr B Analyt Technol Biomed Life Sci. 2008;871(2):164–73.
52. Psychogios N, Hau DD, Peng J, Guo AC, Mandal R, Bouatra S, et al. The human serum metabolome. Flower D, éditeur. PLoS ONE. 2011;6(2):e16957.

53. Bouatra S, Aziat F, Mandal R, Guo AC, Wilson MR, Knox C, et al. The human urine metabolome. PLoS One. 2013;8(9):e73076.
54. Wishart DS, Feunang YD, Marcu A, Guo AC, Liang K, Vázquez-Fresno R, et al. HMDB 4.0: the human metabolome database for 2018. Nucleic Acids Res. 2018;46(D1):D608–17.
55. Xia J, Wishart DS. Web-based inference of biological patterns, functions and pathways from metabolomic data using MetaboAnalyst. Nat Protoc. 2011;6(6):743–60.
56. Emwas AH, Roy R, McKay RT, Ryan D, Brennan L, Tenori L, et al. Recommendations and standardization of biomarker quantification using NMR-based metabolomics with particular focus on urinary analysis. J Proteome Res. 2016;15(2):360–73.
57. Liu KH, Nellis M, Uppal K, Ma C, Tran V, Liang Y, et al. Reference standardization for quantification and harmonization of large-scale metabolomics. Anal Chem. 2020;92(13):8836–44.
58. Lindon JC, Keun HC, Ebbels TM, Pearce JM, Holmes E, Nicholson JK. The consortium for metabonomic toxicology (COMET): aims, activities and achievements. Pharmacogenomics. 2005;6(7):691–9.
59. Sumner LW, Amberg A, Barrett D, Beale MH, Beger R, Daykin CA, et al. Proposed minimum reporting standards for chemical analysis Chemical Analysis Working Group (CAWG) Metabolomics Standards Initiative (MSI). Metabolomics. 2007;3(3):211–21.
60. Sud M, Fahy E, Cotter D, Azam K, Vadivelu I, Burant C, et al. Metabolomics workbench: an international repository for metabolomics data and metadata, metabolite standards, protocols, tutorials and training, and analysis tools. Nucleic Acids Res. 2016;44(D1):D463–70.
61. Haug K, Cochrane K, Nainala VC, Williams M, Chang J, Jayaseelan KV, et al. MetaboLights: a resource evolving in response to the needs of its scientific community. Nucleic Acids Res. 2020;48(D1):D440–4.
62. Salek RM, Neumann S, Schober D, Hummel J, Billiau K, Kopka J, et al. COordination of Standards in MetabOlomicS (COSMOS): facilitating integrated metabolomics data access. Metabolomics. 2015;11(6):1587–97.
63. Rocca-Serra P, Salek RM, Arita M, Correa E, Dayalan S, Gonzalez-Beltran A, et al. Data standards can boost metabolomics research, and if there is a will, there is a way. Metabolomics. 2016;12(1):14.
64. Lazorthes G, Campan L. Hypothermia in the treatment of craniocerebral traumatism. J Neurosurg. 1958;15(2):162–7.
65. Bucher L, Buruschkin R, Kenyon DM, Stenton K, Treseder S. Improving outcomes with therapeutic hypothermia. Dimens Crit Care Nurs. 2013;32(3):147–51.
66. González-Ibarra FP, Varon J, López-Meza EG. Therapeutic hypothermia: critical review of the molecular mechanisms of action. Front Neurol. 2011;2:4.
67. Liu J, Litt L, Segal MR, Kelly MJ, Yoshihara HA, James TL. Outcome-related metabolomic patterns from ^{1}H/^{31}P NMR after mild hypothermia treatments of oxygen—glucose deprivation in a neonatal brain slice model of asphyxia. J Cereb Blood Flow Metab. 2011;31(2):547–59.
68. Vallerand AL, Zamecnik J, Jones PJ, Jacobs I. Cold stress increases lipolysis, FFA Ra and TG/FFA cycling in humans. Aviat Space Environ Med. 1999;70(1):42–50.
69. Marion DW, Obrist WD, Earlier PM, Penrod LE, Darby JM. The use of moderate therapeutic hypothermia for patients with severe head injuries: a preliminary report. J Neurosurg. 1993;79(3):354–62.
70. Fanos V, Antonucci R, Barberini L, Noto A, Atzori L. Clinical application of metabolomics in neonatology. J Matern Fetal Neonatal Med. 2012;25(sup1):104–9.
71. Fujita J. Cold shock response in mammalian cells. J Mol Microbiol Biotechnol. 1999;1(2):243–55.
72. Kozłowska M, Kortas J, Żychowska M, Antosiewicz J, Żuczek K, Perego S, et al. Beneficial effects of whole-body cryotherapy on glucose homeostasis and amino acid profile are associated with a reduced myostatin serum concentration. Sci Rep. 2021;11(1):7097.
73. Angus SA, Henderson WR, Banoei MM, Molgat-Seon Y, Peters CM, Parmar HR, et al. Therapeutic hypothermia attenuates physiologic, histologic, and metabolomic markers of injury in a porcine model of acute respiratory distress syndrome. Physiol Rep. 2022;10(9):e15286.

74. Yang H, Shan W, Zhu F, Wu J, Wang Q. Ketone bodies in neurological diseases: focus on neuroprotection and underlying mechanisms. Front Neurol. 2019;10:585.
75. Gandhi S, Khushu S, Tripathi R. Current metabolomic methodologies & their application to thermal stress. Curr Metab. 2014;1(4):335–52.
76. Gandhi S, Bhonsle S, Koundal S, et al. High resolution ^{1}H NMR approach to study the effects of cold stress on the metabolism of rat renal tissue. In: ISMRM Proc, vol. 2369; 2012.
77. Grosser N, Oberle S, Berndt G, Erdmann K, Hemmerle A, Schröder H. Antioxidant action of l-alanine: heme oxygenase-1 and ferritin as possible mediators. Biochem Biophys Res Commun. 2004;314(2):351–5.
78. Fields PG, Fleurat-Lessard F, Lavenseau L, Febvay G, Peypelut L, Bonnot G. The effect of cold acclimation and deacclimation on cold tolerance, trehalose and free amino acid levels in Sitophilus granarius and Cryptolestes ferrugineus (Coleoptera). J Insect Physiol. 1998;44(10):955–65.
79. Venero C, Borrell J. Rapid glucocorticoid effects on excitatory amino acid levels in the hippocampus: a microdialysis study in freely moving rats. Eur J Neurosci. 1999;11(7):2465–73.
80. Gandhi S, Devi MM, Pal S, Tripathi RP, Khushu S. Metabolic regulatory variations in rats due to acute cold stress & Tinospora Cordifolia intervention: high resolution ^{1}H NMR approach. Metabolomics. 2012;8(3):444–53.
81. Gibala MJ, Tarnopolsky MA, Graham TE. Tricarboxylic acid cycle intermediates in human muscle at rest and during prolonged cycling. Am J Physiol Endocrinol Metab. 1997;272(2):E239–44.
82. Dumas ME, Barton RH, Toye A, Cloarec O, Blancher C, Rothwell A, et al. Metabolic profiling reveals a contribution of gut microbiota to fatty liver phenotype in insulin-resistant mice. Proc Natl Acad Sci U S A. 2006;103(33):12511–6.

Metabolites, Bioactive Compounds, and Browning: Unveiling the Therapeutic Potential of Whole-Body Cryostimulation for Metabolic Health

8

Raffaella Cancello

The relationship between food intake and cold exposure is complex and can be influenced by individual characteristics (sex, age, weight, fitness level, etc.), environmental factors, and pathological state. While cold exposure is commonly believed to stimulate appetite, two historical studies, one conducted by Lewis et al. (1960) in the Arctic and the other by Milan and Rodahl (1961) in the Antarctic, do not support the idea that cold exposure directly leads to a persistent increased food intake [1, 2]. Interestingly, both studies showed a significant increase in body weight between the end of summer, when subjects arrived from warmer climates, and the beginning of winter [1, 2]. However, during the colder months, the body weight remained stable, indicating that food intake was not excessive and appetite was not overly stimulated [2]. These findings suggest that the cold temperature, by itself, does not appear to have a direct influence on increasing food intake. However, the effect of cold exposure on appetite can vary among individuals and may depend on different factors including duration and intensity of exposure. At present, there are no data on food intake rate after whole-body cryotherapy sessions.

Previous research has established a connection between nutrition and thermal tolerance in larvae, particularly concerning cold resistance. Studies with *Drosophila* spp. larvae have shown that diets varying in protein and carbohydrate content can significantly impact the ability to resist chilling [3]. In some cases, cold tolerance in species like *Drosophila melanogaster* was directly linked to specific nutrients in the larvae's diet (e.g., proline) and in the adults' diet (e.g., NaCl and KCl), or nutrients

R. Cancello (✉)
Laboratory of Nutrition and Obesity Research, Obesity Unit, Department of Endocrine and Metabolic Diseases, IRCCS Istituto Auxologico Italiano, Milan, Italy
e-mail: r.cancello@auxologico.it

P. Capodaglio (ed.), *Whole-Body Cryostimulation*,
https://doi.org/10.1007/978-3-031-18545-8_8

93

mediated by gut bacteria in tephritid flies (e.g., *Bactrocera dorsalis*: arginine and proline) [4–6]. These nutritional metabolites are believed to influence freezing temperature and ion regulation, acting as protein and membrane stabilizers, thus preventing cellular damage during cold stress. Additionally, the quantity and composition of lipids acquired by larvae during development may also affect the cold tolerance of adults (e.g., cholesterol) [6]. However, using the protein-fat-fiber diet (PFFD) and a simple experimental setup, researchers were unable to demonstrate a clear association between larval diet and adult cold tolerance [6, 7]. Despite this, the marginal effect observed on male flies' recovery from chilling suggests that larval diet may indeed impact the tolerance to cold. Such research could provide valuable insights into the mechanisms underlying thermal adaptation and could have implications for species' survival and responses to changing environmental conditions.

The most frequently used animal model to investigate human physiology and pathophysiology is rodents (mice and rats). When mice living at a thermoneutral temperature (TN) of 30 °C are transferred to the typical room temperature (RT) of 22 °C, an immediate cold response is observed [8–10]. This response includes increases in various physiological processes such as heat production through shivering, food intake, heart rate, sympathetic nervous system tone, and metabolic rate [10–12]. However, with prolonged exposure to the typical RT (22 °C) for 2 weeks or longer, mice undergo adaptive changes to meet the increased, chronic thermal demand [10]. As a result, mice in typical animal facilities might show few overt signs of cold stress. A significant increase in food intake is observed when comparing the lowest and highest recommended temperatures of tabulation. This cold-induced hypermetabolism is not unique to rodents and can also be observed in humans under substantial cold stress [13, 14]. However, it is important to note that the chronic nature and magnitude of temperature exposure in research facilities for mice may not accurately reflect the temperature variations experienced by humans. Understanding these differences is essential when interpreting research findings and considering the relevance of animal models to human physiology in cold-related studies.

Exploring compounds found in nutrients that may offer potential benefits or properties similar to cold exposure, certain ones have been studied for their ability to mimic aspects of cold-induced effects. However, it is crucial to understand that these compounds cannot fully replace the physiological responses triggered by environmental cold exposure, and their effects may be limited in comparison. Individual responses may vary, and further research is necessary to comprehend the complete extent of these effects. There is a growing body of evidence showing that different metabolites are crucial in responding to cold stress as well as some bioactive compounds found in foods can activate or inhibit different types of TRP channels (see Chap. 2) and influence the related physiological processes activated by cold stimulus.

Diet Metabolites Regulating Browning

Free fatty acids (FFAs) constitute a significant class of endogenous mitochondrial uncouplers, operating through various mechanisms. They directly stimulate mitochondrial respiration in intact isolated brown adipocytes or mitochondria isolated from these cells [15–18], having a direct impact on the activity of Uncoupling Protein 1 (UCP-1). Studies using liposomes enriched in UCP-1 revealed that FFAs serve as a required co-factor for UCP-1-catalyzed proton transport [19], suggesting that the uncoupling effect of FFAs may rely on this channel. It is now widely accepted that, in the presence of specific FFAs, UCP-1 facilitates the electrophoretic transport of protons and selective anions. Other studies have indicated that FFAs, such as palmitate, can physically interact with UCP-1, leading to a change in the protein conformation and ultimately inducing mitochondrial uncoupling [18, 20]. However, some experiments have challenged these conclusions, proposing instead that FFAs can directly act as mitochondrial uncouplers even in the absence of UCP-1, though conflicting results have also been reported [21]. In addition to FFAs a considerable number of metabolites have been described to influence brown adipose tissue (BAT) activity or white adipose tissue (WAT) browning, such as *N*-acetyl aspartate [22, 23], bile acids [24, 25], creatine [26] or ceramides [27].

Glucose uptake, glycolysis, and lactate oxidation are essential processes in brown adipose tissue (BAT) to replenish the tricarboxylic acid cycle (TCA), providing reducing equivalents for the electron transport chain and supporting the regeneration of lipid stores [28–30]. Additionally, systemic succinate has been suggested to stimulate BAT activity [31]. Glucose is an important substrate for BAT and beige adipocytes upon cold exposure in mice and men both in fact classical BAT and beige adipocytes are primarily detected via 18-FDG uptake. Moreover, increasing UCP-1 protein levels in human white adipocytes improved glucose utilization [32, 33] and recently, a distinct glycolytic subtype of beige adipocytes (g-beige) was identified [34, 35]. Glucose uptake upon β-adrenergic stimulation is mediated via GLUT-1 via two distinct signaling pathways: Glut1 transcription and de-novo synthesis are increased in a cAMP-dependent manner [36–38]; its translocation to the plasma membrane depends on mTORC2 that is upregulated upon adrenergic stimulation [36]. Glucose uptake and intracellular glycolysis are then crucial for short-term BAT activity maintaining FA oxidation, and synthesizing glycerol-3-phosphate to replenish the intracellular TG pool. BAT glucose uptake was increased after a carbohydrate-rich meal in human subjects [39, 40]. On the other hand, circulating FA levels and uptake in BAT was reduced in the postprandial time compared to the fasted state, suggesting a shift in BAT substrate utilization from glucose to FAs under nutrient scarcity. These findings could explain the low number of 18FDG-PET-positive subjects in most studies, where participants were asked to fast before measurements. It is still under debate whether different fasting regimens lead to metabolic benefits in humans through WAT browning. More studies are needed to investigate the distinct activators of beige adipocytes as well as its applicability in humans with and without a cryostimulus.

Bioactive Compound Agonists for TRPM8

Several natural compounds have been identified as agonists of TRPM8, meaning they can activate the channel and induce cold sensations. These natural TRPM8 agonists are used in various consumer products, topical analgesics, and even in research settings to study the function of TRPM8 channels and their role in sensory perception and to mimic the cold stimulus [41].

Menthol

Menthol is a compound that is known for its cooling and soothing sensation when applied to the skin or mucous membranes. While menthol can provide a sensation of coldness, it does not actually lower body temperature or mimic the physiological effects of cold exposure. When applied topically or consumed orally, menthol activates specific receptors in the body called TRPM8 receptors (detailed in Chap. 2), which are responsible for sensing cold sensations. This activation leads to a cooling effect on the skin or mucous membranes, providing a perception of coldness. Menthol is commonly found in various products such as topical analgesics, cough drops, and certain cosmetic and personal care items. It is often used to provide temporary relief from pain, itchiness, and congestion. Menthol can create a refreshing sensation and may temporarily alleviate discomfort, but it does not have the same physiological effects on the body as genuine cold exposure. The cooling sensation from menthol is subjective and may vary among individuals. Some people may find it more intense, while others may be less sensitive to its effects. The minimum menthol concentration required for TRPM8 activation is merely 0.1 μM at cellular level [42] in a pH dependent manner [43]. In addition, submillimolar menthol blocks pain/noxious cold-sensing TRPA1 channels, indicating the inverse agonist/antagonist relationship between the two cold-sensing channels, and this could be another explanation for the analgesic action of menthol [44]. There is evidence that stimulation of TRPM8 by menthol mediates brown adipocytes thermogenesis, which could constitute a feasible method of treating obesity [45–47]. Menthol can now be chemically synthesized, rather than extracted from corn mint, and about 50% of menthol in market is artificial, while 50% is natural from mint. Therefore, it is reasonable that diet-induced obesity and glucose abnormalities could be ameliorated by menthol treatment and menthol-induced TRPM8 activation could mimic cold stimulation-induced thermogenesis representing an intriguing approach to treat human obesity and related metabolic disorders.

Eucalyptol

Eucalyptol, also known as 1,8-cineole, is a natural organic compound that is commonly found in the essential oils of various eucalyptus species [48]. It is a colorless liquid with a pleasant and minty aroma, which contributes to the characteristic scent of eucalyptus. Eucalyptol can activate TRP channels, specifically TRPM8. TRPM8 is also known as the cold and menthol receptor and eucalyptol cooling effects and the minty sensation is attributed to its interaction with this receptor. It has also been found to have GABAergic effects, thanks to interaction with GABA receptors in the brain [49]. Eucalyptol has been shown to bind to nicotinic acetylcholine receptors, which are involved in the transmission of nerve signals in the central and peripheral nervous systems and to activate PPARs, the group of nuclear receptors that regulate gene expression and play a role in lipid metabolism and anti-inflammatory responses [50]. Eucalyptol has been widely studied for its properties and is known for its various therapeutic benefits. Eucalyptol is a potent bronchodilator and mucolytic agent, making it effective in easing respiratory issues such as coughs, congestion, and bronchitis. It helps to loosen mucus and alleviate breathing difficulties and possesses anti-inflammatory properties helping to reduce inflammation. Additionally, it has analgesic properties, providing relief from pain and discomfort. Eucalyptol exhibits strong antimicrobial and antiseptic actions, making it effective against various bacteria and fungi in vitro. It is often used to treat minor cuts, wounds, and skin infections. The inhalation of eucalyptol is believed to promote mental clarity and alertness. It can help alleviate mental fatigue and improve concentration [50–57].

Several studies have investigated the impact of eucalyptol on appetite and food intake. Eucalyptol pleasant aroma and flavor may influence sensory perception and appetite. Some research suggests that the aroma of eucalyptol or eucalyptus might be associated with a sense of fullness and reduced appetite, potentially leading to decreased food intake. However, the precise mechanisms by which eucalyptol affects appetite are not fully understood, and further research is necessary to establish a direct link between eucalyptol and food intake regulation. Regarding weight loss, scientific evidence supporting the notion that eucalyptol alone can lead to significant weight loss or appetite suppression is limited. It is essential to approach any claims regarding eucalyptol's weight loss effects with caution until more robust research can substantiate such claims.

Borneol

Borneol is a natural bicyclic organic compound found in various plants, including several species of the genus *Blumea* and the tree *Dryobalanops aromatica* (Borneo camphor) [58]. It is known for its characteristic minty, camphor-like aroma. Borneol has been studied for its interactions with various biological targets, including the TRPM8 receptor [59, 60]. It has been studied for its diverse pharmacological effects, including its potential to mimic certain aspects of cold exposure, also known as "cold mimic" effects. Borneol has been shown to increase heat production in the body, similar to what is observed during cold exposure. This thermogenic effect is thought to be mediated through the activation of brown adipose tissue (BAT) and the induction of mitochondrial uncoupling, leading to increased energy expenditure. It has been reported to influence various metabolic parameters, including glucose and lipid metabolism [61]. It may enhance glucose uptake in cells and improve insulin sensitivity, which could be beneficial in conditions like diabetes or metabolic syndrome [61, 62]. Borneol has been investigated for its potential neuroprotective properties, which could be relevant in conditions involving neurodegeneration or brain injury [63] mimicking the effects of cold exposure which could be relevant in conditions associated with cold-induced pain, such as arthritis or musculoskeletal discomfort. The mechanisms and effects of borneol action are complex and may vary depending on the context and dosage. Further research is needed to fully understand the potential benefits and limitations of borneol as a "cold mimic" and its possible applications in therapeutic settings.

Geraniol

Geraniol (3,7-dimethylocta-trans-2,6-dien-1-ol) is an acyclic monoterpene with a water solubility of 100 mg/L at 25 °C and an n-octanol/water partition coefficient of 2.65 [64]. It is abundant in essential oils extracted from lemongrass, rose, lavender and other aromatic plants. It is known to exert a wide spectrum of pharmacological activities, namely antimicrobial, anti-inflammatory, antioxidant and neuroprotective effects [64]. Its potential therapeutics include anti-inflammatory, antioxidant, neuroprotective and anticancer effects, often evidenced following oral administration of doses ranging from 50 mg/kg to more than 200 mg/kg. The potential clinical use of geraniol appears promising, and the knowledge of in vivo pharmacokinetics and bioavailability data are essential to design appropriate geraniol formulations and plan adequate therapeutic protocols [65, 66]. Geraniol treatment produces an increase in intracellular Ca^{2+} levels in mTRPM8-HEK293 cells [67]. Geraniol ameliorates carbohydrate metabolism and restores glucose homeostasis by altering the activities of enzymes involved in glucose production and utilization [68]. It also protects pancreatic β-cells and exhibits significant insulinotrophic activity in experimental diabetic rats [68]. In addition, immunohistochemical staining of pancreas confirms insulin secretion from remnant pancreatic β-cells in geraniol-treated diabetic rats. This suggests that geraniol exerts significant antidiabetic properties [68–70]; however, further studies are essential to understand the plausible molecular mechanism of geraniol in diabetes.

Bioactive Compound Agonists for TRPA1

Health benefits that might be associated to the stimulation of TRPA1 are various, as it has been shown to be expressed in numerous tissues as pancreatic β-cells, intestinal enteroendocrine cells, dorsal root ganglia (DRG) sensory neurons or skin. Moreover, TRPA1 is activated by a broad variety of natural molecules and has been associated to various physiological mechanisms as well as to the pungent, tingling, irritation and burning experience from their consumption [71]. The TRPA1 ion channel is detailed in Chap. 2. TRPA1 can be activated by various chemical compounds, including isothiocyanates found in wasabi, mustard, and horseradish, as well as thiosulfinates like diallyl sulfide and diallyl disulfide found in garlic and onion from the *Allium* genus [71]. Certain unsaturated aldehydes and irritant compounds from cigarette smoke can also elicit a response from TRPA1 [72]. In the family of alkylamides, compounds like hydroxy-α-sanshool from Sichuan and Melegueta peppers and garlic components (diallyl sulfide, diallyl disulfide, and diallyl trisulfide) can activate TRPA1 [73]. Additionally, some vanilloids, which were initially considered agonists of the TRPV sub-family, have also been found to activate TRPA1, such as ethyl-vanillin, 6-shogaol, and 6-paradol [71]. Thymol, carvacrol, 1′S-1′-acetoxychavicol acetate, cinnamaldehyde, thymoquinone and iso-thiocyanates are natural agonists of TRPA1.

Thymol

Thymol is a natural monoterpenoid phenol that is found in the essential oils of various plants, most notably in thyme (*Thymus vulgaris*) [74]. It is known for its strong aromatic and medicinal properties and has been used for centuries in traditional medicine for its therapeutic effects [74]. Some of the properties and potential benefits of thymol include the antimicrobial and anti-inflammatory properties, which can help reduce inflammation and associated symptoms in various conditions. It can help inhibit the growth and proliferation of various pathogens, making it useful in treating infections [75]. Thymol possesses antioxidant activity, which helps neutralize free radicals and reduce oxidative stress in the body. This antioxidant potential contributes to its potential health benefits [75]. Thymol is commonly used as an expectorant and bronchodilator. It can help promote the clearance of mucus from the respiratory tract and ease breathing difficulties. Thymol has been used traditionally to alleviate digestive issues such as indigestion, gas, and bloating [75]. It may help relax gastrointestinal smooth muscles and improve digestion. Thymol has been reported to have analgesic properties, providing pain relief, and antispasmodic effects, which can help relieve muscle spasms and cramps.

Thymol has been shown to activate TRPA1 at micromolar concentrations, leading to intracellular calcium flux [76]. Whilst the actual mechanism involved is not clear, thymol appears to directly activate TRPA1 and the action can be blocked by camphor. Thymol appears to have a faster activation than other TRPA1 agonists such as cinnamaldehyde, suggesting thymol acts via a different mechanism or binding site [76]. In addition, thymol has a bimodal effect, both activating and inhibiting TRPA1 receptor at high concentrations [76]. This activation of TRPA1 may explain the role thymol can play in pain relief [77]. Alongside TRPA1, TRPM8 has also been shown to be activated by thymol in a manner similar to menthol. Activation of TRPM8 by thymol may mean it also has an anti-inflammatory effect [78]. Some studies suggest that thymol may have anticancer properties and could inhibit the growth of certain cancer cells [79]. However, further research is needed to establish its role in cancer therapy. Thymol is widely used as a flavoring agent in the food and beverage industry due to its pleasant aroma and taste. It is also commonly used in various personal care products, such as mouthwashes and toothpaste, for its antimicrobial and breath-freshening properties.

Carvacrol

Carvacrol is a natural monoterpenoid phenol that is found in the essential oils of various plants, particularly in oregano and thyme. It is known for its strong aromatic and medicinal properties and has been used for its therapeutic effects in traditional medicine for many years. When carvacrol comes into contact with TRPA1, it can activate the channel and lead to the generation of nerve impulses that signal pain and discomfort [80, 81]. This activation of TRPA1 by carvacrol is believed to contribute to its pungent and irritating sensation, similar to that of other natural compounds like mustard oil and cinnamaldehyde, which are also known TRPA1 agonists. The interaction between carvacrol and TRPA1 has been studied for its potential therapeutic applications, particularly in the context of pain management and inflammation [82]. By modulating TRPA1 activity, carvacrol may have implications for conditions involving pain, such as migraine headaches and inflammatory disorders. However, further research is needed to fully understand the specific mechanisms and potential therapeutic uses of carvacrol in relation to TRPA1. Carvacrol has shown promising effects in preclinical studies; however, its application as a therapeutic agent requires more investigation, including clinical trials, to determine its safety and efficacy in humans. Specific research to the direct impact of carvacrol on browning of adipose tissue is limited.

1′S-1′-Acetoxychavicol Acetate (ACA)

The 1′-acetoxychavicol acetate (ACA) is an acetate ester that is chavicol acetate substituted by an acetoxy group at position 1′. It has a role as a plant metabolite, is a natural NF-κB inhibitor and an antineoplastic agent [83]. The ACA is a natural product found in *Alpinia conchigera*, *Apis cerana*, and *Alpinia galangal* (Thai Ginger) [84]. In vitro ACA did not activate TRPV1-expressing human embryonic kidney (HEK) cells, but strongly activated TRPA1-expressing HEK cells [85]. ACA was more potent than allyl isothiocyanate, the typical TRPA1 agonist [85], with a lower EC50 value than allyl isothiocyanate (AITC, pungency in mustard oil), a representative TRPA1 agonist. The ingestion of ACA prevents visceral fat accumulation in mice fed with a high saturated fat diet and increases the levels of the heat-generating protein, UCP1, in BAT [86, 87]. These results suggested a possible effect of ACA on weight reduction through sympathetic nervous system activation. In high-fat-high sucrose-fed rat model, body and visceral fat mass tend to be lower in the ACA group than in the control group. Ohnishi et al. (2012) suggest that ACA inhibits cellular lipid accumulation through the downregulation of PPARγ and C/EBPα via phosphorylation of AMPK in 3 T3-L1 adipocytes [86]. The beneficial effects of ACA against diet-induced obesity are promising, and the diet inclusion of foods containing ACA deserves further investigations.

Cinnamaldehyde

One specific TRPA1 agonist, cinnamaldehyde, found in cinnamon oil, has been associated with positive impacts on metabolism [88–90]. Studies have shown its potential to improve insulin sensitivity and reduce liver fat in obese mice, lower blood glucose levels in diabetic mice, and reduce body weight gain in obese mice [91]. In human studies, cinnamaldehyde ingestion has been linked to increased post-prandial energy expenditure and fat oxidation [92]. Cuminaldehyde, a compound found in cumin and structurally similar to cinnamaldehyde, has demonstrated anti-obesity and anti-hyperglycemic effects in animal models [93]. Cumin seed oil has also been shown to improve insulin sensitivity in patients with type II diabetes. The activation of TRPA1 is hypothesized to be involved in these effects, as it has been shown to contribute to thermogenesis [93]. To investigate further, researchers have studied the response of TRPA1 to cuminaldehyde, as well as other natural aldehydes such as anisaldehyde and tiglic aldehyde. These investigations aimed to understand the potential involvement of TRPA1 activation in the observed metabolic effects of these compounds but the data are limited [94].

It's important to note that while the research shows promising results, the specific mechanisms and implications of TRPA1 activation on metabolism and other physiological processes require further investigation. As with any bioactive compound, caution should be exercised, and further studies, including clinical trials, are needed to fully understand the potential therapeutic applications of these compounds.

Thymoquinone

Thymoquinone is a monoterpene diketone with a boiling point of 230–232 °C. It is the major monoterpene present in the essential oil of *Nigella sativa* seeds, which has a history of use as a folk medicine for various diseases, including eczema, asthma, bronchitis, and inflammation [93]. Thymoquinone exhibits several biological activities, such as anti-tumor, cytotoxic and immunopotentiating, anti-inflammatory, as well as respiratory stimulatory effects [95]. Quinones, including thymoquinone, can react with cellular nucleophiles like thiols or amines. Thymoquinone is believed to activate TRPA1 through covalent protein modification [96, 97]. Thymoquinone's ability to interact with TRPA1 through covalent binding suggests that it may be involved in sensory perception and potentially contribute to its reported biological activities [97]. However, further research is needed to fully understand the mechanisms of action and the implications of TRPA1 activation by thymoquinone in various physiological processes and disease conditions. The biological effects of thymoquinone are likely multifaceted, involving interactions with various molecular targets and pathways.

Isothiocyanates

Isothiocyanates are membrane-permeable electrophiles that form adducts with thiols and primary amines, suggesting that covalent modification, rather than classical lock-and-key binding, accounts for their agonist properties [98, 99]. They are a class of chemical compounds that are commonly found in cruciferous vegetables, such as broccoli, cauliflower, cabbage, and mustard greens responsible for the pungent flavor and characteristic aroma of these vegetables [99]. One notable property of isothiocyanates is their ability to activate the transient receptor potential ankyrin 1

(TRPA1) ion channel [100, 101]. When isothiocyanates come into contact with TRPA1-expressing nerve fibers, they can covalently bind to cysteine residues in the channel's protein structure, leading to the generation of nerve impulses that signal pain and discomfort. This activation of TRPA1 by isothiocyanates is responsible for the pungent and irritating sensation experienced when consuming cruciferous vegetables [99]. Beyond the sensory perception, TRPA1 activation by isothiocyanates has been implicated in various biological activities. For example, it may play a role in the potential health benefits associated with consuming cruciferous vegetables, such as anti-inflammatory and anticancer effects [99]. Some studies suggest that the activation of TRPA1 by isothiocyanates can trigger cellular responses that contribute to these beneficial properties.

Conclusion

While research indicates potential benefits of TRPs agonists for adipose tissue thermogenic activation and browning, the evidence is still emerging, and the mechanisms involved are not fully understood. In addition to the bioactive molecules and compounds described, there are other highly effective synthetic ones with promising applications. Since a balanced diet rich in a variety of nutrient-dense foods, along with regular physical activity, remains the foundation for the overall metabolic health, the chapter was focused on the natural ones. The whole-body cryotherapy intervention coupled with a controlled diet that includes bioactive compounds would probably need to be integrated in future research. What remains unclear is how frequently, how intense, how long and what type of cold is required to elicit significant metabolic improvements. A concerted effort is needed to move towards a more integrated perspective that simultaneously examines thermogenic activation and metabolic response improvements.

References

1. Lewis HE, Masterton JP, Rosenbaum S. Body weight and skinfold thickness of men on a polar expedition. Clin Sci. 1960;19:551–61.
2. Milan FA, Rodahl K. Caloric requirements of man in the antarctic. J Nutr. 1961;75(2):152–6. https://doi.org/10.1093/jn/75.2.152.
3. Andersen LH, Kristensen TN, Loeschcke V, Toft S, Mayntz D. Protein and carbohydrate composition of larval food affects tolerance to thermal stress and desiccation in adult Drosophila melanogaster. J Insect Physiol. 2010;56(4):336–40. https://doi.org/10.1016/j.jinsphys.2009.11.006.
4. Mitchell KA, Boardman L, Clusella-Trullas S, Terblanche JS. Effects of nutrient and water restriction on thermal tolerance: a test of mechanisms and hypotheses. Comp Biochem Physiol A Mol Integr Physiol. 2017;212:15–23. https://doi.org/10.1016/j.cbpa.2017.06.019.
5. Nyamukondiwa C, Terblanche JS. Thermal tolerance in adult Mediterranean and natal fruit flies (Ceratitis capitata and Ceratitis rosa): effect of age, gender and feeding status. J Therm Biol. 2009;34(8):406–14.

6. Andersen LH, Kristensen TN, Loeschcke V, et al. Protein and carbohydrate composition of larval food affects tolerance to thermal stress and desiccation in adult Drosophila melanogaster. J Insect Physiol. 2010;56(4):336–40.

7. Ben-Yosef M, Altman Y, Nemni-Lavi E, Papadopoulos NT, Nestel D. Larval nutritional-stress and tolerance to extreme temperatures in the peach fruit fly, Bactrocera zonata (Diptera: Tephritidae). Fly (Austin). 2023;17(1):2157161. https://doi.org/10.1080/1933693 4.2022.2157161.

8. Weldon CW, Mnguni S, Démares F, du Rand EE, Malod K, Manrakhan A, Nicolson SW. Adult diet does not compensate for impact of a poor larval diet on stress resistance in a tephritid fruit fly. J Exp Biol. 2019;222(Pt 6):jeb192534. https://doi.org/10.1242/jeb.192534.

9. Axsom JE, Nanavati AP, Rutishauser CA, Bonin JE, Moen JM, Lakatta EG. Acclimation to a thermoneutral environment abolishes age-associated alterations in heart rate and heart rate variability in conscious, unrestrained mice. Geroscience. 2020;42(1):217–32. https://doi.org/10.1007/s11357-019-00126-7.

10. Cannon B, Nedergaard J. Brown adipose tissue: function and physiological significance. Physiol Rev. 2004;84(1):277–359. https://doi.org/10.1152/physrev.00015.2003.

11. Nedergaard J, Cannon B. Brown adipose tissue as a heat-producing thermoeffector. Handb Clin Neurol. 2018;156:137–52. https://doi.org/10.1016/B978-0-444-63912-7.00009-6.

12. Cannon B, Nedergaard J. Nonshivering thermogenesis and its adequate measurement in metabolic studies. J Exp Biol. 2011;214(Pt 2):242–53. https://doi.org/10.1242/jeb.050989.

13. Johnson RE, Kark RM. Environment and food intake in man. Science. 1947;105(2728):378–9. https://doi.org/10.1126/science.105.2728.378.

14. Qian S, Yan S, Pang R, Zhang J, Liu K, Shi Z, Wang Z, Chen P, Zhang Y, Luo T, Hu X, Xiong Y, Zhou Y. A temperature-regulated circuit for feeding behavior. Nat Commun. 2022;13(1):4229. https://doi.org/10.1038/s41467-022-31917-w.

15. Di Paola M, Lorusso M. Interaction of free fatty acids with mitochondria: coupling, uncoupling and permeability transition. Biochim Biophys Acta. 2006;1757(9-10):1330–7. https://doi.org/10.1016/j.bbabio.2006.03.024.

16. Bukowiecki LJ, Folléa N, Lupien J, Paradis A. Metabolic relationships between lipolysis and respiration in rat brown adipocytes. The role of long chain fatty acids as regulators of mitochondrial respiration and feedback inhibitors of lipolysis. J Biol Chem. 1981;256:12840–8.

17. Wojtczak L, Schönfeld P. Effect of fatty acids on energy coupling processes in mitochondria. Biochim Biophys Acta. 1993;1183:41–57. https://doi.org/10.1016/0005-2728(93)90004-Y.

18. Divakaruni AS, Humphrey DM, Brand MD. Fatty acids change the conformation of uncoupling protein 1 (UCP1). J Biol Chem. 2012;287:36845–53. https://doi.org/10.1074/jbc. M112.381780.

19. Hoang T, Smith MD, Jelokhani-Niaraki M. Expression, folding, and proton transport activity of human uncoupling protein-1 (UCP1) in lipid membranes: evidence for associated functional forms. J Biol Chem. 2013;288(51):36244–58. https://doi.org/10.1074/jbc. M113.509935.

20. Breen EP, Gouin SG, Murphy AF, Haines LR, Jackson AM, Pearson TW, Murphy PV, Porter RK. On the mechanism of mitochondrial uncoupling protein 1 function. J Biol Chem. 2006;281(4):2114–9. https://doi.org/10.1074/jbc.M511575200.

21. Demine S, Renard P, Arnould T. Mitochondrial uncoupling: a key controller of biological processes in physiology and diseases. Cell. 2019;8(8):795. https://doi.org/10.3390/cells8080795.

22. Prokesch A, Pelzmann HJ, Pessentheiner AR, Huber K, Madreiter-Sokolowski CT, Drougard A, Schittmayer M, Kolb D, Magnes C, Trausinger G, Graier WF, Birner-Gruenberger R, Pospisilik JA, Bogner-Strauss JG. N-acetylaspartate catabolism determines cytosolic acetyl-CoA levels and histone acetylation in brown adipocytes. Sci Rep. 2016;6:23723. https://doi.org/10.1038/srep23723.

23. Pessentheiner AR, Pelzmann HJ, Walenta E, Schweiger M, Groschner LN, Graier WF, Kolb D, Uno K, Miyazaki T, Nitta A, Rieder D, Prokesch A, Bogner-Strauss JG. NAT8L (N-acetyltransferase 8-like) accelerates lipid turnover and increases energy expenditure

in brown adipocytes. J Biol Chem. 2013;288(50):36040–51. https://doi.org/10.1074/jbc. M113.491324.

24. Broeders EP, Nascimento EB, Havekes B, Brans B, Roumans KH, Tailleux A, Schaart G, Kouach M, Charton J, Deprez B, Bouvy ND, Mottaghy F, Staels B, van Marken Lichtenbelt WD, Schrauwen P. The bile acid chenodeoxycholic acid increases human brown adipose tissue activity. Cell Metab. 2015;22(3):418–26. https://doi.org/10.1016/j.cmet.2015.07.002.

25. Watanabe M, Houten SM, Mataki C, Christoffolete MA, Kim BW, Sato H, Messaddeq N, Harney JW, Ezaki O, Kodama T, Schoonjans K, Bianco AC, Auwerx J. Bile acids induce energy expenditure by promoting intracellular thyroid hormone activation. Nature. 2006;439(7075):484–9. https://doi.org/10.1038/nature04330.

26. Kazak L, Rahbani JF, Samborska B, Lu GZ, Jedrychowski MP, Lajoie M, Zhang S, Ramsay L, Dou FY, Tenen D, Chouchani ET, Dzeja P, Watson IR, Tsai L, Rosen ED, Spiegelman BM. Ablation of adipocyte creatine transport impairs thermogenesis and causes diet-induced obesity. Nat Metab. 2019;1(3):360–70. https://doi.org/10.1038/s42255-019-0035-x.

27. Chaurasia B, Kaddai VA, Lancaster GI, Henstridge DC, Sriram S, Galam DL, Gopalan V, Prakash KN, Velan SS, Bulchand S, Tsong TJ, Wang M, Siddique MM, Yuguang G, Sigmundsson K, Mellet NA, Weir JM, Meikle PJ, Bin M, Yassin MS, Shabbir A, Shayman JA, Hirabayashi Y, Shiow ST, Sugii S, Summers SA. Adipocyte ceramides regulate subcutaneous adipose browning, inflammation, and metabolism. Cell Metab. 2016;24(6):820–34. https://doi.org/10.1016/j.cmet.2016.10.002.

28. Klepac K, Georgiadi A, Tschöp M, Herzig S. The role of brown and beige adipose tissue in glycaemic control. Mol Asp Med. 2019;68:90–100. https://doi.org/10.1016/j.mam.2019.07.001.

29. Kim KH, Kim YH, Son JE, Lee JH, Kim S, Choe MS, Moon JH, Zhong J, Fu K, Lenglin F, Yoo JA, Bilan PJ, Klip A, Nagy A, Kim JR, Park JG, Hussein SM, Doh KO, Hui CC, Sung HK. Intermittent fasting promotes adipose thermogenesis and metabolic homeostasis via VEGF-mediated alternative activation of macrophage. Cell Res. 2017;27(11):1309–26. https://doi.org/10.1038/cr.2017.126.

30. Jeong JH, Chang JS, Jo YH. Intracellular glycolysis in brown adipose tissue is essential for optogenetically induced nonshivering thermogenesis in mice. Sci Rep. 2018;8(1):6672. https://doi.org/10.1038/s41598-018-25265-3.

31. Mills EL, Pierce KA, Jedrychowski MP, Garrity R, Winther S, Vidoni S, Yoneshiro T, Spinelli JB, Lu GZ, Kazak L, Banks AS, Haigis MC, Kajimura S, Murphy MP, Gygi SP, Clish CB, Chouchani ET. Accumulation of succinate controls activation of adipose tissue thermogenesis. Nature. 2018;560(7716):102–6. https://doi.org/10.1038/s41586-018-0353-2.

32. Min SY, Kady J, Nam M, Rojas-Rodriguez R, Berkenwald A, Kim JH, Noh HL, Kim JK, Cooper MP, Fitzgibbons T, Brehm MA, Corvera S. Human 'brite/beige' adipocytes develop from capillary networks, and their implantation improves metabolic homeostasis in mice. Nat Med. 2016;22(3):312–8. https://doi.org/10.1038/nm.4031.

33. Tews D, Pula T, Funcke JB, Jastroch M, Keuper M, Debatin KM, Wabitsch M, Fischer-Posovszky P. Elevated UCP1 levels are sufficient to improve glucose uptake in human white adipocytes. Redox Biol. 2019;26:101286. https://doi.org/10.1016/j.redox.2019.101286.

34. Chen Y, Ikeda K, Yoneshiro T, Scaramozza A, Tajima K, Wang Q, Kim K, Shinoda K, Sponton CH, Brown Z, Brack A, Kajimura S. Thermal stress induces glycolytic beige fat formation via a myogenic state. Nature. 2019;565(7738):180–5. https://doi.org/10.1038/s41586-018-0801-z.

35. Zu Y, Pahlavani M, Ramalingam L, Jayarathne S, Andrade J, Scoggin S, Festuccia WT, Kalupahana NS, Moustaid-Moussa N. Temperature-dependent effects of eicosapentaenoic acid (EPA) on browning of subcutaneous adipose tissue in ucp1 knockout male mice. Int J Mol Sci. 2023;24(10):8708. https://doi.org/10.3390/ijms24108708.

36. Dallner OS, Chernogubova E, Brolinson KA, Bengtsson T. Beta3-adrenergic receptors stimulate glucose uptake in brown adipocytes by two mechanisms independently of glucose transporter 4 translocation. Endocrinology. 2006;147(12):5730–9. https://doi.org/10.1210/en.2006-0242.

37. Shimizu Y, Nikami H, Tsukazaki K, Machado UF, Yano H, Seino Y, Saito M. Increased expression of glucose transporter GLUT-4 in brown adipose tissue of fasted rats after cold exposure. Am J Phys. 1993;264(6 Pt 1):E890–5. https://doi.org/10.1152/ajpendo.1993.264.6.E890.

38. Olichon-Berthe C, Van Obberghen E, Le Marchand-Brustel Y. Effect of cold acclimation on the expression of glucose transporter Glut 4. Mol Cell Endocrinol. 1992;89(1–2):11–8. https://doi.org/10.1016/0303-7207(92)90205-k.

39. Din MU, Saari T, Raiko J, Kudomi N, Maurer SF, Lahesmaa M, Fromme T, Amri EZ, Klingenspor M, Solin O, Nuutila P, Virtanen KA. Postprandial oxidative metabolism of human brown fat indicates thermogenesis. Cell Metab. 2018;28(2):207–216.e3. https://doi.org/10.1016/j.cmet.2018.05.020.

40. Blondin DP, Labbé SM, Phoenix S, Guérin B, Turcotte ÉE, Richard D, Carpentier AC, Haman F. Contributions of white and brown adipose tissues and skeletal muscles to acute cold-induced metabolic responses in healthy men. J Physiol. 2015;593(3):701–14. https://doi.org/10.1113/jphysiol.2014.283598.

41. LeGay CM, Gorobets E, Iftinca M, Ramachandran R, Altier C, Derksen DJ. Natural-product-derived transient receptor potential melastatin 8 (TRPM8) channel modulators. Org Lett. 2016;18(11):2746–9. https://doi.org/10.1021/acs.orglett.6b01222.

42. Xu L, Han Y, Chen X, Aierken A, Wen H, Zheng W, Wang H, Lu X, Zhao Z, Ma C, Liang P, Yang W, Yang S, Yang F. Molecular mechanisms underlying menthol binding and activation of TRPM8 ion channel. Nat Commun. 2020;11(1):3790. https://doi.org/10.1038/s41467-020-17582-x.

43. Andersson DA, Chase HW, Bevan S. TRPM8 activation by menthol, icilin, and cold is differentially modulated by intracellular pH. J Neurosci. 2004;24(23):5364–9. https://doi.org/10.1523/JNEUROSCI.0890-04.2004.

44. Karashima Y, Damann N, Prenen J, Talavera K, Segal A, Voets T, Nilius B. Bimodal action of menthol on the transient receptor potential channel TRPA1. J Neurosci. 2007;27(37):9874–84. https://doi.org/10.1523/JNEUROSCI.2221-07.2007.

45. Ma S, Yu H, Zhao Z, Luo Z, Chen J, Ni Y, Jin R, Ma L, Wang P, Zhu Z, Li L, Zhong J, Liu D, Nilius B, Zhu Z. Activation of the cold-sensing TRPM8 channel triggers UCP1-dependent thermogenesis and prevents obesity. J Mol Cell Biol. 2012;4(2):88–96. https://doi.org/10.1093/jmcb/mjs001.

46. Sakellariou P, Valente A, Carrillo AE, Metsios GS, Nadolnik L, Jamurtas AZ, Koutedakis Y, Boguszewski C, Andrade CM, Svensson PA, Kawashita NH, Flouris AD. Chronic l-menthol-induced browning of white adipose tissue hypothesis: a putative therapeutic regime for combating obesity and improving metabolic health. Med Hypotheses. 2016;93:21–6. https://doi.org/10.1016/j.mehy.2016.05.006.

47. Jiang C, Zhai M, Yan D, Li D, Li C, Zhang Y, Xiao L, Xiong D, Deng Q, Sun W. Dietary menthol-induced TRPM8 activation enhances WAT "browning" and ameliorates diet-induced obesity. Oncotarget. 2017;8(43):75114–26. https://doi.org/10.18632/oncotarget.20540.

48. Seol GH, Kim KY. Eucalyptol and its role in chronic diseases. Adv Exp Med Biol. 2016;929:389–98. https://doi.org/10.1007/978-3-319-41342-6_18.

49. Ceremuga TE, McClellan CB, Green XC, Heber BE, Jolly ML, Malone TB, Schaaf JL, Isaacs AP. Investigation of the anxiolytic and antidepressant effects of eucalyptol (1,8-Cineole), a compound from eucalyptus, in the adult male Sprague-Dawley rat. AANA J. 2017;85(4):277–84.

50. Jarvis GE, Barbosa R, Thompson AJ. Noncompetitive inhibition of 5-HT3 receptors by citral, linalool, and eucalyptol revealed by nonlinear mixed-effects modeling. J Pharmacol Exp Ther. 2016;356(3):549–62. https://doi.org/10.1124/jpet.115.230011.

51. Worth H, Schacher C, Dethlefsen U. Concomitant therapy with Cineole (Eucalyptole) reduces exacerbations in COPD: a placebo-controlled double-blind trial. Respir Res. 2009;10(1):69. https://doi.org/10.1186/1465-9921-10-69.

52. Juergens LJ, Worth H, Juergens UR. New perspectives for mucolytic, anti-inflammatory and adjunctive therapy with 1,8-cineole in COPD and asthma: review on the new therapeutic approach. Adv Ther. 2020;37(5):1737–53. https://doi.org/10.1007/s12325-020-01279-0.

53. Yin C, Liu B, Wang P, Li X, Li Y, Zheng X, Tai Y, Wang C, Liu B. Eucalyptol alleviates inflammation and pain responses in a mouse model of gout arthritis. Br J Pharmacol. 2020;177(9):2042–57. https://doi.org/10.1111/bph.14967.

54. Arooj B, Asghar S, Saleem M, Khalid SH, Asif M, Chohan T, Khan IU, Zubair HM, Yaseen HS. Anti-inflammatory mechanisms of eucalyptol rich Eucalyptus globulus essential oil alone and in combination with flurbiprofen. Inflammopharmacology. 2023;31(4):1849–62. https://doi.org/10.1007/s10787-023-01237-6.

55. Kennedy-Feitosa E, Cattani-Cavalieri I, Barroso MV, Romana-Souza B, Brito-Gitirana L, Valenca SS. Eucalyptol promotes lung repair in mice following cigarette smoke-induced emphysema. Phytomedicine. 2019;55:70–9. https://doi.org/10.1016/j.phymed.2018.08.012.

56. Merghni A, Belmamoun AR, Urcan AC, Bobiş O, Lassoued MA. 1,8-Cineol (Eucalyptol) Disrupts membrane integrity and induces oxidative stress in methicillin-resistant Staphylococcus aureus. Antioxidants. 2023;12(7):1388. https://doi.org/10.3390/antiox12071388.

57. Bhowal M, Gopal M. Eucalyptol: safety and pharmacological profile. J Pharm Sci. 2015;5:125–31.

58. Mei Y, Li L, Fan L, Fan W, Liu L, Zhang F, Hu Z, Wang K, Yang L, Wang Z. The history, stereochemistry, ethnopharmacology and quality assessment of borneol. J Ethnopharmacol. 2023;300:115697. https://doi.org/10.1016/j.jep.2022.115697.

59. Wang S, Zhang D, Hu J, Jia Q, Xu W, Su D, Song H, Xu Z, Cui J, Zhou M, Yang J, Xiao J. A clinical and mechanistic study of topical borneol-induced analgesia. EMBO Mol Med. 2017;9(6):802–15. https://doi.org/10.15252/emmm.201607300.

60. Chen GL, Lei M, Zhou LP, Zeng B, Zou F. Borneol is a TRPM8 agonist that increases ocular surface wetness. PLoS One. 2016;11(7):e0158868. https://doi.org/10.1371/journal.pone.0158868.

61. Madhuri K, Naik PR. Ameliorative effect of borneol, a natural bicyclic monoterpene against hyperglycemia, hyperlipidemia and oxidative stress in streptozotocin-induced diabetic Wistar rats. Biomed Pharmacother. 2017;96:336–47. https://doi.org/10.1016/j.biopha.2017.09.122.

62. Hong L, Li X, Bao Y, Duvall CL, Zhang C, Chen W, Peng C. Preparation, preliminary pharmacokinetic and brain targeting study of metformin encapsulated W/O/W composite submicron emulsions promoted by borneol. Eur J Pharm Sci. 2019;133:160–6. https://doi.org/10.1016/j.ejps.2019.03.019.

63. Yu B, Yao Y, Zhang X, Ruan M, Zhang Z, Xu L, Liang T, Lu J. Synergic neuroprotection between Ligusticum Chuanxiong Hort and Borneol against ischemic stroke by neurogenesis via modulating reactive astrogliosis and maintaining the blood-brain barrier. Front Pharmacol. 2021;12:666790. https://doi.org/10.3389/fphar.2021.666790.

64. Pavan B, Dalpiaz A, Marani L, Beggiato S, Ferraro L, Canistro D, Paolini M, Vivarelli F, Valerii MC, Comparone A, De Fazio L, Spisni E. Geraniol pharmacokinetics, bioavailability and its multiple effects on the liver antioxidant and xenobiotic-metabolizing enzymes. Front Pharmacol. 2018;9:18. https://doi.org/10.3389/fphar.2018.00018.

65. Mączka W, Wińska K, Grabarczyk M. One hundred faces of geraniol. Molecules. 2020;25(14):3303. https://doi.org/10.3390/molecules25143303.

66. Ben AR. Potential effects of geraniol on cancer and inflammation-related diseases: a review of the recent research findings. Molecules. 2023;28(9):3669. https://doi.org/10.3390/molecules28093669.

67. Calixto JB, Kassuya CA, André E, Ferreira J. Contribution of natural products to the discovery of the transient receptor potential (TRP) channels family and their functions. Pharmacol Ther. 2005;106(2):179–208. https://doi.org/10.1016/j.pharmthera.2004.11.008.

68. Babukumar S, Vinothkumar V, Sankaranarayanan C, Srinivasan S. Geraniol, a natural monoterpene, ameliorates hyperglycemia by attenuating the key enzymes of carbohydrate metabolism in streptozotocin-induced diabetic rats. Pharm Biol. 2017;55(1):1442–9. https://doi.org/10.1080/13880209.2017.1301494.

69. Bharate SS, Bharate SB. Modulation of thermoreceptor TRPM8 by cooling compounds. ACS Chem Neurosci. 2012;3(4):248–67. https://doi.org/10.1021/cn300006u.

70. Gandhi GR, Hillary VE, Antony PJ, Zhong LLD, Yogesh D, Krishnakumar NM, Ceasar SA, Gan RY. A systematic review on anti-diabetic plant essential oil compounds: dietary sources, effects, molecular mechanisms, and safety. Crit Rev Food Sci Nutr. 2023:1–20. https://doi.org/10.1080/10408398.2023.2170320.
71. Stinson RJ, Morice AH, Sadofsky LR. Modulation of transient receptor potential (TRP) channels by plant derived substances used in over-the-counter cough and cold remedies. Respir Res. 2023;24(1):45. https://doi.org/10.1186/s12931-023-02347-z.
72. Simon SA, Liedtke W. How irritating: the role of TRPA1 in sensing cigarette smoke and aerogenic oxidants in the airways. J Clin Invest. 2008;118(7):2383–6. https://doi.org/10.1172/JCI36111.
73. Riera CE, Menozzi-Smarrito C, Affolter M, Michlig S, Munari C, Robert F, Vogel H, Simon SA, le Coutre J. Compounds from Sichuan and Melegueta peppers activate, covalently and non-covalently, TRPA1 and TRPV1 channels. Br J Pharmacol. 2009;157(8):1398–409. https://doi.org/10.1111/j.1476-5381.2009.00307.x.
74. Hazzit M, Baaliouamer A, Faleiro ML, Miguel MG. Composition of the essential oils of *Thymus* and *Origanum* species from Algeria and their antioxidant and antimicrobial activities. J Agric Food Chem. 2006;54:6314–632.
75. Gabbai-Armelin PR, Sales LS, Ferrisse TM, De Oliveira AB, De Oliveira JR, Giro EMA, Brighenti FL. A systematic review and meta-analysis of the effect of thymol as an anti-inflammatory and wound healing agent: a review of thymol effect on inflammation and wound healing: a review of thymol effect on inflammation and wound healing. Phytother Res. 2022;36(9):3415–43. https://doi.org/10.1002/ptr.7541.
76. Lee SP, Buber MT, Yang Q, Cerne R, Cortés RY, Sprous DG, Bryant RW. Thymol and related alkyl phenols activate the hTRPA1 channel. Br J Pharmacol. 2008;153(8):1739–49. https://doi.org/10.1038/bjp.2008.85.
77. Xu ZH, Wang C, Fujita T, Jiang CY, Kumamoto E. Action of thymol on spontaneous excitatory transmission in adult rat spinal substantia gelatinosa neurons. Neurosci Lett. 2015;606:94–9. https://doi.org/10.1016/j.neulet.2015.08.042.
78. Wang W, Wang H, Zhao Z, Huang X, Xiong H, Mei Z. Thymol activates TRPM8-mediated Ca^{2+} influx for its antipruritic effects and alleviates inflammatory response in Imiquimod-induced mice. Toxicol Appl Pharmacol. 2020;407:115247. https://doi.org/10.1016/j.taap.2020.115247.
79. Islam MT, Khalipha ABR, Bagchi R, Mondal M, Smrity SZ, Uddin SJ, Shilpi JA, Rouf R. Anticancer activity of thymol: a literature-based review and docking study with Emphasis on its anticancer mechanisms. IUBMB Life. 2019;71(1):9–19. https://doi.org/10.1002/iub.1935.
80. Shen J, Shan J, Zhong L, Liang B, Zhang D, Li M, Tang H. Dietary phytochemicals that can extend longevity by regulation of metabolism. Plant Foods Hum Nutr. 2022;77(1):12–9. https://doi.org/10.1007/s11130-021-00946-z.
81. Mukaiyama M, Usui T, Nagumo Y. Non-electrophilic TRPA1 agonists, menthol, carvacrol and clotrimazole, open epithelial tight junctions via TRPA1 activation. J Biochem. 2020;168(4):407–15. https://doi.org/10.1093/jb/mvaa057.
82. Alvarenga EM, Souza LK, Araújo TS, Nogueira KM, Sousa FB, Araújo AR, Martins CS, Pacífico DM. Carvacrol reduces irinotecan-induced intestinal mucositis through inhibition of inflammation and oxidative damage via TRPA1 receptor activation. Chem Biol Interact. 2016;260:129–40. https://doi.org/10.1016/j.cbi.2016.11.009.
83. Baradwaj RG, Rao MV, Senthil KT. Novel purification of 1′S-1′-Acetoxychavicol acetate from Alpinia galanga and its cytotoxic plus antiproliferative activity in colorectal adenocarcinoma cell line SW480. Biomed Pharmacother. 2017;91:485–93. https://doi.org/10.1016/j.biopha.2017.04.114.
84. Ramanunny AK, Wadhwa S, Gulati M, Vishwas S, Khursheed R, Paudel KR, Gupta S, Porwal O, Alshahrani SM, Jha NK, Chellappan DK, Prasher P, Gupta G, Adams J, Dua K, Tewari D, Singh SK. Journey of Alpinia galanga from kitchen spice to nutraceutical to folk

medicine to nanomedicine. J Ethnopharmacol. 2022;291:115144. https://doi.org/10.1016/j.jep.2022.115144.

85. Narukawa M, Koizumi K, Iwasaki Y, Kubota K, Watanabe T. Galangal pungent component, 1′-acetoxychavicol acetate, activates TRPA1. Biosci Biotechnol Biochem. 2010;74(8):1694–6. https://doi.org/10.1271/bbb.100133.

86. Ohnishi R, Matsui-Yuasa I, Deguchi Y, Yaku K, Tabuchi M, Munakata H, Akahoshi Y, Kojima-Yuasa A. 1′-acetoxychavicol acetate inhibits adipogenesis in 3T3-L1 adipocytes and in high fat-fed rats. Am J Chin Med. 2012;40(6):1189–204. https://doi.org/10.1142/S0192415X12500887.

87. Kojima-Yuasa A, Matsui-Yuasa I. Pharmacological effects of 1′-acetoxychavicol acetate, a major constituent in the rhizomes of Alpinia galanga and Alpinia conchigera. J Med Food. 2020;23(5):465–75. https://doi.org/10.1089/jmf.2019.4490.

88. Alpizar YA, Gees M, Sanchez A, Apetrei A, Voets T, Nilius B, Talavera K. Bimodal effects of cinnamaldehyde and camphor on mouse TRPA1. Pflugers Arch. 2013;465(6):853–64. https://doi.org/10.1007/s00424-012-1204-x.

89. Kataoka Y, Kenny GP, Nishiyasu T, Amano T, Mündel T, Zheng H, Lei TH, Watanabe K, Fujii N. TRPA1 channel activation with cinnamaldehyde induces cutaneous vasodilation through NOS, but Not COX and KCa channel, mechanisms in humans. J Cardiovasc Pharmacol. 2022;79(3):375–82. https://doi.org/10.1097/FJC.0000000000001188.

90. Zhu R, Liu H, Liu C, Wang L, Ma R, Chen B, Li L, Niu J, Fu M, Zhang D, Gao S. Cinnamaldehyde in diabetes: a review of pharmacology, pharmacokinetics and safety. Pharmacol Res. 2017;122:78–89. https://doi.org/10.1016/j.phrs.2017.05.019.

91. Wang P, Yang Y, Wang D, Yang Q, Wan J, Liu S, Zhou P, Yang Y. Cinnamaldehyde ameliorates vascular dysfunction in diabetic mice by activating Nrf2. Am J Hypertens. 2020;33(7):610–9. https://doi.org/10.1093/ajh/hpaa024.

92. Camacho S, Michlig S, de Senarclens-Bezençon C, Meylan J, Meystre J, Pezzoli M, Markram H, le Coutre J. Anti-obesity and anti-hyperglycemic effects of cinnamaldehyde via altered ghrelin secretion and functional impact on food intake and gastric emptying. Sci Rep. 2015;5:7919. https://doi.org/10.1038/srep07919.

93. Legrand C, Merlini JM, de Senarclens-Bezençon C, Michlig S. New natural agonists of the transient receptor potential Ankyrin 1 (TRPA1) channel. Sci Rep. 2020;10(1):11238. https://doi.org/10.1038/s41598-020-68013-2.

94. Kaur J, Kumar V, Kumar V, Shafi S, Khare P, Mahajan N, Bhadada SK, Kondepudi KK, Bhunia RK, Kuhad A, Bishnoi M. Combination of TRP channel dietary agonists induces energy expending and glucose utilizing phenotype in HFD-fed mice. Int J Obes. 2022;46(1):153–61. https://doi.org/10.1038/s41366-021-00967-3.

95. Malik S, Singh A, Negi P, Kapoor VK. Thymoquinone: a small molecule from nature with high therapeutic potential. Drug Discov Today. 2021;26(11):2716–25. https://doi.org/10.1016/j.drudis.2021.07.013.

96. Shi MM, Kugelman A, Iwamoto T, Tian L, Forman HJ. Quinone-induced oxidative stress elevates glutathione and induces gamma-glutamylcysteine synthetase activity in rat lung epithelial L2 cells. J Biol Chem. 1994;269:26512–7.

97. Songa Y, Wagner BA, Witmer JR, Lehmlera HJ, Buettnera GR. Nonenzymatic displacement of chlorine and formation of free radicals upon the reaction of glutathione with PCB quinines. Proc Natl Acad Sci U S A. 2009;106:9725–30.

98. Uchida K, Miura Y, Nagai M, Tominaga M. Isothiocyanates from Wasabia japonica activate transient receptor potential ankyrin 1 channel. Chem Senses. 2012;37:809–18.

99. Vanduchova A, Anzenbacher P, Anzenbacherova E. Isothiocyanate from broccoli, sulforaphane, and its properties. J Med Food. 2019;22(2):121–6. https://doi.org/10.1089/jmf.2018.0024.

100. Sandor Z, Dekany A, Kelemen D, Bencsik T, Papp R, Bartho L. The TRPA1 Activator Allyl Isothiocyanate (AITC) contracts human jejunal muscle: pharmacological analysis. Basic Clin Pharmacol Toxicol. 2016;119(3):341–2. https://doi.org/10.1111/bcpt.12574.

101. Ohashi N, Tashima K, Namiki T, Horie S. Allyl isothiocyanate, an activator of TRPA1, increases gastric mucosal blood flow through calcitonin gene-related peptide and adrenomedullin in anesthetized rats. J Pharmacol Sci. 2023;151(4):187–94. https://doi.org/10.1016/j.jphs.2023.02.002.

Possible Applications of Cold Stimulus in Obesity and Diabetes

9

Saverio Cinti

Introduction

In mammals, the adipose tissues are contained in a true organ: the adipose organ [1]. It consists of a subcutaneous and a visceral component (Fig. 9.1). This organ contain two types of tissues: white adipose tissue (WAT) and brown adipose tissue (BAT), which together contribute to the formation of subcutaneous and visceral components [1]. In adult humans, WAT is the predominant tissue type (Fig. 9.2), composed by spherical adipocytes containing a large unilocular lipid droplet, which releases fatty acids during intervals between meals (Fig. 9.3a). Its primary function is thus related to the organism's nutritional needs. Additionally, WAT secretes several hormones/cytokines which predominantly act on the brain, influencing behaviours necessary for food search and intake. The first and last, in chronological order of identification are leptin [2] and asprosin [3]. Leptin is the hormone that plays a crucial role in regulating energy balance and body weight at hypothalamic level. It is primarily secreted by white adipose tissue (WAT) cells, and its levels in the bloodstream is directly related to the amount of body fat. The more adipose tissue an individual has, the more leptin is produced from adipocytes. Leptin acts mainly on the hypothalamus in the brain, which is the centre for appetite and energy expenditure control. When leptin levels rise, it signals to the brain that the body has sufficient energy stores, leading to decreased appetite and increased energy expenditure. In contrast, lower leptin levels signal a state of energy deficit, which results in increased appetite and reduced energy expenditure. Leptin is an essential hormone in maintaining body weight and preventing obesity. In cases of leptin deficiency or leptin resistance, individuals may experience uncontrolled appetite, overeating and weight gain. Leptin also plays a role in various other physiological processes, such as fertility, immune function and bone metabolism [2].

S. Cinti (✉)
Centre of Obesity, Marche Polytechnic University, Ancona, Italy

P. Capodaglio (ed.), *Whole-Body Cryostimulation*,
https://doi.org/10.1007/978-3-031-18545-8_9

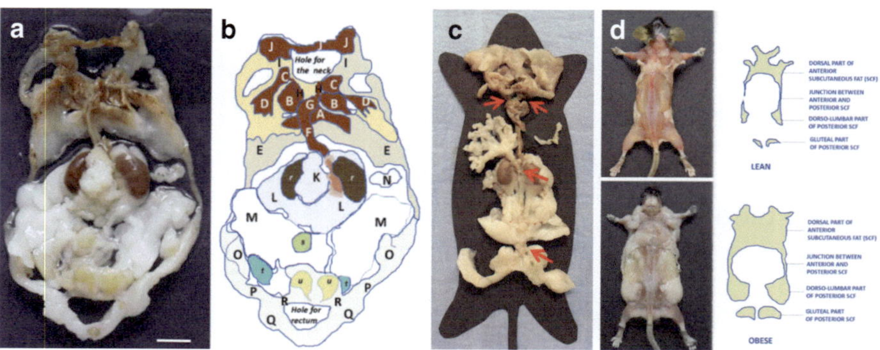

Fig. 9.1 (**a**) Anatomical preparation of the adipose organ (male C57BL/6 adult lean mouse). White (WAT) and brown (BAT) adipose tissues are recognizable by their specific colours. (**b**) Scheme legend: A: interscapular BAT (SC), B: subscapular BAT (SC), C: supraclavicular BAT (SC), D: axillary BAT (SC), E: axillo-thoracic WAT (SC), F and G: periaortic mediastinal BAT (V), H: SVC, I: cervical subcutaneous WAT (SC), J: cervical subcutaneous BAT (SC), K: mesenteric WAT (V), L: perirenal-retroperitoneal WAT-BAT (V), M: epididymal WAT (V), N: omental WAT (V), O: dorso-lumbar WAT (SC), P: inguinal WAT (SC), Q: gluteal WAT (SC). A + B + C + D + E + I + J: anterior subcutaneous part of adipose organ. O + P + Q: posterior subcutaneous part of the adipose organ. F + G + K + L + M + N: visceral part of the adipose organ. *r* kidney, *s* urinary bladder, *u* preputial glands, *SC* subcutaneous, *V* visceral. (**c**) Anatomical preparation of the adipose organ (female C57BL/6 adult lean mouse) as a unitary structure laying on a template. (**d**) Dorsal view of adult C57BL6 female mice after skin removal. Anterior and posterior subcutaneous parts of the adipose organ are visible in both lean (upper panel) and obese animals. Bar: 8 mm in **a** and **b**, 13 mm in **c** and 40 mm in **d** (*From: Giordano A* et al. *The Adipose Organ Is a Unitary Structure in Mice and Humans. Biomedicines. 2022 Sep 14;10(9):2275.* https://doi. org/10.3390/biomedicines10092275. *PMID: 36140375; PMCID: PMC9496043*)

Asprosin is the last recently discovered hormone primarily secreted by white adipose tissue (WAT) and plays a significant role in regulating glucose metabolism and appetite [3]. It was first identified in 2016 and has since garnered attention in the field of metabolic research. When asprosin levels increase, it stimulates the liver to release more glucose, leading to elevated blood glucose levels. This effect is particularly important during fasting periods when the body needs to maintain adequate blood glucose levels for energy production. Moreover, asprosin has been found to have an impact on appetite regulation. High levels of asprosin have been associated with increased feelings of hunger and enhanced food intake. The hormone acts on the hypothalamus in the brain, which is the central regulator of appetite and energy balance, to promote hunger and influence eating behaviours. Abnormal levels of asprosin have been linked to certain metabolic disorders, including insulin resistance and type 2 diabetes. It is important to note that asprosin is a relatively new area of study, and scientists continue to investigate its functions and potential implications for human health.

In contrast to WAT, BAT is composed of smaller multilocular adipocytes containing numerous characteristic mitochondria (Fig. 9.3b). Brown adipose tissue (BAT) mitochondria are specialized organelles found in brown adipocytes, unique compared to those found in other tissues due to their abundance and the presence of a

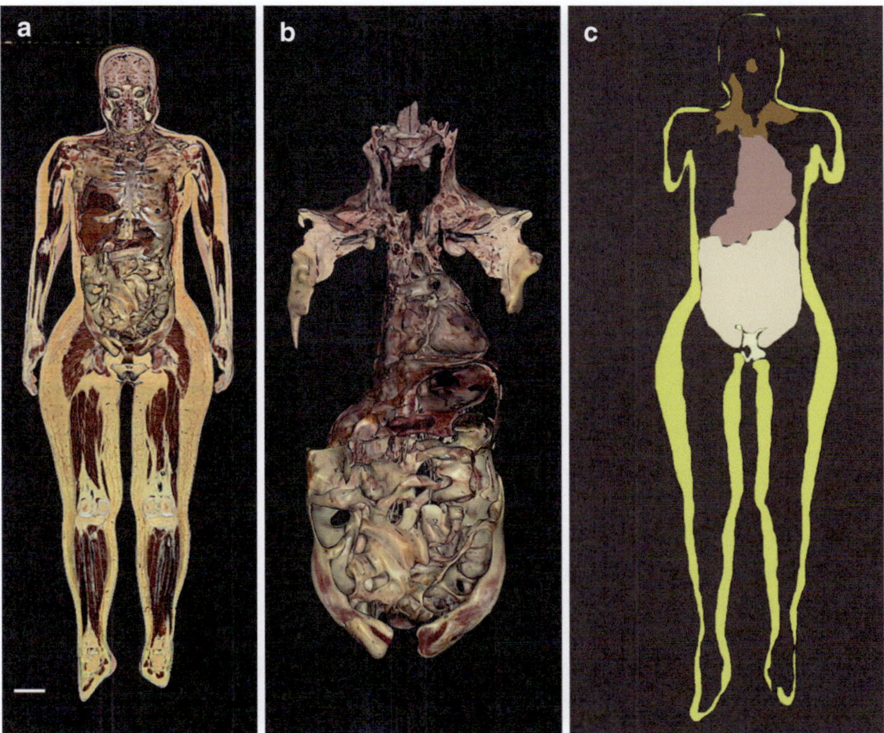

Fig. 9.2 Representative images showing the whole adipose organ in a coronal section of a virtual cadaver (left panel), the 3D reconstruction of isolated visceral fat in connection with the supraclavicular-axillary part of the adipose organ (middle panel), and the evidenced visceral (brown, beige and pale white) and subcutaneous (yellow) parts of the adipose organ (right panel). Bar: 65 mm in **a**, 35 mm in **b** and 75 mm in **c** (*From: Giordano A* et al. *The Adipose Organ Is a Unitary Structure in Mice and Humans. Biomedicines. 2022 Sep 14;10(9):2275.* https://doi.org/10.3390/biomedicines10092275. *PMID: 36140375; PMCID: PMC9496043*)

specific protein called uncoupling protein 1 (UCP1) [4]. The primary function of BAT mitochondria is to generate heat through a process called non-shivering thermogenesis. This process is crucial for maintaining body temperature, especially in response to cold exposure. The UCP1, which is located in the inner mitochondrial membrane and it is also known as thermogenin because it uncouples the process of electron transport chain and ATP synthesis from the mitochondrial respiration, causing the energy produced during cellular respiration to be dissipated as heat instead of being used to generate ATP (adenosine triphosphate). When the body is exposed to cold temperatures or when activated through other stimuli (such as certain hormones or factors), BAT is stimulated to release fatty acids stored in its cells. These fatty acids are transported to the mitochondria, where they undergo a process of thermogenesis. UCP1 facilitates the transport of protons across the inner mitochondrial membrane, creating a proton gradient and dissipating the energy as heat rather than storing it as ATP. This results in heat production, which helps to warm

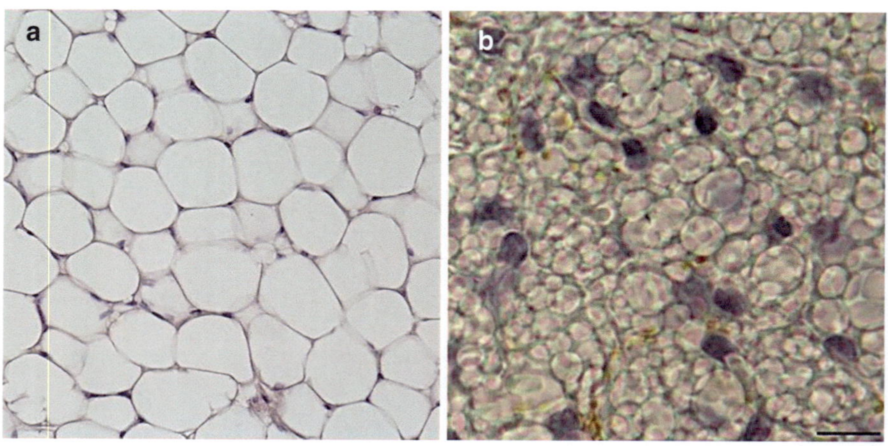

Fig. 9.3 Light microscopy of WAT (**a**) and BAT (**b**). Bar = 35 μm in **a** and 12 μm in **b**

the body. The BAT can be activated through different mechanisms, including exposure to cold temperatures (cold-induced thermogenesis), sympathetic nervous system activation and certain hormones (such as norepinephrine) [4]. The presence of abundant mitochondria with UCP1 in brown adipocytes is what gives brown adipose tissue its distinctive brown colour, hence the name 'brown adipose tissue'. The study of BAT and its mitochondria is of great interest in metabolic research and efforts to contrast obesity and related metabolic disorders.

Both WAT and BAT possess a fascinating property called trans-differentiation [5]. When exposed to chronic cold, WAT can undergo a transformation into BAT, thereby enhancing thermogenesis. This process allows the body to generate more heat to maintain its temperature in cold conditions dissipating energy. Conversely, under conditions of chronic positive energy balance, BAT can convert into WAT, increasing the adipose organ's capacity for storing energy. This adaptive response is essential as it prepares the body for potential fasting periods, during which stored energy becomes crucial for sustaining physiological functions.

Overall, the ability of WAT and BAT to transdifferentiate underscores the remarkable plasticity of adipose tissue in response to environmental and physiological cues, contributing to the body's ability to adapt to varying energy needs [5].

The Adipose Organ in Obesity

Obesity in mammals refers to a condition where an individual accumulates excessive body fat, leading to an increase in body weight beyond what is considered healthy or normal for their age, sex and height. Obesity is a complex and multifactorial condition that can arise from a combination of genetic, environmental, behavioural and physiological factors. Obesity is associated with a wide range of health risks and complications, including an increased risk of developing type 2 diabetes, cardiovascular diseases, certain cancers, joint problems and other chronic conditions.

The adipose organ in obesity primarily consists of white adipose tissue (WAT) expansion. In particular, white adipocytes undergo hypertrophy and hyperplasia. The hypertrophic state contributes to chronic low-grade inflammation, with infiltrating macrophages playing a crucial role [6, 7]. Hypertrophic adipocytes release chemo-attractants (particularly MCP1 and Hp), which attract macrophages to the adipose tissue. Additionally, adipocytes secrete the cytokine IL-1β, which triggers an autocrine mechanism resulting in the secretion of a protein called sFRP4. This protein negatively affects insulin secretion [8].

As adipocytes enlarge, they reach a critical death size (CDS), leading to the cell death. Visceral adipocytes tend to reach their CDS earlier than subcutaneous adipocytes due to their lower CDS [9, 10]. The 'debris' from dead adipocytes, primarily composed of residual lipids, needs to be cleared, and macrophages surround this debris, forming characteristic crown-like structures (CLS) [9]. However, the volume of macrophages is much smaller than the size of the lipid droplets they need to reabsorb, leading to chronic inflammation. During their activity, macrophages secrete various cytokines (TNFα, IL-6, iNOS) and other factors (resistin, adipsin, RBP4, several miRNAs), which have secondary effects [6, 7, 11–14]. These effects include interference with insulin receptor activity, leading to insulin resistance [14]. Insulin resistance results in hyperproduction of insulin, but its effect is blocked by an increased density of noradrenergic fibres in the Langerhans islets, leading to inhibition of insulin secretion [15–17]. As a consequence, obesity is closely linked to the development of type 2 diabetes. Furthermore, the lower CDS of visceral adipocytes and the consequent higher density of CLS inflammation explain the well-known fact that visceral obesity is associated with worse clinical consequences than subcutaneous obesity [18]. Overall, these interconnected processes in the obese adipose organ provide insights into the complex relationship between obesity and type 2 diabetes, shedding light on the mechanisms underlying their close association.

The hyperplasia refers to an increase in the number of fat cells number within the body's adipose tissue. In the context of obesity, it is one of the physiological mechanisms that contribute to the excessive accumulation of body fat. Initially, adipocytes can expand to accommodate this extra energy (hypertrophy); however, when the capacity of individual fat cells is reached, the body starts creating new adipocytes through a process called hyperplasia. As for the hypertrophy, the hyperplasia of adipocytes is an adaptive response of the body to an excess of calories and energy storage. However, the continuous expansion of adipose tissue can lead to ectopic fat deposition. Ectopic fat deposition in obesity refers to the abnormal accumulation of fat in tissues and organs other than adipose tissue, like the liver, skeletal muscles, heart and pancreas. This ectopic fat accumulation can have significant health implications and contribute to metabolic dysfunction. Non-alcoholic fatty liver disease (NAFLD) is a condition characterized by the accumulation of fat in the liver cells. In obesity, the liver can become overwhelmed with excess fat, leading to NAFLD, which can progress to more severe conditions like non-alcoholic steatohepatitis (NASH) and liver fibrosis. Obesity can lead to increased fat accumulation in skeletal muscles. This intramuscular fat, also known as intramyocellular lipid (IMCL), can impair muscle insulin sensitivity and contribute to insulin resistance, a hallmark of type 2 diabetes. Ectopic fat deposition in the myocardium (heart muscle) is associated with obesity and can contribute to cardiovascular disease risk and fat accumulation in the pancreas may impair its ability to produce insulin, further contributing to deterioration of the insulin-secreting capacity and islet inflammation, contributing to insulin resistance and type 2 diabetes onset. The degree of liver fat accumulation showed strong correlations with obesity-related parameters, while the degree of pancreatic fat accumulation was weakly or not associated with these parameters. These results suggest that pancreatic fat accumulation has a different aetiology from liver fat accumulation.

The presence of ectopic fat can disrupt the normal functioning of these organs and tissues, leading to various metabolic abnormalities. For example, insulin resistance in skeletal muscles and the liver can result in impaired glucose regulation, while ectopic fat in the heart can affect cardiac function and increase the risk of heart disease.

Importantly not all the individuals living with obesity develop ectopic fat deposition, and the distribution of fat storage can vary among individuals based on genetic and lifestyle factors. However, the presence of ectopic fat is associated with an increased risk of metabolic syndrome, type 2 diabetes, cardiovascular disease and other obesity-related health complications.

Therapeutic Perspectives of Cold-Induced Adipocyte Transdifferentiation

The transdifferentiation property of the adipose organ offers a promising therapeutic strategy: browning of the obese adipose tissue [1]. The most natural and physiologic approach to induce WAT-BAT conversion is through chronic cold exposure. Recent studies have demonstrated that individuals living in cold-exposed regions tend to have larger amounts of BAT, even in areas of the adipose organ is typically composed of WAT [19, 20]. Additionally, research has explored the potential of β3 adrenoceptor agonists in curbing obesity and type 2 diabetes in small mammals [21–23]. In this context, new β3 agonists, such as mirabegron, have been developed. An experimental study administering a single oral dose of mirabegron (200 mg) to 12 young lean volunteers showed BAT activation similar to that achieved through a cold exposure test (2 h at 14 °C) as evidenced by significant glucose uptake during PET analyses [24]. Further investigations involving chronic administration of mirabegron in 14 healthy women with a BMI of 25.4 kg/m^2, using a daily dose of 100 mg for 4 weeks, demonstrated increased BAT activity, metabolism, beneficial lipoprotein biomarkers and improved insulin secretion and sensitivity. Importantly, these positive effects were observed without any changes in body weight or composition [25]. These findings suggest that browning the adipose organ using β3 agonists like mirabegron may hold promise as a therapeutic approach for obesity and type 2 diabetes. Such strategies aim to increase thermogenesis and metabolic activity in adipose tissue, potentially improving metabolic health without the need for weight loss.

Cold stimulus has shown potential applications in the management and treatment of obesity and diabetes. Cold exposure has been shown to influence appetite-regulating hormones such as leptin and ghrelin, which may help reduce food intake and promote weight loss in obese individuals. Controlling appetite is crucial for managing obesity and preventing excessive calorie consumption [26]. Cold exposure has been associated with reduced inflammation, which is often elevated in obesity and diabetes. By reducing inflammation, cold stimulus may help alleviate some of the complications associated with these conditions.

Whole-body cryotherapy (WBC), which involves exposing the body to extremely cold temperatures, has gained popularity as a potential therapy for obesity and diabetes. In 37 menopausal women exposed to 20 WBC sessions (-130 °C, 3 min each), a significant decrease in glucose concentration was reported and the changes in asprosin circulating concentration positively correlated with changes in glucose concentration. Asprosin concentration before WBC correlated positively with metabolic disorder risk factor levels, and the change in asprosin concentration after 20 WBC correlated negatively with metabolic disorder risk factor levels: fasting glucose, AIP, and the leptin/adiponectin index. While more research is needed, this kind of study suggests that WBC may positively impact metabolism and insulin sensitivity [27].

Conclusion

In conclusion, the potential benefits of chronic cold exposure or treatments simulating such exposure are significant in the context of contrasting obesity and type 2 diabetes. By inducing WAT-BAT trans-differentiation and activating BAT, these approaches hold promise as perspective therapies for addressing these prevalent health conditions. Embracing the concept of using cold to harness the body's natural mechanisms might pave the way for innovative and effective treatments for obesity and type 2 diabetes. Further research in this area is essential to fully understand and maximize the therapeutic potential of these approaches.

References

1. Cinti S. Adipose organ development and remodeling. Compr Physiol. 2018;8(4):1357–431. https://doi.org/10.1002/cphy.c170042. PMID: 30215863.
2. Friedman JM. Leptin and the endocrine control of energy balance. Nat Metab. 2019;1(8):754–64. https://doi.org/10.1038/s42255-019-0095-y.
3. Romere C, Duerrschmid C, Bournat J, Constable P, Jain M, Xia F, Saha PK, Del Solar M, Zhu B, York B, Sarkar P, Rendon DA, Gaber MW, LeMaire SA, Coselli JS, Milewicz DM, Sutton VR, Butte NF, Moore DD, Chopra AR. Asprosin, a fasting-induced glucogenic protein hor-

mone. Cell. 2016;165(3):566–79. https://doi.org/10.1016/j.cell.2016.02.063. Epub 2016 Apr 14. PMID: 27087445; PMCID: PMC4852710.

4. Cannon B, Nedergaard J. Brown adipose tissue: function and physiological significance. Physiol Rev. 2004;84(1):277–359. https://doi.org/10.1152/physrev.00015.2003. PMID: 14715917.

5. Cinti S. Adipocyte differentiation and transdifferentiation: plasticity of the adipose organ. J Endocrinol Invest. 2002;25(10):823–35. https://doi.org/10.1007/BF03344046. PMID: 12508945.

6. Xu H, Barnes GT, Yang Q, Tan G, Yang D, Chou CJ, Sole J, Nichols A, Ross JS, Tartaglia LA, Chen H. Chronic inflammation in fat plays a crucial role in the development of obesity-related insulin resistance. J Clin Invest. 2003;112(12):1821–30. https://doi.org/10.1172/JCI19451. PMID: 14679177; PMCID: PMC296998.

7. Weisberg SP, McCann D, Desai M, Rosenbaum M, Leibel RL, Ferrante AW Jr. Obesity is associated with macrophage accumulation in adipose tissue. J Clin Invest. 2003;112(12):1796–808. https://doi.org/10.1172/JCI19246. PMID: 14679176; PMCID: PMC296995.

8. Mahdi T, Hänzelmann S, Salehi A, Muhammed SJ, Reinbothe TM, Tang Y, Axelsson AS, Zhou Y, Jing X, Almgren P, Krus U, Taneera J, Blom AM, Lyssenko V, Esguerra JL, Hansson O, Eliasson L, Derry J, Zhang E, Wollheim CB, Groop L, Renström E, Rosengren AH. Secreted frizzled-related protein 4 reduces insulin secretion and is overexpressed in type 2 diabetes. Cell Metab. 2012;16(5):625–33. https://doi.org/10.1016/j.cmet.2012.10.009. PMID: 23140642.

9. Cinti S, Mitchell G, Barbatelli G, Murano I, Ceresi E, Faloia E, Wang S, Fortier M, Greenberg AS, Obin MS. Adipocyte death defines macrophage localization and function in adipose tissue of obese mice and humans. J Lipid Res. 2005;46(11):2347–55. https://doi.org/10.1194/jlr. M500294-JLR200. Epub 2005 Sep 8. PMID: 16150820.

10. Murano I, Barbatelli G, Parisani V, Latini C, Muzzonigro G, Castellucci M, Cinti S. Dead adipocytes, detected as crown-like structures, are prevalent in visceral fat depots of genetically obese mice. J Lipid Res. 2008;49(7):1562–8. https://doi.org/10.1194/jlr.M800019-JLR200. Epub 2008 Apr 3. PMID: 18390487.

11. Camastra S, Vitali A, Anselmino M, Gastaldelli A, Bellini R, Berta R, Severi I, Baldi S, Astiarraga B, Barbatelli G, Cinti S, Ferrannini E. Muscle and adipose tissue morphology, insulin sensitivity and beta-cell function in diabetic and nondiabetic obese patients: effects of bariatric surgery. Sci Rep. 2017;7(1):9007. https://doi.org/10.1038/s41598-017-08444-6. Erratum in: Sci Rep. 2018 May 22;8(1):8177. PMID: 28827671; PMCID: PMC5566429.

12. Mori MA, Raghavan P, Thomou T, Boucher J, Robida-Stubbs S, Macotela Y, Russell SJ, Kirkland JL, Blackwell TK, Kahn CR. Role of microRNA processing in adipose tissue in stress defense and longevity. Cell Metab. 2012;16(3):336–47. https://doi.org/10.1016/j. cmet.2012.07.017. PMID: 22958919; PMCID: PMC3461823.

13. Mori MA, Ludwig RG, Garcia-Martin R, Brandão BB, Kahn CR. Extracellular miRNAs: from biomarkers to mediators of physiology and disease. Cell Metab. 2019;30(4):656–73. https://doi.org/10.1016/j.cmet.2019.07.011. Epub 2019 Aug 22. PMID: 31447320; PMCID: PMC6774861.

14. Hotamisligil GS. Inflammation, metaflammation and immunometabolic disorders. Nature. 2017;542(7640):177–85. https://doi.org/10.1038/nature21363. PMID: 28179656.

15. Giannulis I, Mondini E, Cinti F, Frontini A, Murano I, Barazzoni R, Barbatelli G, Accili D, Cinti S. Increased density of inhibitory noradrenergic parenchymal nerve fibers in hypertrophic islets of Langerhans of obese mice. Nutr Metab Cardiovasc Dis. 2014;24(4):384–92. https://doi.org/10.1016/j.numecd.2013.09.006. Epub 2013 Oct 23. PMID: 24462047; PMCID: PMC4082304.

16. Cinti F, Bouchi R, Kim-Muller JY, Ohmura Y, Sandoval PR, Masini M, Marselli L, Suleiman M, Ratner LE, Marchetti P, Accili D. Evidence of β-cell dedifferentiation in human type 2 diabetes. J Clin Endocrinol Metab. 2016;101(3):1044–54. https://doi.org/10.1210/jc.2015-2860. Epub 2015 Dec 29. PMID: 26713822; PMCID: PMC4803182.

17. Cinti F, Mezza T, Severi I, Suleiman M, Cefalo CMA, Sorice GP, Moffa S, Impronta F, Quero G, Alfieri S, Mari A, Pontecorvi A, Marselli L, Cinti S, Marchetti P, Giaccari A. Noradrenergic

fibers are associated with beta-cell dedifferentiation and impaired beta-cell function in humans. Metabolism. 2021;114:154414. https://doi.org/10.1016/j.metabol.2020.154414. Epub 2020 Oct 28. PMID: 33129839.

18. Björntorp P, Rosmond R. Visceral obesity and diabetes. Drugs. 1999;58(Suppl 1):13–8; discussion 75–82. PMID: 10576519. https://doi.org/10.2165/00003495-199958001-00005.

19. Jespersen NZ, Feizi A, Andersen ES, Heywood S, Hattel HB, Daugaard S, Peijs L, Bagi P, Feldt-Rasmussen B, Schultz HS, Hansen NS, Krogh-Madsen R, Pedersen BK, Petrovic N, Nielsen S, Scheele C. Heterogeneity in the perirenal region of humans suggests presence of dormant brown adipose tissue that contains brown fat precursor cells. Mol Metab. 2019;24:30–43. https://doi.org/10.1016/j.molmet.2019.03.005. Epub 2019 Mar 15. PMID: 31079959; PMCID: PMC6531810.

20. Efremova A, Senzacqua M, Venema W, Isakov E, Di Vincenzo A, Zingaretti MC, Protasoni M, Thomski M, Giordano A, Cinti S. A large proportion of mediastinal and perirenal visceral fat of Siberian adult people is formed by UCP1 immunoreactive multilocular and paucilocular adipocytes. J Physiol Biochem. 2020;76(2):185–92. https://doi.org/10.1007/s13105-019-00721-4. Epub 2019 Dec 18. PMID: 31853729.

21. De Matteis R, Arch JR, Petroni ML, Ferrari D, Cinti S, Stock MJ. Immunohistochemical identification of the beta(3)-adrenoceptor in intact human adipocytes and ventricular myocardium: effect of obesity and treatment with ephedrine and caffeine. Int J Obes Relat Metab Disord. 2002;26(11):1442–50. https://doi.org/10.1038/sj.ijo.0802148. PMID: 12439645.

22. Ghorbani M, Himms-Hagen J. Appearance of brown adipocytes in white adipose tissue during CL 316,243-induced reversal of obesity and diabetes in Zucker fa/fa rats. Int J Obes Relat Metab Disord. 1997;21(6):465–75. https://doi.org/10.1038/sj.ijo.0800432. PMID: 9192230.

23. Fisher MH, Amend AM, Bach TJ, Barker JM, Brady EJ, Candelore MR, Carroll D, Cascieri MA, Chiu SH, Deng L, Forrest MJ, Hegarty-Friscino B, Guan XM, Hom GJ, Hutchins JE, Kelly LJ, Mathvink RJ, Metzger JM, Miller RR, Ok HO, Parmee ER, Saperstein R, Strader CD, Stearns RA, MacIntyre DE, et al. A selective human beta3 adrenergic receptor agonist increases metabolic rate in rhesus monkeys. J Clin Invest. 1998;101(11):2387–93. https://doi.org/10.1172/JCI2496. PMID: 9616210; PMCID: PMC508828.

24. Cypess AM, Weiner LS, Roberts-Toler C, Franquet Elía E, Kessler SH, Kahn PA, English J, Chatman K, Trauger SA, Doria A, Kolodny GM. Activation of human brown adipose tissue by a β3-adrenergic receptor agonist. Cell Metab. 2015;21(1):33–8. https://doi.org/10.1016/j.cmet.2014.12.009. PMID: 25565203; PMCID: PMC4298351.

25. O'Mara AE, Johnson JW, Linderman JD, Brychta RJ, McGehee S, Fletcher LA, Fink YA, Kapuria D, Cassimatis TM, Kelsey N, Cero C, Sater ZA, Piccinini F, Baskin AS, Leitner BP, Cai H, Millo CM, Dieckmann W, Walter M, Javitt NB, Rotman Y, Walter PJ, Ader M, Bergman RN, Herscovitch P, Chen KY, Cypess AM. Chronic mirabegron treatment increases human brown fat, HDL cholesterol, and insulin sensitivity. J Clin Invest. 2020;130(5):2209–19. https://doi.org/10.1172/JCI131126. PMID: 31961826; PMCID: PMC7190915.

26. Ivanova YM, Blondin DP. Examining the benefits of cold exposure as a therapeutic strategy for obesity and type 2 diabetes. J Appl Physiol (1985). 2021;130(5):1448–59. https://doi.org/10.1152/japplphysiol.00934.2020.

27. Wiecek M, Szymura J, Sproull J, Szygula Z. Decreased blood Asprosin in hyperglycemic menopausal women as a result of whole-body cryotherapy regardless of metabolic syndrome. J Clin Med. 2019;8(9):1428. https://doi.org/10.3390/jcm8091428. PMID: 31510055; PMCID: PMC6780623.

Part II

Applications in Clinical Conditions

Fibromyalgia

Federica Verme, Paolo Piterà, Jacopo Maria Fontana,
Giorgia Varallo, Alessandra Scarpa, Stefania Cattaldo,
Stefania Mai, and Paolo Capodaglio

Fibromyalgia: Overview and Clinical Manifestations

Fibromyalgia (FM) is a medical debilitating condition characterised by chronic widespread musculoskeletal pain [1]. Severe fatigue, morning stiffness, sleep disturbances (including insomnia, frequent awakenings and non-restorative sleep),

F. Verme (✉) · P. Piterà · J. M. Fontana
Research Laboratory in Biomechanics, Rehabilitation and Ergonomics, IRCCS Istituto
Auxologico Italiano, Piancavallo (Verbania), Italy
e-mail: f.verme@auxologico.it; p.pitera@auxologico.it; j.fontana@auxologico.it

G. Varallo
Department of Medicine and Surgery, University of Parma, Parma, Italy
e-mail: giorgia.varallo@unipr.it

A. Scarpa
Psychology Research Laboratory, IRCCS Istituto Auxologico Italiano, Milan, Italy
e-mail: a.scarpa@auxologico.it

S. Cattaldo
Laboratory of Clinical Neurobiology, IRCCS Istituto Auxologico Italiano,
Piancavallo (Verbania), Italy
e-mail: s.cattaldo@auxologico.it

S. Mai
Laboratory of Metabolic Research, IRCCS Istituto Auxologico Italiano,
Piancavallo (Verbania), Italy
e-mail: s.mai@auxologico.it

P. Capodaglio
Research Laboratory in Biomechanics, Rehabilitation and Ergonomics, IRCCS Istituto
Auxologico Italiano, Piancavallo (Verbania), Italy

Physical Medicine and Rehabilitation, Department of Surgical Sciences, University of Torino,
Torino, Italy
e-mail: p.capodaglio@auxologico.it; paolo.capodaglio@unito.it

P. Capodaglio (ed.), *Whole-Body Cryostimulation*,
https://doi.org/10.1007/978-3-031-18545-8_10

autonomic disturbances, hypersensitivity to external stimuli, memory deficits and psychological and cognitive symptoms may also be present, reducing people's quality of life and limiting social, occupational and recreational activities [2–4].

Pain is the main symptom characterising this condition: patients often describe it as neuropathic pain, and its type, location and severity depend on certain modulating factors, such as work activities, comorbidities, temperature variations, physical and mental stress [2, 3]. In addition, patients with FM often report depressive symptomatology [4, 5], which could be ascribed to chronic pain and its related limitations [6, 7].

In some studies, patients with FM reported lower threshold and tolerance for pain [8, 9], hyperalgesia and allodynia [10], a slower cognitive processing speed [11], a cortical or subcortical increase in pain processing compared with healthy subjects [12] and evidence of the presence of polyneuropathy in both small and large fibres [13]. Emerging evidence on FM suggests a neurogenic common origin characterised by increased activation in brain areas dedicated to pain, altered connectivity and reduced brain activity. Moreover, hypotheses on the pathogenesis of FM include central sensitisation to pain and impairments of endogenous pain-inhibiting mechanisms [2].

In terms of prevalence, FM is the third most common musculoskeletal condition, affecting about 0.2 and 6.6% of people worldwide and being more common in women aged 20–55 years old [2, 14–17]. Due to the associated comorbidities and access to healthcare, it represents a major economic burden on society [18]. A number of predisposing factors are known, including genetic, stressful or traumatic events, viral infections and obesity, but the aetiology of FM and the underlying cause of FM-related alterations are not fully unravelled.

Given the lack of biomarkers, FM diagnosis is exclusively clinical [2], although the results of a recently published study show that a subset of fibromyalgia patients have elevated levels of anti-satellite glia cell immunoglobulin G antibodies, and these antibodies are related to more severe FM symptoms [19]. The classification and diagnostic criteria of FM are currently based on the 2016 revisions to the 2010/2011 American College of Rheumatology (ACR) diagnostic criteria [20] and on the ACTTION-APS Pain Taxonomy diagnostic criteria [21].

FM requires a multidisciplinary therapeutic approach including pharmacological treatments and non-pharmacological measures [2, 22]. The very first step in managing patients with FM is educating them in understanding their illness before they are prescribed any medications and encouraging them to exercise regularly, follow a balanced diet and to develop their own techniques and approaches to improve their quality of life [2]. There is no gold standard pharmacological treatment; therefore, a combination of drugs, usually antidepressants, anticonvulsants, anti-inflammatories and antioxidants, can be employed [2, 23, 24]. Non-pharmacological treatment measures include physiotherapy, aerobic and anaerobic training, and psychotherapy, including cognitive-behavioural interventions, biofeedback and psychological support [2, 25, 26].

Whole-Body Cryostimulation

The physiological effects of whole-body cryostimulation (WBC) exposure have been extensively discussed in previous chapters. Due to its anti-inflammatory, antioxidant, analgesic and exercise-mimicking effects [27, 28], WBC is known to be effective in reducing pain and inflammatory status, improving several metabolic mechanisms such as thermogenesis, lipid profile, insulin sensitivity and glucose utilisation [15, 29], but also depression, anxiety [30] and sleep quality [31]. Cycles of WBC have been shown to reduce fatigue, disease activity and pain in patients with rheumatic (rheumatoid arthritis [32], ankylosing spondylitis [33] and polymyalgia rheumatica [34]), metabolic [29, 35] and neurological conditions [36], and post-COVID-19 condition [37, 38]. Inflammation is also a mediating pathway to neuroprogression in depression [39], being co-morbid depression very common among FM patients, with a lifetime prevalence of 62–86% [40, 41]. For all those reasons, WBC has been proposed as a promising adjunct treatment for FM due to its effects on the main FM symptoms [15]. The following paragraphs provide a detailed analysis and explanation of how the WBC acts on these specific aspects of FM.

Clinical Effects

Chronic pain is the most common symptom associated with FM, greatly affecting patients' quality of life. Pain is a complex phenomenon, being pain perception influenced by genetic, environmental, societal, physiological and psychological factors [15, 42]. Two neural pathways are involved in pain transmission: ascending pathways carry sensory information, including nociceptive signals, through peripheral nerves towards the spinal cord and brain for processing, whereas the nerves going down from the brain to the periphery via the spinal cord comprise the descending pathways, sending modulatory (excitatory and/or inhibitory) signals to the reflex organs. These physical and noxious chemical signals are detected by nociceptors, specialised peripheral sensory neurons activated by thermal, mechanical and chemical stimuli [15, 42].

As mentioned above, FM is considered a central sensitivity syndrome [43]. In FM, ascending and descending pathways regulating pain signals operate abnormally causing central sensitisation, which is a mechanism of neuronal signal amplification within the central nervous system that leads to increased pain perception [44, 45]. For this reason, patients with FM present a lower pain threshold that leads to widespread hyperalgesia and allodynia, conditions that have been confirmed in clinical studies using functional neuroimaging or measuring alterations in neurotransmitter levels that influence sensory transmission and pain [43, 46–48].

A recent study by Varallo et al. [7] showed that the implementation of ten sessions of WBC over 2 weeks to patients with FM and obesity produced additional benefits in terms of pain, depressive symptoms, disease impact and sleep quality.

Most of the studies included in Fontana et al. scoping review [15] hypothesised that WBC could be effective in relieving pain and/or inflammatory processes in FM patients, with the aim of managing the disease's main symptoms and thus improving health-related quality of life. These studies tested the effectiveness of WBC as a therapeutic tool and its practicability for clinical routine in FM.

All studies considered the effect of WBC on pain relief. Bettoni et al. carried out two studies on the efficacy and safety of WBC in FM patients showing the superiority of WBC compared with the use of antioxidant and analgesic agents alone on pain, fatigue reduction [49] and quality of life, compared with subjects with FM not treated with WBC [17]. However, physical activity, also used to treat FM, may have masked these results by opposing the vasodilation induced by it to the vasoconstriction induced by WBC. In the randomised cross-over trial of Rivera et al., the individuals' Visual Analogue Scale (VAS) and Fibromyalgia Impact Questionnaire (FIQ) scores did not return to baseline after the first treatment with WBC due to too short wash-out periods, so that only results of the first sequence could be reported [50]. The results of the first period showed a significant effect of WBC on pain (VAS) and disease impact (FIQ score). Vitenet et al. reported that WBC (10 sessions over 8 days) significantly improved health-reported quality of life [51], although the sample size was limited, including only 11 patients undergoing WBC.

The study of Metzger et al. reported a decreased pain intensity and a short-term pain relief of about 90 minutes after cold application [52], but did not include a control group receiving a regular rehabilitation programme. Therefore, the reduction in pain could be due not only to the analgesic effect of WBC, but also to the parallel effect of rehabilitation. However, they described some adjustment time before reaching maximum pain relief, in their case after about 2 weeks (half of the treatment). Interestingly, most patients rated the effect of WBC as not very effective in the context of the overall treatment, perhaps also due to the session conditions (temperature -105 °C and 2–3 patients in the room).

A prospective controlled study by Klemm et al. included patients on stable pharmacological and nonpharmacological treatment before and during the study, excluding physical activity as a possible confounder of the reduced level of pain found after WBC treatment, but there was no control group not on WBC treatment [53].

WBC and other conventional thermotherapy techniques were compared in two studies for effectiveness. Kurzeja et al. [54] investigated the effect of thermotherapy with WBC (-110 °C) alone compared with mud bath ($+40$ °C) and hot air ($+42$ °C) combined in the daily shift. In both therapy groups, pain intensity was substantially reduced, with no significant differences between groups. However, pain scores in the WBC group were lower, and patients reported pain relief for 2–3 h after cold exposure. WBC may also provide better results in combination with physiotherapy than with steam therapy in terms of pain, fatigue and sleep problems. The improvement in these symptoms could be attributed to the systemic response and serotonin levels stimulated by WBC, although these results are not complete due to the lack of information on the temperature used, the inhomogeneous population in terms of age and sex, and the lack of data confirming the results and conclusions [55].

Duration of Effects

The duration of the effects of WBC was insufficiently evaluated, as only two groups performed follow-up investigations. Vitenet et al. [51] performed 10 WBC sessions on 24 FM patients in addition to usual care over a duration of 8 days and observed that the positive effects assessed by the physical and mental composite scores of SF-36 lasted for at least 1 month following intervention. Klemm et al. [53] showed that 3 months after discontinued treatment the effects of WBC on pain and disease activity were no longer reduced. Specifically, they demonstrated that serial WBC (between 6 and 10 sessions in a maximum of 3 weeks) elicited effects for more than 1 month after the end of WBC treatment, then decreasing gradually to null effect after 3 months.

To ascertain the duration of clinical-functional benefits after a WBC cycle (10 treatments), our group (Verme et al., unpublished data) carried out 10-min follow-up telephone interviews, which included six sections aimed at investigating patients' well-being status, use of pain/anti-inflammatory medications, pain level, fatigue, sleep quality and psychological aspects (mood, anxiety, and depression). Nineteen patients (n = 19) with FM and obesity successfully completed the telephone interview. 18 out of 19 (95%) patients reported having felt better after completing their 10 treatments, and that these benefits lasted over time (4 months on average). Almost all patients ($n = 18$) were taking pain medications or anti-inflammatory drugs before undergoing cryostimulation, and 10 out of 18 patients (55%) reported reducing or discontinuing the use of these drugs for an average of 5 months after completing the treatments. In addition, 18 patients (95%) reported improvement on the numeric pain rating scale (NPRS) score after completing the 10 treatments, with an average score of 4.19 on the NPRS post-WBC, compared to the recorded mean score of 8.33 pre-WBC ($p = 0.000$), which lasted an average of 4 months. Most patients ($n = 17$, 89%) noted increased energy and decreased fatigue in performing daily life activities, even for 3–4 months after treatment discontinuation. Among the patients we interviewed, 14 reported having poor sleep quality before starting WBC. 10 out of 14 patients (71%) improved their sleep quality, particularly decreased night wakings and claimed waking up more rested, with positive effects lasting for 4 months on average. Lastly, the effects of WBC on mood and anxiety were investigated: 11 patients (58%) reported having felt better in terms of mood and anxiety episodes after WBC until the widespread pain recurred, which was usually after 4 months.

These preliminary data suggest a positive effect of a WBC cycle on pain, fatigue, sleep quality, state of well-being and psychological aspects (mood and anxiety), with an average duration of effects of 4 months after the intervention, making WBC also a promising tool for long-term management of fibromyalgia symptoms. However, it must be considered that patients referred to our facility underwent a multidisciplinary rehabilitation programme that included nutritional interventions, physiotherapy and physical activity, making it difficult to estimate the extent to which WBC actually contributed to symptom management. Future research will aim to implement follow-up interviews to assess the long-term effects of WBC and to include control groups in research protocols.

Molecular Effects

Besides pain sensitivity, pain inhibition or pain amplification, FM pathogenesis is also the result of an imbalance between pro- and anti-inflammatory cytokines, genetic predisposition and triggering environmental factors, such as mechanical/physical trauma or injury and psychosocial stressors which ultimately lead to pain and impaired pain processing [15].

The role of neurological inflammation in FM is increasingly recognised, as there is growing evidence that in fibromyalgia inflammatory mechanisms of neurogenic origin occur in the peripheral tissues, spinal cord and brain, involving a variety of neuropeptides, chemokines and cytokines and the activation of both the innate and adaptive immune systems [56]. In a review by O'Mahony et al., significant differences were found in the peripheral blood cytokine profiles of FM patients compared with healthy controls, even though the profile of FM patients includes pro-inflammatory (TNF-α, IL-6 and IL-8), anti-inflammatory cytokines (IL-10) and also chemokine (eotaxin) signatures [57].

A number of neuropeptides involved in neuroinflammation and various pro-inflammatory cytokines, such as IL-1β, IL-6, IL-8 and tumour necrosis factor α (TNF-α), have been found to be elevated in animal models of neuropathic pain and in the cerebrospinal fluid (CSF), peripheral tissues and blood of patients with chronic neuropathic pain conditions, including FM. Furthermore, pharmacologically decreasing or inhibiting these pro-inflammatory cytokines can prevent, reduce or reverse pain (allodynia and hyperalgesia), as demonstrated in both animal models and clinical studies [43, 56, 58].

The induction and maintenance of pain as well as the occurrence of many clinical features of FM (such as swelling, dysesthesia, skin manifestations, fluid retention and increased levels of fibronectin, which is a tissue marker of endothelial activation) are therefore thought to be influenced by an imbalance of pro- and anti-inflammatory cytokines as a result of a neuroinflammatory condition generating descending pathways that affect predominant FM symptoms, such as pain, fatigue and cognitive impairment. Moreover, environmental triggers and the physiological mechanisms related to stress and emotions are the upstream driving mechanism of neurogenic inflammation in FM [15, 43, 56]. In fact, it has been established that FM may have an imbalance in cytokine production and secretion. A systematic review with meta-analysis by Uçeyler et al. showed that FM patients have higher serum levels of IL-1 receptor antagonist, IL-6 and IL-8, and higher plasma levels of IL-8, compared to controls [59], while two studies of Lubkowska et al. showed how WBC affects the inflammatory status by inducing an imbalance towards the anti-inflammatory side, as shown by an increase in levels of IL-6 (which can act both as a pro-inflammatory and anti-inflammatory cytokine) and IL-10, an anti-inflammatory cytokine, after consecutive sessions of cryotherapy [60, 61]. Furthermore, WBC seems to improve the oxidative status in a dose-dependent way already after a limited number of sessions [62, 63]. The clinical and molecular effects of WBC were combined in the study by Klemm et al. [53] in which a significant reduction in pain and disease activity was observed after serial sessions of WBC. In this study, patients with FM had significantly different levels of IL-1, IL-6, TNF-α and IL-10 at each reading point and showed a significantly different response compared with healthy controls in terms of changes in IL-1, -6, and -10 over time to WBCs. In particular, FM patients had higher levels of IL-1, -6, -10 and TNF-α at baseline than healthy subjects. After three and six sessions, the levels of IL-1, IL-6 and IL-10 decreased significantly and stabilised up to 3 months after stopping WBC treatment. TNF-α levels of FM patients and healthy controls were not affected by WBC. Therefore, although the levels of IL-1, IL-6 and IL-10 in FM patients were higher than in healthy controls after 6 sessions of WBC and 3 months after the last session of WBC, their significant long-term alteration confirms the overall beneficial effects of WBC [15].

Gene Expression

Gene expression was also poorly covered, as only one group provided a couple of studies in the form of abstracts. The first study [64] analysed changes in gene expression in peripheral blood cells of FM patients subjected to a series of three exposures to WBC over 3 days, correlating the reduction in pain intensity with transcripts that were found to be significantly changed already after a single exposure to WBC. Most of the down-regulated transcripts belonged to a group of noncoding RNAs (small nucleolar RNA, SNORD), while the up-regulated transcripts were a few specific genes (PBX1, SFRP2, MAP2K3 and SLC25A39) involved in various physiological and pathological cellular processes that act as internal signals controlling various levels of gene expression. However, the sample size and homogeneity were rather limited, as only 10 patients were studied. Another study by the same group examined changes in gene expression of specific genes (CCL4, TGFBR3, CD69 and MAP2K3) identified as significantly regulated in the peripheral blood cells of 22 patients with FM who underwent a series of three exposures to WBC over 3 days [65]. The expression levels of two proteins produced by T-lymphocyte activation, CCL4 and CD69, were significantly reduced after the third exposure from baseline. In contrast, the expression of MAP2K3, a protein activated by cytokines and environmental stress in vivo, was increased in 13 patients, while expression levels in the other 9 patients remained almost unchanged. Interestingly, the changes in gene expression were found to be statistically significant after the third cold exposure, although they were already evident after the first cold exposure. The down-regulation of the membrane proteoglycan TGFBR3 (that can also function as a co-receptor with other TGF-β receptors) observed in the pilot study could not be confirmed in the larger cohort. Unfortunately, both studies do not provide further speculation or discussion of the results [15].

Conclusive Remarks

This chapter summarises the current understanding of the role of WBC as an adjuvant treatment for FM. We are aware of the following limitations:

1. The molecular mechanisms and regulation of gene expression underlying the reported positive effects of WBC have not been fully reviewed, since only changes in a few inflammatory markers and genes have been observed.
2. The inconsistency of the reported results could be attributed to the lack of standardised protocols for the use of WBC in the treatment of FM (in terms of temperature, number of sessions, exposure time and sample collection time). In this regard, many of the studies we reviewed included confounding factors such as physical activity and pharmacological treatment, which are crucial in the modulation of a number of pain-related parameters (such as anti-inflammatory and antioxidants).
3. The quality of the articles was significantly reduced by the lack of properly designed randomised controlled trials, a blinding method, or adequate control groups within the researched papers. In general, the modest amount of published literature, the low quality of the studies and information provided, the absence of standard protocols and the small irregular sample sizes make it difficult to compare results between studies.

Therefore, randomised control trials are needed to confirm and strengthen the significance of WBC-induced clinical changes and identify its effects at the molecular level. Despite important limitations of the available studies, growing scientific evidence indicates that WBC effectively reduces FM symptoms (Fig. 10.1). Particularly due to its rapid anti-inflammatory effect, WBC has the potential to boost rehabilitation programmes in achieving functional outcomes

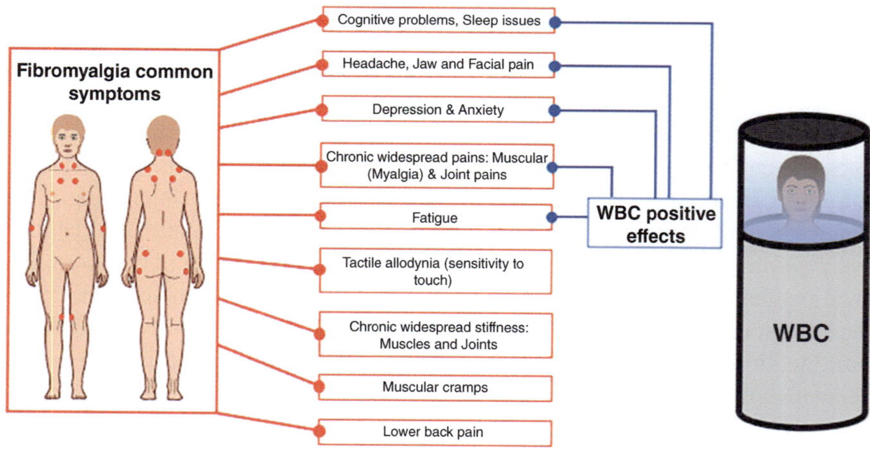

Fig. 10.1 Summary of the positive effects of WBC on FM common symptoms

in FM patients, which seems attractive in terms of the cost-effectiveness of rehabilitation. Furthermore, the high compliance and highly positive perception of the treatment reported by FM patients in most studies, as well as in our personal experience (based on our preliminary data), seem to make WBC a preferred component of the rehabilitation programme, which appears crucial in the long-term management of this chronic condition.

References

1. Bhargava J, Hurley JA. Fibromyalgia. StatPearls; 2023.
2. Sarzi-Puttini P, Giorgi V, Marotto D, Atzeni F. Fibromyalgia: an update on clinical characteristics, aetiopathogenesis and treatment. Nat Rev Rheumatol. 2020;16:645–60.
3. Koroschetz J, Rehm SE, Gockel U, Brosz M, Freynhagen R, Tölle TR, Baron R. Fibromyalgia and neuropathic pain—differences and similarities. A comparison of 3057 patients with diabetic painful neuropathy and fibromyalgia. BMC Neurol. 2011;11:55.
4. Gormsen L, Rosenberg R, Bach FW, Jensen TS. Depression, anxiety, health-related quality of life and pain in patients with chronic fibromyalgia and neuropathic pain. Eur J Pain. 2010;14:127.e1–8.
5. Bennett RM, Jones J, Turk DC, Russell IJ, Matallana L. An internet survey of 2,596 people with fibromyalgia. BMC Musculoskelet Disord. 2007;8:27.
6. Harris S, Morley S, Barton SB. Role loss and emotional adjustment in chronic pain. Pain. 2003;105:363–70.
7. Varallo G, Piterà P, Fontana JM, Gobbi M, Arreghini M, Giusti EM, Franceschini C, Plazzi G, Castelnuovo G, Capodaglio P. Is whole-body cryostimulation an effective add-on treatment in individuals with fibromyalgia and obesity? A randomized controlled clinical trial. J Clin Med. 2022;11:4324.
8. de la Coba P, Bruehl S, Galvez-Sánchez CM, Reyes Del Paso GA. Slowly repeated evoked pain as a marker of central sensitization in fibromyalgia: diagnostic accuracy and reliability in comparison with temporal summation of pain. Psychosom Med. 2018;80:573–80.
9. de la Coba P, Bruehl S, Moreno-Padilla M, Reyes Del Paso GA. Responses to slowly repeated evoked pain stimuli in fibromyalgia patients: evidence of enhanced pain sensitization. Pain Med. 2017;18:1778–86.
10. Maugars Y, Berthelot J-M, Le Goff B, Darrieutort-Laffite C. Fibromyalgia and associated disorders: from pain to chronic suffering, from subjective hypersensitivity to hypersensitivity syndrome. Front Med (Lausanne). 2021;8:666914.
11. Montoro CI, Duschek S, de Guevara CML, Fernández-Serrano MJ, Reyes del Paso GA. Aberrant cerebral blood flow responses during cognition: implications for the understanding of cognitive deficits in fibromyalgia. Neuropsychology. 2015;29:173–82.
12. Gracely RH, Petzke F, Wolf JM, Clauw DJ. Functional magnetic resonance imaging evidence of augmented pain processing in fibromyalgia. Arthritis Rheum. 2002;46:1333–43.
13. Martínez-Lavín M. Fibromyalgia and small fiber neuropathy: the plot thickens! Clin Rheumatol. 2018;37:3167–71.
14. da Silva Almeida DO, Pontes-Silva A, Dibai-Filho AV, Costa-de-Jesus SF, Avila MA, Fidelis-de-Paula-Gomes CA. Women with fibromyalgia (ACR criteria) compared with women diagnosed by doctors and women with osteoarthritis: cross-sectional study using functional and clinical variables. Int J Rheum Dis. 2023;26:2278. https://doi.org/10.1111/1756-185X.14720.
15. Fontana JM, Gobbi M, Piterà P, Giusti EM, Capodaglio P. Whole-body cryostimulation in fibromyalgia: a scoping review. Appl Sci. 2022;12:4794.
16. Marques AP, de Sousa do Espírito Santo A, Berssaneti AA, Matsutani LA, Yuan SLK. Prevalence of fibromyalgia: literature review update. Rev Bras Reumatol Eng Ed. 2017;57:356–63.

17. Bettoni L, Bonomi FG, Zani V, Manisco L, Indelicato A, Lanteri P, Banfi G, Lombardi G. Effects of 15 consecutive cryotherapy sessions on the clinical output of fibromyalgic patients. Clin Rheumatol. 2013;32:1337–45.

18. Berger A, Dukes E, Martin S, Edelsberg J, Oster G. Characteristics and healthcare costs of patients with fibromyalgia syndrome. Int J Clin Pract. 2007;61:1498–508.

19. Krock E, Morado-Urbina CE, Menezes J, et al. Fibromyalgia patients with elevated levels of anti–satellite glia cell immunoglobulin G antibodies present with more severe symptoms. Pain. 2023;164:1828–40.

20. Wolfe F, Clauw DJ, Fitzcharles M-A, Goldenberg DL, Häuser W, Katz RL, Mease PJ, Russell AS, Russell IJ, Walitt B. 2016 revisions to the 2010/2011 fibromyalgia diagnostic criteria. Semin Arthritis Rheum. 2016;46:319–29.

21. Arnold LM, Bennett RM, Crofford LJ, et al. AAPT diagnostic criteria for fibromyalgia. J Pain. 2019;20:611–28.

22. Briones-Vozmediano E, Vives-Cases C, Ronda-Pérez E, Gil-González D. Patients' and professionals' views on managing fibromyalgia. Pain Res Manag. 2013;18:19–24.

23. Giorgi V, Sirotti S, Romano ME, Marotto D, Ablin JN, Salaffi F, Sarzi-Puttini P. Fibromyalgia: one year in review 2022. Clin Exp Rheumatol. 2022;40:1065–72.

24. Moore RA, Fisher E, Häuser W, Bell RF, Perrot S, Bidonde J, Makri S, Straube S. Pharmacological therapies for fibromyalgia (fibromyalgia syndrome) in adults—an overview of Cochrane reviews. Cochrane Database Syst Rev. 2021. https://doi.org/10.1002/14651858.CD013151.pub2.

25. Rolls C, Prior Y. Non-pharmacological interventions for people with fibromyalgia: a systematic review. Rheumatology. 2018;57:key075.509.

26. Hassett AL, Williams DA. Non-pharmacological treatment of chronic widespread musculoskeletal pain. Best Pract Res Clin Rheumatol. 2011;25:299–309.

27. Lombardi G, Ziemann E, Banfi G. Whole-body cryotherapy in athletes: from therapy to stimulation. An updated review of the literature. Front Physiol. 2017;8:258.

28. Sadura-Sieklucka T, Sołtysiuk B, Karlicka A, Sokołowska B, Kontny E, Księżopolska-Orłowska K. Effects of whole body cryotherapy in patients with rheumatoid arthritis considering immune parameters. Reumatologia. 2019;57:320–5.

29. Fontana JM, Bozgeyik S, Gobbi M, Piterà P, Giusti EM, Dugué B, Lombardi G, Capodaglio P. Whole-body cryostimulation in obesity. A scoping review. J Therm Biol. 2022;106:103250.

30. Rymaszewska J, Ramsey D, Chładzińska-Kiejna S. Whole-body cryotherapy as adjunct treatment of depressive and anxiety disorders. Arch Immunol Ther Exp (Warsz). 2008;56:63–8.

31. Bouzigon R, Ravier G, Dugue B, Grappe F. The use of whole-body cryostimulation to improve the quality of sleep in athletes during high level standard competitions. Br J Sports Med. 2014;48:572.

32. Hirvonen HE, Mikkelsson MK, Kautiainen H, Pohjolainen TH, Leirisalo-Repo M. Effectiveness of different cryotherapies on pain and disease activity in active rheumatoid arthritis. A randomised single blinded controlled trial. Clin Exp Rheumatol. 2006;24:295–301.

33. Romanowski MW, Straburzyńska-Lupa A. Is the whole-body cryotherapy a beneficial supplement to exercise therapy for patients with ankylosing spondylitis? J Back Musculoskelet Rehabil. 2020;33:185–92.

34. Verme F, Scarpa A, Varallo G, Piterà P, Capodaglio P, Fontana JM. Effects of whole-body cryostimulation on pain management and disease activity in active rheumatic polymyalgia: a case-report. Biomedicines. 2023;11:1594.

35. Kozłowska M, Kortas J, Żychowska M, Antosiewicz J, Żuczek K, Perego S, Lombardi G, Ziemann E. Beneficial effects of whole-body cryotherapy on glucose homeostasis and amino acid profile are associated with a reduced myostatin serum concentration. Sci Rep. 2021;11:7097.

36. Miller E, Kostka J, Włodarczyk T, Dugué B. Whole-body cryostimulation (cryotherapy) provides benefits for fatigue and functional status in multiple sclerosis patients. A case-control study. Acta Neurol Scand. 2016;134:420–6.

37. Gobbi M, Trotti G, Tanzi M, Kasap F, Piterà P, Capodaglio P. Post-COVID symptoms and whole-body cryotherapy: a case report. J Rehabil Med Clin Commun. 2022;5:1000075.
38. Piterà P, Gobbi M, Fontana JM, Cattaldo S, Massucci M, Capodaglio P. Whole-body cryostimulation: a rehabilitation booster in post-COVID patients? A case series. Appl Sci. 2022;12:4830.
39. Berk M, Williams LJ, Jacka FN, et al. So depression is an inflammatory disease, but where does the inflammation come from? BMC Med. 2013;11:200.
40. Veltri A, Scarpellini P, Piccinni A, Conversano C, Giacomelli C, Bombardieri S, Bazzichi L, Dell'Osso L. Methodological approach to depressive symptoms in fibromyalgia patients. Clin Exp Rheumatol. 2012;30:136–42.
41. Bradley LA. Pathophysiology of fibromyalgia. Am J Med. 2009;122:S22.
42. Yam MF, Loh YC, Tan CS, Khadijah Adam S, Abdul Manan N, Basir R. General pathways of pain sensation and the major neurotransmitters involved in pain regulation. Int J Mol Sci. 2018;19:2164.
43. Siracusa R, Paola RD, Cuzzocrea S, Impellizzeri D. Fibromyalgia: pathogenesis, mechanisms, diagnosis and treatment options update. Int J Mol Sci. 2021;22:3891.
44. Muir WW, Woolf CJ. Mechanisms of pain and their therapeutic implications. J Am Vet Med Assoc. 2001;219:1346–56.
45. Latremoliere A, Woolf CJ. Central sensitization: a generator of pain hypersensitivity by central neural plasticity. J Pain. 2009;10:895–926.
46. O'Brien AT, Deitos A, Triñanes Pego Y, Fregni F, Carrillo-de-la-Peña MT. Defective endogenous pain modulation in fibromyalgia: a meta-analysis of temporal summation and conditioned pain modulation paradigms. J Pain. 2018;19:819–36.
47. Clauw DJ. Fibromyalgia: a clinical review. JAMA. 2014;311:1547–55.
48. Harris RE, Clauw DJ. Imaging central neurochemical alterations in chronic pain with proton magnetic resonance spectroscopy. Neurosci Lett. 2012;520:192–6.
49. Bettoni L, Bonomi FG, Zani V, Indelicato A, Banfi G. THU0347 efficacy and safety of whole body cryotherapy in fibromyalgic patients. Ann Rheum Dis. 2013;71:273.
50. Rivera J, Tercero MJ, Salas JS, Gimeno JH, Alejo JS. The effect of cryotherapy on fibromyalgia: a randomised clinical trial carried out in a cryosauna cabin. Rheumatol Int. 2018;38:2243–50.
51. Vitenet M, Tubez F, Marreiro A, Polidori G, Taiar R, Legrand F, Boyer FC. Effect of whole body cryotherapy interventions on health-related quality of life in fibromyalgia patients: a randomized controlled trial. Complement Ther Med. 2018;36:6–8.
52. Metzger D, Zwingmann C, Protz W, Jäckel WH. [Whole-body cryotherapy in rehabilitation of patients with rheumatoid diseases—pilot study]. Rehabilitation (Stuttg). 2000;39:93–100.
53. Klemm P, Becker J, Aykara I, Asendorf T, Dischereit G, Neumann E, Müller-Ladner U, Lange U. Serial whole-body cryotherapy in fibromyalgia is effective and alters cytokine profiles. Adv Rheumatol. 2021;61:3.
54. Kurzeja R, Gutenbrunner C, Krohn-Grimberghe B. Primäre Fibromyalgie: Vergleich der Kältekammertherapie mit zwei klassischen Wärmetherapieverfahren. Aktuelle Rheumatologie. 2003;28:158–63.
55. Sundaram VM. To compare the effectiveness of whole body cryotherapy against steam therapy in patients with chronic fibromyalgia. Physiotherapy. 2015;101:e988–9.
56. Littlejohn G, Guymer E. Neurogenic inflammation in fibromyalgia. Semin Immunopathol. 2018;40:291–300.
57. O'Mahony LF, Srivastava A, Mehta P, Ciurtin C. Is fibromyalgia associated with a unique cytokine profile? A systematic review and meta-analysis. Rheumatology (Oxford). 2021;60:2602–14.
58. Hung AL, Lim M, Doshi TL. Targeting cytokines for treatment of neuropathic pain. Scand J Pain. 2017;17:287–93.
59. Uçeyler N, Häuser W, Sommer C. Systematic review with meta-analysis: cytokines in fibromyalgia syndrome. BMC Musculoskelet Disord. 2011;12:245.
60. Lubkowska A, Szyguła Z, Chlubek D, Banfi G. The effect of prolonged whole-body cryostimulation treatment with different amounts of sessions on chosen pro- and anti-inflammatory cytokines levels in healthy men. Scand J Clin Lab Invest. 2011;71:419–25.

61. Lubkowska A, Szygula Z, Klimek AJ, Torii M. Do sessions of cryostimulation have influence on white blood cell count, level of IL6 and total oxidative and antioxidative status in healthy men? Eur J Appl Physiol. 2010;109:67–72.
62. Lubkowska A, Dołęgowska B, Szyguła Z. Whole-body cryostimulation—potential beneficial treatment for improving antioxidant capacity in healthy men—significance of the number of sessions. PLoS One. 2012;7:e46352.
63. Wojciak G, Szymura J, Szygula Z, Gradek J, Wiecek M. The effect of repeated whole-body cryotherapy on Sirt1 and Sirt3 concentrations and oxidative status in older and young men performing different levels of physical activity. Antioxidants (Basel). 2020;10:37.
64. Drynda S, Mika O, Koczan D, Kekow J. AB0661 Impact of whole-body cryotherapy on transcriptome of peripheral blood cells in patients with fibromyalgia. Ann Rheum Dis. 2014;72:A990–1.
65. Drynda S, Mika O, Kekow J. THU0313 Impact of whole-body cryotherapy on gene expression of peripheral blood cells in patients with fibromyalgia. Ann Rheum Dis. 2015;74:309.

Obesity

11

Jacopo Maria Fontana, Paolo Piterà, Federica Verme, Riccardo Cremascoli, Amelia Brunani, Stefania Cattaldo, Stefania Mai, Alessandra Milesi, Laura Bianchi, Federica Galli, Federica La Pilusa, Francesca Tiburzi, Raffaella Cancello, and Paolo Capodaglio

J. M. Fontana (✉) · P. Piterà · F. Verme · A. Brunani
Research Laboratory in Biomechanics, Rehabilitation and Ergonomics, IRCCS Istituto
Auxologico Italiano, Piancavallo (Verbania), Italy
e-mail: j.fontana@auxologico.it; p.pitera@auxologico.it; f.verme@auxologico.it;
brunani@auxologico.it

R. Cremascoli
Department of Neurology and Neurorehabilitation, IRCCS Istituto Auxologico Italiano,
Piancavallo (Verbania), Italy

Department of Neurosciences, University of Turin, Turin, Italy
e-mail: r.cremascoli@auxologico.it

S. Cattaldo · A. Milesi
Laboratory of Clinical Neurobiology, IRCCS Istituto Auxologico Italiano,
Piancavallo (Verbania), Italy
e-mail: s.cattaldo@auxologico.it; a.milesi@auxologico.it

S. Mai
Laboratory of Metabolic Research, IRCCS Istituto Auxologico Italiano,
Piancavallo (Verbania), Italy
e-mail: s.mai@auxologico.it

L. Bianchi · F. Galli · F. La Pilusa · F. Tiburzi
Neurophysiopathology Unit, IRCCS Istituto Auxologico Italiano,
Piancavallo (Verbania), Italy

R. Cancello
Obesity Unit, Laboratory of Nutrition and Obesity Research, Department of Endocrine and
Metabolic Diseases, IRCCS Istituto Auxologico Italiano, Milan, Italy
e-mail: r.cancello@auxologico.it

P. Capodaglio
Research Laboratory in Biomechanics, Rehabilitation and Ergonomics, IRCCS Istituto
Auxologico Italiano, Piancavallo (Verbania), Italy

Physical Medicine and Rehabilitation, Department of Surgical Sciences,
University of Torino, Torino, Italy
e-mail: p.capodaglio@auxologico.it; paolo.capodaglio@unito.it

P. Capodaglio (ed.), *Whole-Body Cryostimulation*,
https://doi.org/10.1007/978-3-031-18545-8_11

Obesity: Overview and Clinical Manifestations

Currently available treatments for the management of obesity struggle to provide clinically significant weight loss and reduction of the chronic low-grade inflammatory state in order to reduce obesity-related complications [1]. Such options include behavioural changes, adapted physical activity, nutrition therapy, psychological support, web-related digital interventions, pharmacotherapy, and bariatric surgery [1–3]. Those complementary approaches, aimed to achieve and maintain clinically meaningful weight loss, can be applied according to an escalation strategy based on the presence and severity of comorbidities [3]. Pharmacological therapies have so far offered auxiliary treatments with moderate effects on weight loss [4, 5], but new drugs now available promise to be game changers. However, patients' compliance with prescriptions remains a relevant issue in terms of long-term weight control and health-related benefits [4, 6, 7].

In the absence of a structured intervention, relapses of this chronic remitting disease are likely to occur [1, 8]. Low-grade inflammation is a key feature of dysmetabolic conditions and, thereby, long-term approaches focused on both induction of weight loss and stimulation of the anti-inflammatory response should be adopted [1, 2, 9]. Regular exercise has been shown to increase energy expenditure and reduce chronic inflammation by decreasing mononuclear cell production of pro-inflammatory cytokines [10], hypoxia, oxidative stress [11], serum leukocyte [12] and release of cell adhesion molecules [13], stimulating the production of mediators by immune cells and tissue (i.e. skeletal muscle) with anti-inflammatory properties [14], myokine [15] and adipose tissue lipolysis [16, 17]. The combination of a calorie restriction diet with exercise has been found effective in reducing serum concentrations of markers of chronic inflammation such as C-reactive protein (CRP), tumour necrosis factor-alpha (TNFα) and interleukin 6 (IL-6) in adults with overweight and obesity with active lifestyles [18]. This also leads to a negative energy balance and triggers cascades of metabolic and neurohormonal adaptive mechanisms that limit systemic inflammation [1, 17]. However, the induced weight loss is modest and the dropout rate from physical training programmes is high, due to either musculoskeletal or motivational issues [19, 20].

Therefore, it appears of paramount importance to find effective add-on intervention strategies that can raise the chances of reaching the goals of established weight loss and improved inflammatory status. On the basis of the limited data available in the literature so far, WBC is emerging as a promising adjuvant intervention in the treatment of obesity able to reduce at the same time systemic inflammation, oxidative stress, abdominal obesity and body mass.

The aim of this chapter is to provide an up-to-date picture of the evidence supporting the beneficial effects of WBC in patients with obesity.

Clinical Effects

The cryogenic stimulus has widely acknowledged anti-inflammatory/antioxidant properties, mimicking an exercise-induced effect [21, 22]. This aspect is of particular interest in patients with metabolic conditions who present with chronic low-grade inflammatory status and often with reduced physical capacity that hinders adherence to physical activity programmes and exerts interesting metabolic effects. Sudden changes in muscle and skin temperature result (see Chap. 1) in lower fatigue sensation and mood improvement with a possible positive impact on depression and sleep quality [23]. However, there is a range of individual responses to cold due to inter-individual differences, such as body size, BMI, fitness level, amount of subcutaneous fat and gender [24–26]. After repeated exposures to WBC, the following effects have been measured: improvement of inflammatory and metabolic profile [21], enhancement of the antioxidant system [27], improvement of insulin sensitivity [28], increase of brown adipose tissue (BAT) volume percentage, decreased percentage of adipose tissue [29], enhanced secretion of endorphins [30] and slowed-down nerve conduction velocity [31].

Haematological Parameters

A limited number of papers have taken into consideration the effects of WBC on patients with obesity focusing on haematological markers, metabolic parameters, lipid and endocrine profile, antioxidant enzyme activities and inflammatory and cellular stress response [27, 29, 32–36]. Haematological parameters outside the health reference range are diagnostic for a variety of pathologies including obesity [37]. Several works described the effect of WBC on haematological parameters in patients with obesity, but the results are inconsistent due to variations in methodological factors, such as sample size, number of sessions, temperature exposure, class of obesity and timing of blood sample collection. Ziemann et al. reported no significant variation 24 h after 10 sessions of WBC in white blood cells, red blood cells (RBC) and haematocrit (Hct). Most of the values and differences initially observed between the groups were maintained, suggesting that cardiorespiratory fitness level and, probably, obesity class (not specifically described in the groups) were not influenced by WBC [36]. Wyrostek et al. described statistically significant differences (in terms of the reference range) in red blood cell parameters [RBC, Hct, mean corpuscular volume (MCV), mean corpuscular haemoglobin concentration (MCHC) and mean platelet volume (MPV)]. They reported a decrease in RBC, MCV and Hct and an increase in MCHC in the high-body fat group (HBF) and a decrease in Hct, MCV and MPV and an increase in RBC and MCHC in the normal-body fat group (NBF) after 10 and 20 sessions [35].

On the other hand, the study by Lubkowska et al. showed a decrease in RBC, Hb, Hct and leukocytes (this latter only temporarily) accompanied by an increase in MCH, MCHC and RDW [33]. However, the study cohort with obesity and overweight was subjected to two sets of 20 daily WBC sessions for 6 months in combination with a physical training programme that may have influenced the outcomes associated with WBC.

Dulian et al. only investigated the effect of WBC on iron metabolism. Hepcidin, an iron regulatory hormone that can inhibit iron transport from cells by blocking ferroportin, decreased after 10 sessions of WBC, but no changes in iron and ferritin concentrations were detected [32]. Thus, based on these results, WBC seems to exert a general positive effect on these subjects regardless of their fitness level or their obesity class.

Regarding the immune system, WBC showed no detrimental effects on immune cells. No significant changes in white blood cell parameters were noticed in subjects with obesity undergoing 10 [35, 36] or 20 WBC sessions [29]. However, Lubkowska et al. observed a transient decrease in the number of white blood cells at the end of the experiment, which could be due to the combination of WBC and physical training and not due to the heterogeneity of the study group, as this is a general effect [33]. Finally, one study observed decreased leukocyte mRNA expression of two genes encoding heat shock protein after WBC in patients with normal body mass (NBM) and high body mass (HBM with obesity). The mRNA expression of HSPA1A and HSPB1 decreased gradually with the number of cryostimulation sessions. A significant difference was found in the expression of HSPA1A after 20 sessions (NBM > HBM) and for HSPB1 at baseline and after 20 sessions (HBM > NBM), suggesting that this reduction may affect adipose tissue and could be related to fat reduction [34].

In summary, a decrease in haemoglobinisation, possibly associated with increased haemolysis, is a specific but temporary feature of WBC treatment. Similar results have also been reported from studies not conducted in obesity/overweight cohorts [22, 38, 39], indicating that they may simply reflect a temporary physiological adaptation. Furthermore, it is also important to consider that haematological changes could be influenced by the number of WBC sessions, as shown by Szygula et al. in a study conducted on physically active students [40]. A temporary decrease in Hb, Hct and RBC after 10 sessions remained consistently low until 20 sessions, then increased after the 30th session, possibly due to a resumption of erythropoiesis.

Overall, it seems that 10 and 20 sessions of WBC are safe for patients with different classes of obesity; therefore, the possibility of increasing the number of treatments should be further explored in future studies.

Inflammatory Response

Quantification of the inflammatory response has been widely used to determine the degree of inflammation in various conditions including obesity which is characterised by a chronic low-grade inflammatory status [17, 41, 42]. Previous studies have described the local and systemic anti-inflammatory effects of WBC [43–45], but only four studies have focused on different inflammatory markers of patients with obesity, including TNFα [36, 46], IL-6 [9, 29, 32], IL-10 [36] and CRP [29, 32, 34], before and after WBC. Ziemann et al. [36] found a correlation between TNFα trends and cardiorespiratory fitness. In general, baseline TNFα values were elevated, most likely due to low-grade systemic inflammation. The authors compared the results obtained in participants with low (LCF) and high cardiorespiratory fitness (HCF), reporting a significant decrease in TNFα concentration in subjects with obesity after ten 3-min WBC sessions at $-110\ °C$. This result was more pronounced in patients with LCF than those with HCF, correlating with cardiorespiratory fitness, as the difference was more pronounced in LCFs than HCFs.

Similarly, a significant progressive reduction in TNFα was reported between 10 and 20 WBC in patients with class I (IOb) and class II (IIOb) obesity by Pilch et al. [46]. However, the reduction was not followed by increased ADP levels, usually inhibited by TNFα in adipocytes [47].

In patients with inflammatory rheumatic diseases [48] and in professional tennis players [45], the decrease in TNFα concentrations was comparable to that previously reported after performing low-intensity exercise [49]. Banfi et al. [43] reported increased concentrations of anti-inflammatory cytokines and a decrease in the pro-inflammatory cytokines/chemokines, IL-2 and IL-8 in peripheral blood as a consequence of local and systemic analgesic effects of WBC.

IL-6 has a dual mode of action. It can act as a pro-inflammatory cytokine and as an anti-inflammatory myokine depending on (1) its production site, (2) the stimulation pathway that enabled its release and (3) its basal concentration [50]. Chronic inflammatory conditions are characterised by mildly elevated levels of IL-6 that play a role in systemic inflammation, i.e. by stimulating other anti-inflammatory cytokines such as IL-10 and inhibiting the production of the pro-inflammatory cytokine TNFα [49].

In individuals with obesity, IL-6 concentration positively correlates with visceral adipose tissue mass, BMI and waist circumference [51]. In addition, it can have a metabolic effect that stimulates lipolysis and fat oxidation [52]. Increased levels of IL-6 may also originate from the contracting muscle and act as an anti-inflammatory mediator [53], but some studies have demonstrated increased IL-6 concentrations after WBC: in postmenopausal women with obesity and metabolic syndrome (MetS) after 10 and 20 sessions of WBC [29]; in professional tennis players exposed to 10 sessions of WBC, twice a day for 5 days, in combination with moderate intensity physical training [45]; and in two separate groups of clinically healthy untrained men [54, 55] where the blood concentration was increased above baseline after the first and the tenth exposure [55]. However, in two different studies conducted on men with obesity, 10 sessions of WBC did not significantly alter IL-6 concentrations [32, 36], whereas its decrease after 10 sessions was reported only in LCF subjects with obesity and not in the HCF group with obesity [36]. IL-10 is an anti-inflammatory cytokine with multiple and pleiotropic effects in immunoregulation and inflammation, and it was found to be increased in rugby players after 5 sessions of WBC [43] and in HCF and LCF subjects with obesity after 10 sessions with a sustained increase that lasted 24 h after the last session. Interestingly, baseline values of IL-10 in the LCF were already significantly higher, maybe as an enhanced defensive response to low-grade systemic inflammation. Similarly, in subjects with obesity, CRP concentrations at baseline, also correlated with BMI, were higher in subjects with obesity than in those without obesity [51], again reiterating that obesity is characterised by a higher inflammatory state. Therefore, it would be expected that the anti-inflammatory effect of cold would decrease the level of CRP, which usually increases rapidly in response to inflammation. This is shown in two studies:

the work of Dulian et al. reported that the decline in CRP levels was similar in both the low fitness (LFL) and the high fitness (HFL) level group with obesity regardless of the number of sessions (either 1 or 10) [32] while in the study of Pournot, a similar decrease was observed in well-trained athletes exposed to five sessions of WBC for up to 96 h after exercise [56]. However, in two other studies, WBC did not induce significant CRP levels: in men or menopausal women with obesity, regardless of their body mass (high or normal) or comorbidity with metabolic syndrome, and in 20-year-old men without obesity, regardless of their fitness level after 10 WBC treatments [57].

In general, even if the findings are not always in line, WBC appears to yield an anti-inflammatory effect that is highly correlated with the fitness level in individuals with obesity.

Body Composition

Measurement of body composition may vary in precision according to the technique used and the population characteristics, and in some cases, studies report the participants' body composition at baseline without describing the technique used for their quantification. Unfortunately, in two articles, body composition was assessed to describe only the population sample in terms of the amount of fat and lean mass but no data were collected after WBC [29, 34]. Więcek et al. reported a significant reduction in waist, hips and abdominal circumference, waist-to-height ratio, triceps and abdominal skinfold thickness in one group of women with overweight and two groups of menopausal women with obesity, healthy and with MetS, after 10 WBC sessions. After 20 sessions of WBC, these effects intensified. Moreover, a significant reduction in body mass, BMI, absolute total body fat and leg fat was also achieved. Particularly the MetS group showed a significant reduction in the percentage of total, trunk and android fat [29], but a comparison between weight groups, especially between subjects with IOb and IIOb, could not be made because there was no clear differentiation by BMI.

Similarly, in the work by Pilch et al., a significant decrease in fat mass, percentage of body fat, waist/hip circumference and BMI was reported after 20 sessions of WBC in males with IOb with high body mass [34]. However, no changes in body composition in IOb men were found after 10 sessions by Ziemann et al. [36] while no significant changes in body weight, waist-hip ratio, BMI, body fat mass, skeletal muscle and subcutaneous fat mass after 40 WBC exposures associated with an intensive exercise programme were reported by Lubkowska et al. [33]. However, the group included subjects with an average BMI greater than 30, probably consisting of both IOb and IIOb.

Finally, the Pilch group's latest study [46] found the greatest changes in subcutaneous fat tissue thickness significantly reduced in the IOb group reproducing their previous results [34], in contrast to the findings of the Lubkowska's [33] and Ziemann's [36] groups.

The results regarding body composition are heterogeneous in the analysed studies, partly due to the presence of confounding interventions, such as dietary therapy and physical activity, and the absence of a control group. However, they all suggest that WBC may lead to a reduction in adipose tissue and circumferences in different regions of the body.

Preliminary results from our group (Fontana et al. unpublished data) at two different temperatures, −55 °C (considered 'non-cryogenic') and −110 °C, showed that cooler temperature (−110 °C) is more effective in reducing waist circumference than non-cryogenic temperature (−55 °C), suggesting greater cold-induced fat redistribution in the −110 °C group, which could be secondary to the conversion of WAT to BAT and an increase in BAT volume and activity. Furthermore, higher subcutaneous fat in individuals with obesity could cause lower heat loss [58] by slowing the increase in metabolic rate compared with individuals without obesity. This would explain the different effects of WBC on body composition at different BMIs.

Lipid Profile and Adipokines

Visceral obesity is strongly associated with dyslipidaemia characterised by high plasma triglycerides, LDL cholesterol and low HDL cholesterol [33, 59].

Since lipids are the preferred fuel source for thermogenesis, one would expect a change in their profile after WBC, as cold exposure activates white adipose tissue (WAT) and brown adipose tissue (BAT) [28, 60]. However, Pilch et al. reported no significant changes in the lipid profile but only a positive trend of recovery in the IOb group [46], while Lubkowska et al. observed a reduction in triglycerides and LDL cholesterol and a modest increase in HDL cholesterol after a 6-month intervention with WBC [33]. Moreover, the heterogeneity of the study group (I/IIOb and overweight) and the exercise programme followed by the study participants may have favoured this trend, since exercise can lower total cholesterol and LDL and increases HDL cholesterol levels.

Moreover, discordant results regarding pro-inflammatory adipokines levels (adiponectin, leptin, visfatin and resistin) after WBC have also been reported [29, 32, 33, 36]. Ziemann et al. showed that 10 WBC sessions influenced the concentration of adipokines resistin and visfatin in relation to the subjects' cardiorespiratory fitness levels which increased at the end of treatments in LCF participants (with both IOb and IIOb) and, in contrast, decreased significantly in HCF subjects with only IOb. Adiponectin and leptin were not affected [36]. Interestingly, irisin, a recently discovered exercise-induced myokine that stimulates browning of WAT and promotes thermogenesis [22, 61], increased in all participants with IOb and IIOb 24 h after the first and the tenth session of WBC [32]. In particular, irisin concentrations increased significantly by 20% only in the LFL subjects with IOb and IIOb, decreasing in subjects with an HFL with only IOb [32]. An increase in irisin was also reported: in women with obesity and MetS; in healthy women after 1 and 10 sessions of WBC, where the level further increased to return to baseline after 20 sessions [29]. Lubkowska et al. found an elevation only in visfatin levels after 6 months

[33]. No changes in adiponectin, resistin and leptin concentrations were observed after WBC exposures. Again, in these studies, the heterogeneity of the study group (subjects with I/IIOb and overweight), the participants' engagement in physical activity during the 6-month programme and the two sets of 20 WBC sessions may have influenced the outcomes. In line with previous published results [62–65], no changes in adiponectin levels between 10 and 20 sessions of WBC in patients with obesity were observed by Pilch et al. However, adiponectin levels in individuals with obesity (especially in those with visceral obesity) were lower than those in lean subjects with a larger individual variability in the IIOb group [46]. Interestingly, they showed a significant decrease in leptin levels only in IOb and IIOb groups between 10 and 20 WBC sessions, but not in the healthy controls.

In summary, adiponectin does not seem to undergo significant changes after WBC, while leptin either decreased or did not change. The decrease observed by Pilch et al. suggests its beneficial effect on metabolism, muscle shivering and glucose uptake [62, 66] through impairment of expression and functional activity of beta-3 adrenergic receptors in obesity [67]. In contrast, the lack of change observed by Lubkowska et al. [33] was not expected. Leptin is known to decrease after physical activity and after body mass loss, so a synergistic effect was expected after WBC.

Regarding visfatin, resistin and irisin, it appears that the initial fitness level and the amount of fat mass may determine the response to treatment, although these are results obtained on subjects with obesity [32, 36]. In a group of patients with IOb and IIOb, reduced fitness and increased adiposity, visfatin, resistin and irisin were found to be significantly increased, whereas their counterparts with only IOb and higher fitness status responded in the opposite way. Preliminary data from our group (Fontana et al. unpublished data) seem to suggest that the metabolic effects of WBC in patients with obesity could be more pronounced as temperatures drop. In fact, $-110\ ^{\circ}C$ appears to induce more pronounced effects than $-55\ ^{\circ}C$ on total cholesterol (-16% vs. -8%, respectively), triglycerides (-20% vs. -9%, respectively), LDL (-24% vs. -10%, respectively), HDL (-12% vs. 6%, respectively) and glucose (-10% vs. -2%, respectively). This is in line with previous time- and dose-response studies [68–70].

It is known that cold exposure increases lipid metabolism, which is the preferred fuel source for thermogenesis. Therefore, a change in lipid profile after WBC can be explained by activation of white adipose tissue (WAT) and brown adipose tissue (BAT) after cold exposure [71]. Most importantly, BAT plays an important role in lowering blood glucose and improving insulin sensitivity in humans, thus helping to reduce insulin resistance and the risk of diseases, including diabetes [72]. Brown adipocytes, after being activated by cold exposure, begin to oxidise their own lipid reserves or fatty acids removed from the circulation and other substrates, e.g. glucose, to produce heat and increase metabolic rate. Thus, the decrease in glucose and HBa1c% (and insulin, although not significantly) that we observed in our preliminary results, indicates a rapid burning of this high-energy compound, a finding in agreement with previous research showing that cold exposure can lower fasting glucose and insulin levels [73].

Energy and Bone Metabolism

We know that energy and bone metabolism interact with each other: bone turnover is strikingly dependent upon energy availability/demand and is regulated by several energy-related hormones, myokines, adipokines and neurotransmitters (i.e. insulin, leptin, adiponectin, epinephrine/norepinephrine) [74]. Therefore, glucose homeostasis, fat metabolism, adipose tissue metabolism and bone remodelling are closely linked and regulate one another in order to maintain energy homeostasis [15]. A study by Straburzyńska-Lupa et al. assessed the effect of acute WBC treatment (24 h after the exposure) on sclerostin levels in healthy young men with different physical fitness levels: a first single WBC exposure induced significant changes in serum sclerostin, which may reflect a 'larger skeleton' able to produce and release more sclerostin [74]. It is also possible to hypothesise a role for WBC-dependent sympathetic activation that induces osteocytes, the main cellular source of sclerostin, to express β-adrenergic receptors, the activation of which is associated in vivo with increased osteoclastogenesis [75]. The acute increase of sclerostin after a single WBC application is of particular interest; however, further studies need to demonstrate a direct effect of adrenergic stimulation on its expression/release. Galliera et al. also reported that in rugby players five WBC sessions stimulated the increase of the OPG-to-RANKL ratio (the resorption-to-formation balance index), which may indicate an osteogenic effect of WBC when associated with adequate training [76]. A recent controlled clinical trial found that WBC led to an increase in bone remodelling (new bone formation) with no parallel increase in bone resorption. Those studies indicate that osteoporosis could benefit from WBC since cold exposure activates specific osteoimmunological biomarkers that are crucial for bone remodelling with no concurrent increase in bone resorption factors. Unfortunately, no studies on subjects with obesity are available so far.

Autonomic Modulation

WBC has been reported to maximise physical recovery after exercise, reduce the ensuing muscle damage and trigger cardiovascular responses leading to an increased vagal drive. As indicated in Chap. 1, the rapid cooling induces a potent skin vasoconstriction, which shifts the blood towards the central region of the body; the ensuing baroreceptor reflex would then be responsible for a depression of the sympathetic activity and an enhancement of the vagal drive. The modulation of the activity of autonomic fibres innervating the heart can be determined noninvasively by measuring the heart rate variability (HRV), i.e. the fluctuations in time between two heartbeats, widely acknowledged as an indicator of cardiac sympathetic and parasympathetic control [77]. In particular, the fraction of the total power in the low-frequency range (LF) reflects both the sympathetic and the parasympathetic drive, while the fraction in the high-frequency range (HF) unveils the parasympathetic drive through the vagus nerve. Sympathovagal balance is commonly expressed by the LF/HF ratio.

A recent meta-analysis highlights that sympathetic activity is markedly and significantly increased in subjects with obesity, even when subjects do not concomitantly present with hypertension, diabetes mellitus, obstructive sleep apnea and MetS, conditions characterised per se by adrenergic activation [78]. This adrenergic overdrive exhibits an early appearance and progression with increasing severity of these conditions. Also, patients with obesity present with chronic low-grade inflammatory status. Inflammation has a negative effect on the autonomic nervous system [79]. The sympathetic nervous system is involved in inflammation via a direct influence of neurotransmitters on immune cells or an indirect effect via regulating blood and lymphatic flows [80]. The parasympathetic nervous system could be also involved in local control of inflammation in rheumatic diseases through the vagus nerve, which has been shown to have anti-inflammatory properties through the action of acetylcholine [81]. Furthermore, it has been reported [82] that patients with inflammatory diseases have an impaired autonomic nervous function. The physiopathological mechanism of this dysfunction could be explained by the presence of circulating anti-neuronal autoantibodies directed against sympathetic and parasympathetic nervous structures [83].

A predominance of parasympathetic drive is commonly observed following WBC. The latter has been found to induce a larger stimulation of the autonomic system compared to partial-body cold exposure (i.e. not exposing the head to cold) [68]. Such modulation of the autonomic nervous system is factually associated with faster post-exercise recovery and promises to help counteract the obesity-related adrenergic overdrive by 'resetting' the sympathovagal balance [83]. Current literature reports that WBC involves the autonomic drive at rest [70, 84, 85], but these studies did not address the effect of exercise. Storniolo et al. recorded electrocardiogram (ECG) in 28 healthy adults who underwent rest, all-out effort on a cycloergometer, 5-min recovery and again rest and evaluated sympathovagal balance by measuring HR variability power in the low- and high-frequency bands. After 3–5 days, WBC was applied and the whole procedure was repeated. They concluded that WBC may be fruitful both for boosting exercise performance and for speeding up post-exercise recovery: an increase in exercise duration and a shortening of the HR recovery after a single session of WBC were indeed found [86]. However, Louis et al. warn about possible physiological habituation to repeated WBC sessions: after 5 WBC daily exposures on subjects without obesity, they recorded a lower autonomic response as compared to day one [70]. This may indicate that WBC protocols should take that into consideration and the 'dose' of cold exposure should be gradually increased within a WBC cycle. Preliminary data from our group on subjects with obesity (Cremascoli et al. unpublished data) show changes in HRV with an increase in parasympathetic tone after the completion of the WBC cycle. The stimulation of the parasympathetic branch appears to be greater at lower temperatures of exposure, with a decrease in systolic blood pressure in acute (clinostatism) and in both systolic and diastolic blood pressure at the end of the WBC cycle. This autonomic modulating effect observed supports the use of WBC as an additional treatment in the multidisciplinary treatment of obesity, a condition characterised by sympathetic overdrive and autonomic unbalance.

Conclusive Remarks

Despite the significant evidence reviewed in this chapter, the molecular mechanisms underlying the reported beneficial effects of WBC in obesity have not been thoroughly investigated yet. The lack of standardised protocols for the use of WBC in the treatment of obesity (temperature, number of sessions, time of exposure and sample collection time varied among studies) may account for the discrepancies reported in the literature.

Also, confounding factors such as physical activity and diet, which have a key role in modulating antioxidant, anti-inflammatory and body composition, were present in most articles. The absence of randomised controlled trials, blinding or proper control groups within the searched papers inevitably reduces the conclusiveness of results. The absence of stratification of participants according to their BMI and class of obesity also continues to be present in most papers. A clear distinction was made only in the work of Pilch and collaborators [27, 34, 46], whereas in other studies, BMI values were averaged (at least for a subgroup of the study), not allowing to understand to which class of obesity the different participants belonged to. In general, the limited literature available, the low quality of the studies, the small sample sizes and the variety of WBC protocols do not allow for proper comparison of outcome measurements among the studies. Therefore, future studies with larger sample sizes and more rigorous methodological study designs are needed to confirm the significance of the physiological changes and identify the effects of WBC at the molecular level. Many of the results obtained in the selected articles do not clearly address the questions of whether the number of WBC sessions should be considered as a function of BMI and whether increasing the number of WBC sessions parallel to an increase in BMI would yield positive results.

The seductive aspect of WBC relies on its triple action: anti-inflammatory/antioxidant, metabolic and modulating of the autonomic system (Fig. 11.1). WBC seems to yield the potential of becoming an adjuvant therapeutic approach to existing strategies, capable of reducing systemic inflammation, abdominal obesity and body mass in individuals with obesity, particularly those with LFL. The efficacy of WBC appears to be directly related to individual body composition, fat mass percentage and initial fitness capacity, mimicking exercise-induced effects. This seems of particular interest in a population with a high dropout rate from exercise programmes for various reasons and is advocated to unveil a new scenario in the treatment of obesity and obesity-related disorders. Patients with obesity often have reduced ability to engage in regular physical activity, one of the mechanisms responsible for the anti-inflammatory response. WBC may therefore represent a feasible alternative to reduce chronic inflammation that underlies most of the obesity-related comorbidities. WBC yields the potential to magnify the short-term results of multidisciplinary interventions aimed at weight loss/improvement of functional and health status and maintaining long-term benefits. This may also lead to a reduction in pharmacological therapies and health costs. More targeted and personalised therapies may also lead to more efficient use of resources for health systems through efficiencies in care delivery.

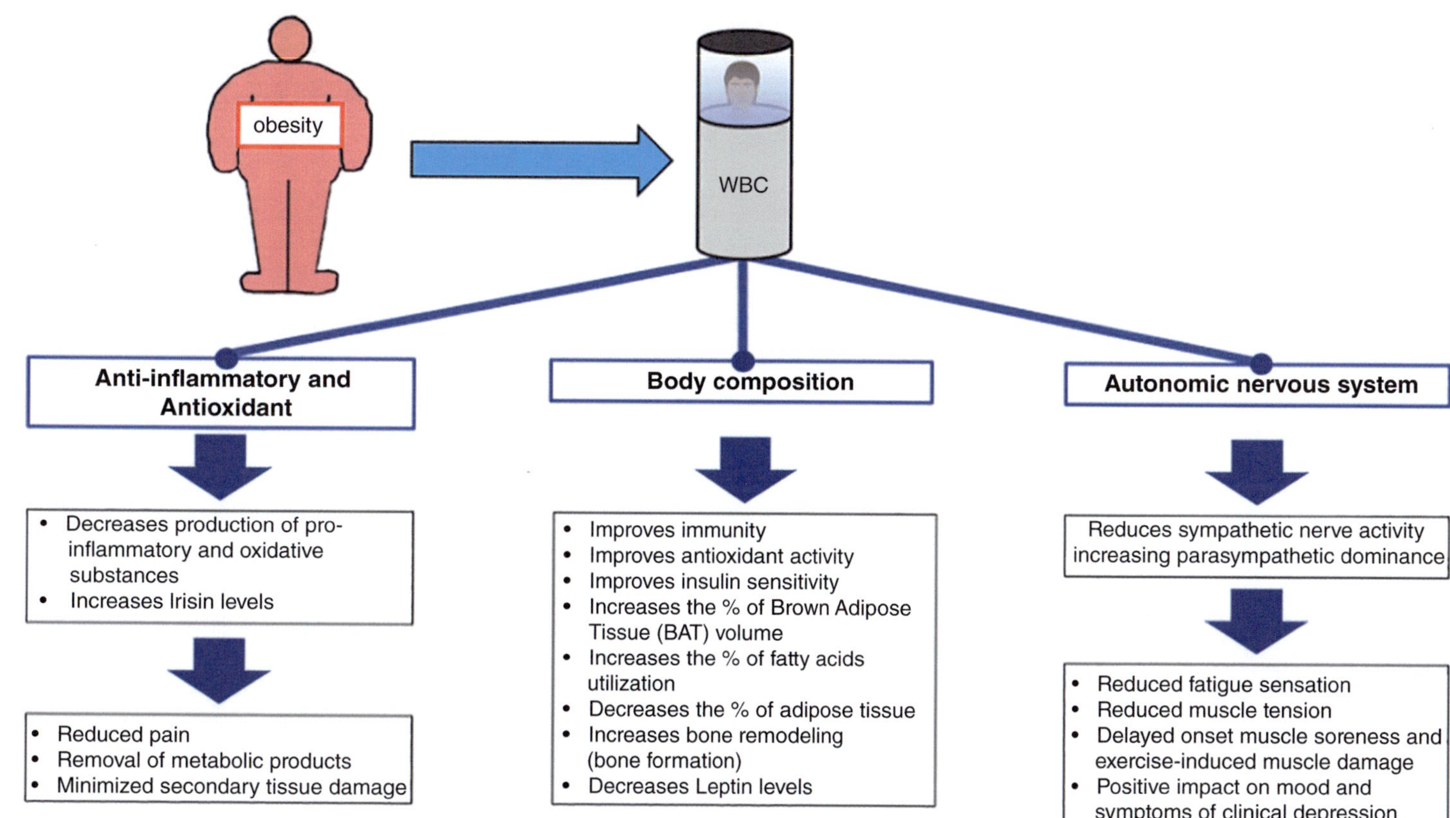

Fig. 11.1 Effects of WBC on obesity

Gender differences will also have to be taken into account: in fact, muscle, bone and fat mass differ between men and women and such gender differences call for personalised WBC protocols. We know that cardiovascular diseases (CVD) have been studied mainly in men, but they are the first cause of mortality and disability in women. Gender differences have obvious relevance to the efficacy and side effect profiles of various treatments in the two sexes, including WBC. Premenopausal women have a lower CVD risk than men; this disappears after menopause with deterioration of glucose homeostasis. The lower risk of type 2 diabetes mellitus (T2DM) and CVD in premenopausal women might have created an important misconception that these diseases are of less importance in women than in men. Women with T2DM have similar CVD risks as men with T2DM, which suggests that the presence of T2DM might offset the protective cardiovascular effects of being female. Sexual dimorphism in adipose tissue, skeletal muscle and liver substrate metabolism contributes considerably to gender differences in tissue-specific insulin sensitivity and cardiometabolic health. Women have a higher adipose tissue mass for a given BMI but store a higher proportion of excess energy in subcutaneous lower body adipose depots. Premenopausal women have a larger capacity to store lipids in skeletal muscle than men matched for age and BMI. However, they are characterised by lower lipid-induced insulin resistance and higher insulin-mediated glucose uptake than men. A better understanding of the physiology of gender differences in adipose tissue distribution, skeletal muscle and liver substrate metabolism would lead to the development of gender-specific treatments of obesity and diabetes, including WBC. Given the limitations of the included studies, the data reviewed in this chapter fail to reach definitive conclusions regarding the efficacy of WBC as an add-on treatment in the management of obesity. Available data are still scanty and inconsistent, and the quality of the studies generally remains low.

References

1. Wharton S, Lau DCW, Vallis M, et al. Obesity in adults: a clinical practice guideline. CMAJ. 2020;192:E875–91.
2. Kuk JL, Ardern CI, Church TS, Sharma AM, Padwal R, Sui X, Blair SN. Edmonton obesity staging system: association with weight history and mortality risk. Appl Physiol Nutr Metab. 2011;36:570–6.
3. Byrne NM, Meerkin JD, Laukkanen R, Ross R, Fogelholm M, Hills AP. Weight loss strategies for obese adults: personalized weight management program vs. standard care. Obesity. 2006;14:1777–88.
4. Glandt M, Raz I. Present and future: pharmacologic treatment of obesity. J Obes. 2011;2011:e636181.
5. Garvey WT, Birkenfeld AL, Dicker D, Mingrone G, Pedersen SD, Satylganova A, Skovgaard D, Sugimoto D, Jensen C, Mosenzon O. Efficacy and safety of Liraglutide 3.0 mg in individuals with overweight or obesity and type 2 diabetes treated with basal insulin: the SCALE insulin randomized controlled trial. Diabetes Care. 2020;43:1085–93.
6. Anderson JW, Konz EC, Frederich RC, Wood CL. Long-term weight-loss maintenance: a meta-analysis of US studies. Am J Clin Nutr. 2001;74:579–84.
7. Castellani W, Ianni L, Ricca V, Mannucci E, Rotella CM. Adherence to structured physical exercise in overweight and obese subjects: a review of psychological models. Eat Weight Disord. 2003;8:1–11.

8. Franco M, Bilal U, Orduñez P, Benet M, Morejón A, Caballero B, Kennelly JF, Cooper RS. Population-wide weight loss and regain in relation to diabetes burden and cardiovascular mortality in Cuba 1980-2010: repeated cross sectional surveys and ecological comparison of secular trends. BMJ. 2013;346:f1515.

9. Ziemann E, Zembroñ-Lacny A, Kasperska A, Antosiewicz J, Grzywacz T, Garsztka T, Laskowski R. Exercise training-induced changes in inflammatory mediators and heat shock proteins in young tennis players. J Sports Sci Med. 2013;12:282–9.

10. Beavers KM, Brinkley TE, Nicklas BJ. Effect of exercise training on chronic inflammation. Clin Chim Acta. 2010;411:785–93.

11. Powers SK, Ji LL, Leeuwenburgh C. Exercise training-induced alterations in skeletal muscle antioxidant capacity: a brief review. Med Sci Sports Exerc. 1999;31:987–97.

12. Adamopoulos S, Parissis J, Kroupis C, Georgiadis M, Karatzas D, Karavolias G, Koniavitou K, Coats AJ, Kremastinos DT. Physical training reduces peripheral markers of inflammation in patients with chronic heart failure. Eur Heart J. 2001;22:791–7.

13. Koh Y, Park J. Cell adhesion molecules and exercise. J Inflamm Res. 2018;11:297–306.

14. Burini RC, Anderson E, Durstine JL, Carson JA. Inflammation, physical activity, and chronic disease: an evolutionary perspective. Sports Med Health Sci. 2020;2:1–6.

15. Kirk B, Feehan J, Lombardi G, Duque G. Muscle, bone, and fat crosstalk: the biological role of myokines, osteokines, and adipokines. Curr Osteoporos Rep. 2020;18:388–400.

16. De Glisezinski I, Crampes F, Harant I, Berlan M, Hejnova J, Langin D, Rivière D, Stich V. Endurance training changes in lipolytic responsiveness of obese adipose tissue. Am J Physiol. 1998;275:E951–6.

17. You T, Berman DM, Ryan AS, Nicklas BJ. Effects of hypocaloric diet and exercise training on inflammation and adipocyte lipolysis in obese postmenopausal women. J Clin Endocrinol Metab. 2004;89:1739–46.

18. Liu Y, Hong F, Lebaka VR, Mohammed A, Ji L, Zhang Y, Korivi M. Calorie restriction with exercise intervention improves inflammatory response in overweight and obese adults: a systematic review and meta-analysis. Front Physiol. 2021;12:754731.

19. Petridou A, Siopi A, Mougios V. Exercise in the management of obesity. Metabolism. 2019;92:163–9.

20. Redman L, Tam C, Covington J, Ravussin E. Little evidence of systemic and adipose tissue inflammation in overweight individuals. Front Genet. 2012;3:58.

21. White GE, Wells GD. Cold-water immersion and other forms of cryotherapy: physiological changes potentially affecting recovery from high-intensity exercise. Extreme Physiol Med. 2013;2:26.

22. Lombardi G, Ziemann E, Banfi G. Whole-body cryotherapy in athletes: from therapy to stimulation. An updated review of the literature. Front Physiol. 2017;8:258.

23. Rymaszewska J, Ramsey D, Chładzińska-Kiejna S. Whole-body cryotherapy as adjunct treatment of depressive and anxiety disorders. Arch Immunol Ther Exp (Warsz). 2008;56:63–8.

24. Castellani JW, Young AJ. Human physiological responses to cold exposure: acute responses and acclimatization to prolonged exposure. Auton Neurosci Basic Clin. 2016;196:63–74.

25. Gordon CJ. The therapeutic potential of regulated hypothermia. Emerg Med J. 2001;18:81–9.

26. Gordon CJ, Fogarty AL, Greenleaf JE, Taylor NAS, Stocks JM. Direct and indirect methods for determining plasma volume during thermoneutral and cold-water immersion. Eur J Appl Physiol. 2003;89:471–4.

27. Pilch W, Wyrostek J, Piotrowska A, Czerwińska-Ledwig O, Zuziak R, Sadowska-Krępa E, Maciejczyk M, Żychowska M. Blood pro-oxidant/antioxidant balance in young men with class II obesity after 20 sessions of whole body cryostimulation: a preliminary study. Redox Rep. 2021;26:10–7.

28. Hanssen MJW, van der Lans AAJJ, Brans B, Hoeks J, Jardon KMC, Schaart G, Mottaghy FM, Schrauwen P, van Marken Lichtenbelt WD. Short-term cold acclimation recruits Brown adipose tissue in obese humans. Diabetes. 2016;65:1179–89.

29. Wiecek M, Szymura J, Sproull J, Szygula Z. Whole-body cryotherapy is an effective method of reducing abdominal obesity in menopausal women with metabolic syndrome. J Clin Med. 2020;9:2797.

30. Leppäluoto J, Westerlund T, Huttunen P, Oksa J, Smolander J, Dugué B, Mikkelsson M. Effects of long-term whole-body cold exposures on plasma concentrations of ACTH, beta-endorphin, cortisol, catecholamines and cytokines in healthy females. Scand J Clin Lab Invest. 2008;68:145–53.
31. Bouzigon R, Dupuy O, Tiemessen I, De Nardi M, Bernard J-P, Mihailovic T, Theurot D, Miller ED, Lombardi G, Dugué BM. Cryostimulation for post-exercise recovery in athletes: a consensus and position paper. Front Sports Act Living. 2021;3:688828.
32. Dulian K, Laskowski R, Grzywacz T, Kujach S, Flis DJ, Smaruj M, Ziemann E. The whole body cryostimulation modifies irisin concentration and reduces inflammation in middle aged, obese men. Cryobiology. 2015;71:398–404.
33. Lubkowska A, Dudzińska W, Bryczkowska I, Dołęgowska B. Body composition, lipid profile, adipokine concentration, and antioxidant capacity changes during interventions to treat overweight with exercise programme and whole-body cryostimulation. Oxid Med Cell Longev. 2015;2015:803197.
34. Pilch W, Wyrostek J, Major P, Zuziak R, Piotrowska A, Czerwińska-Ledwig O, Grzybkowska A, Zasada M, Ziemann E, Żychowska M. The effect of whole-body cryostimulation on body composition and leukocyte expression of HSPA1A, HSPB1, and CRP in obese men. Cryobiology. 2020;94:100–6.
35. Wyrostek J, Piotrowska A, Czerwińska-Ledwig O, Zuziak R, Szyguła Z, Cisoń T, Żychowska M, Pilch W. Complex effects of whole body cryostimulation on hematological markers in patients with obesity. PLoS One. 2021;16:e0249812.
36. Ziemann E, Olek RA, Grzywacz T, Antosiewicz J, Kujach S, Łuszczyk M, Smaruj M, Śledziewska E, Laskowski R. Whole-body cryostimulation as an effective method of reducing low-grade inflammation in obese men. J Physiol Sci. 2013;63:333–43.
37. Purdy JC, Shatzel JJ. The hematologic consequences of obesity. Eur J Haematol. 2021;106:306–19.
38. Banffi G, Krajewska M, Melegati G, Patacchini M. Effects of whole-body cryotherapy on haematological values in athletes. Br J Sports Med. 2008;42:858.
39. Lombardi G, Lanteri P, Porcelli S, Mauri C, Colombini A, Grasso D, Zani V, Bonomi FG, Melegati G, Banfi G. Hematological profile and martial status in Rugby players during whole body cryostimulation. PLoS One. 2013;8:e55803.
40. Szygula Z, Lubkowska A, Giemza C, Skrzek A, Bryczkowska I, Dołęgowska B. Hematological parameters, and hematopoietic growth factors: Epo and IL-3 in response to whole-body cryostimulation (WBC) in military academy students. PLoS One. 2014;9:e93096.
41. Guillot X, Tordi N, Mourot L, Demougeot C, Dugué B, Prati C, Wendling D. Cryotherapy in inflammatory rheumatic diseases: a systematic review. Expert Rev Clin Immunol. 2014;10:281–94.
42. Ramos EJB, Xu Y, Romanova I, Middleton F, Chen C, Quinn R, Inui A, Das U, Meguid MM. Is obesity an inflammatory disease? Surgery. 2003;134:329–35.
43. Banfi G, Melegati G, Barassi A, d'Eril GM. Effects of the whole-body cryotherapy on NTproBNP, hsCRP and troponin I in athletes. J Sci Med Sport. 2009;12:609–10.
44. Stanek A, Wielkoszyński T, Bartuś S, Cholewka A. Whole-body cryostimulation improves inflammatory endothelium parameters and decreases oxidative stress in healthy subjects. Antioxidants (Basel). 2020;9:1308.
45. Ziemann E, Olek RA, Kujach S, Grzywacz T, Antosiewicz J, Garsztka T, Laskowski R. Five-day whole-body cryostimulation, blood inflammatory markers, and performance in high-ranking professional tennis players. J Athl Train. 2012;47:664–72.
46. Pilch W, Piotrowska A, Wyrostek J, Czerwińska-Ledwig O, Ziemann E, Antosiewicz J, Zasada M, Kulesa-Mrowiecka M, Żychowska M. Different changes in adipokines, lipid profile, and TNF-alpha levels between 10 and 20 whole body cryostimulation sessions in individuals with I and II degrees of obesity. Biomedicines. 2022;10:269.
47. Furukawa S, Fujita T, Shimabukuro M, Iwaki M, Yamada Y, Nakajima Y, Nakayama O, Makishima M, Matsuda M, Shimomura I. Increased oxidative stress in obesity and its impact on metabolic syndrome. J Clin Invest. 2004;114:1752–61.

48. Lange U, Uhlemann C, Müller-Ladner U. Serielle Ganzkörperkältetherapie im Criostream bei entzündlich-rheumatischen Erkrankungen. Med Klin. 2008;103:383–8.
49. Petersen AMW, Pedersen BK. The anti-inflammatory effect of exercise. J Appl Physiol (1985). 2005;98:1154–62.
50. Villar-Fincheira P, Sanhueza-Olivares F, Norambuena-Soto I, Cancino-Arenas N, Hernandez-Vargas F, Troncoso R, Gabrielli L, Chiong M. Role of Interleukin-6 in vascular health and disease. Front Mol Biosci. 2021;8:641734.
51. Park HS, Park JY, Yu R. Relationship of obesity and visceral adiposity with serum concentrations of CRP, TNF-α and IL-6. Diabetes Res Clin Pract. 2005;69:29–35.
52. van Hall G, Steensberg A, Sacchetti M, et al. Interleukin-6 stimulates lipolysis and fat oxidation in humans. J Clin Endocrinol Metab. 2003;88:3005–10.
53. Lombardi G, Sanchis-Gomar F, Perego S, Sansoni V, Banfi G. Implications of exercise-induced adipo-myokines in bone metabolism. Endocrine. 2016;54:284–305.
54. Lubkowska A, Szygula Z, Klimek AJ, Torii M. Do sessions of cryostimulation have influence on white blood cell count, level of IL6 and total oxidative and antioxidative status in healthy men? Eur J Appl Physiol. 2010;109:67–72.
55. Lubkowska A, Szyguła Z, Chlubek D, Banfi G. The effect of prolonged whole-body cryostimulation treatment with different amounts of sessions on chosen pro- and anti-inflammatory cytokines levels in healthy men. Scand J Clin Lab Invest. 2011;71:419–25.
56. Pournot H, Bieuzen F, Louis J, Fillard J-R, Barbiche E, Hausswirth C. Time-course of changes in inflammatory response after whole-body cryotherapy multi exposures following severe exercise. PLoS One. 2011;6:e22748.
57. Śliwicka E, Cisoń T, Straburzyńska-Lupa A, Pilaczyńska-Szcześniak Ł. Effects of whole-body cryotherapy on 25-hydroxyvitamin D, irisin, myostatin, and interleukin-6 levels in healthy young men of different fitness levels. Sci Rep. 2020;10:6175.
58. Speakman JR. Chapter 26—Obesity and thermoregulation. In: Romanovsky AA, editor. Handbook of clinical neurology. Elsevier; 2018. pp. 431–443.
59. Martínez Larrad MT, Corbatón Anchuelo A, Fernández Pérez C, Pérez Barba M, Lazcano Redondo Y, Serrano Ríos M, Segovia Insulin Resistance Study Group (SIRSG). Obesity and cardiovascular risk: variations in Visfatin gene can modify the obesity associated cardiovascular risk. Results from the Segovia population based-study. Spain. PLoS One. 2016;11:e0153976.
60. Cheng L, Wang J, Dai H, et al. Brown and beige adipose tissue: a novel therapeutic strategy for obesity and type 2 diabetes mellitus. Adipocyte. 2021;10:48–65.
61. Boström P, Wu J, Jedrychowski MP, et al. A PGC1-α-dependent myokine that drives brown-fat-like development of white fat and thermogenesis. Nature. 2012;481:463–8.
62. Meier U, Gressner AM. Endocrine regulation of energy metabolism: review of pathobiochemical and clinical chemical aspects of leptin, ghrelin, adiponectin, and resistin. Clin Chem. 2004;50:1511–25.
63. Valassi E, Scacchi M, Cavagnini F. Neuroendocrine control of food intake. Nutr Metab Cardiovasc Dis. 2008;18:158–68.
64. Vega GL, Grundy SM. Metabolic risk susceptibility in men is partially related to adiponectin/leptin ratio. J Obes. 2013;2013:e409679.
65. Hotta K, Funahashi T, Arita Y, et al. Plasma concentrations of a novel, adipose-specific protein, adiponectin, in type 2 diabetic patients. Arterioscler Thromb Vasc Biol. 2000;20:1595–9.
66. Ahima RS, Lazar MA. Adipokines and the peripheral and neural control of energy balance. Mol Endocrinol. 2008;22:1023–31.
67. Collins S, Daniel KW, Rohlfs EM, Ramkumar V, Taylor IL, Gettys TW. Impaired expression and functional activity of the beta 3- and beta 1-adrenergic receptors in adipose tissue of congenitally obese (C57BL/6J ob/ob) mice. Mol Endocrinol. 1994;8:518–27.
68. Hausswirth C, Schaal K, Le Meur Y, Bieuzen F, Filliard J-R, Volondat M, Louis J. Parasympathetic activity and blood catecholamine responses following a single partial-body cryostimulation and a whole-body cryostimulation. PLoS One. 2013;8:e72658.
69. Zalewski P, Klawe JJ, Pawlak J, Tafil-Klawe M, Newton J. Thermal and hemodynamic response to whole-body cryostimulation in healthy subjects. Cryobiology. 2013;66:295–302.

70. Louis J, Theurot D, Filliard J-R, Volondat M, Dugué B, Dupuy O. The use of whole-body cryotherapy: time- and dose-response investigation on circulating blood catecholamines and heart rate variability. Eur J Appl Physiol. 2020;120:1733–43.
71. Valgas P, da Silva C, Hernández-Saavedra D, White JD, Stanford KI. Cold and exercise: therapeutic tools to activate brown adipose tissue and combat obesity. Biology. 2019;8:9.
72. Sellers AJ, Pallubinsky H, Rense P, Bijnens W, van de Weijer T, Moonen-Kornips E, Schrauwen P, van Marken Lichtenbelt WD. The effect of cold exposure with shivering on glucose tolerance in healthy men. J Appl Physiol (1985). 2021;130:193–205.
73. Ivanova YM, Blondin DP. Examining the benefits of cold exposure as a therapeutic strategy for obesity and type 2 diabetes. J Appl Physiol (1985). 2021;130:1448–59.
74. Straburzyńska-Lupa A, Cisoń T, Gomarasca M, Babińska A, Banfi G, Lombardi G, Śliwicka E. Sclerostin and bone remodeling biomarkers responses to whole-body cryotherapy (− 110 °C) in healthy young men with different physical fitness levels. Sci Rep. 2021;11:16156.
75. Gerosa L, Lombardi G. Bone-to-brain: a round trip in the adaptation to mechanical stimuli. Front Physiol. 2021;12:623893.
76. Galliera E, Dogliotti G, Melegati G, Corsi Romanelli MM, Cabitza P, Banfi G. Bone remodelling biomarkers after whole body cryotherapy (WBC) in elite rugby players. Injury. 2013;44:1117–21.
77. Heart rate variability. Standards of measurement, physiological interpretation, and clinical use. Task Force of the European Society of Cardiology and the North American Society of Pacing and Electrophysiology. Eur Heart J. 1996;17:354–381.
78. Grassi G, Biffi A, Seravalle G, Trevano FQ, Dell'Oro R, Corrao G, Mancia G. Sympathetic neural overdrive in the obese and overweight state. Hypertension. 2019;74:349–58.
79. Bellocchi C, Carandina A, Montinaro B, Targetti E, Furlan L, Rodrigues GD, Tobaldini E, Montano N. The interplay between autonomic nervous system and inflammation across systemic autoimmune diseases. Int J Mol Sci. 2022;23:2449.
80. Pongratz G, Straub RH. The sympathetic nervous response in inflammation. Arthritis Res Ther. 2014;16:504.
81. Borovikova LV, Ivanova S, Zhang M, Yang H, Botchkina GI, Watkins LR, Wang H, Abumrad N, Eaton JW, Tracey KJ. Vagus nerve stimulation attenuates the systemic inflammatory response to endotoxin. Nature. 2000;405:458–62.
82. Maule S, Quadri R, Mirante D, Pellerito RA, Marucco E, Marinone C, Vergani D, Chiandussi L, Zanone MM. Autonomic nervous dysfunction in systemic lupus erythematosus (SLE) and rheumatoid arthritis (RA): possible pathogenic role of autoantibodies to autonomic nervous structures. Clin Exp Immunol. 1997;110:423–7.
83. Capodaglio P, Cremascoli R, Piterà P, Fontana JM. Whole-body Cryostimulation: a rehabilitation booster. J Rehabil Med Clin Commun. 2022;5:2810.
84. Theurot D, Dugué B, Douzi W, Guitet P, Louis J, Dupuy O. Impact of acute partial-body cryostimulation on cognitive performance, cerebral oxygenation, and cardiac autonomic activity. Sci Rep. 2021;11:7793.
85. Louis J, Schaal K, Bieuzen F, Le Meur Y, Filliard J-R, Volondat M, Brisswalter J, Hausswirth C. Head exposure to cold during whole-body cryostimulation: influence on thermal response and autonomic modulation. PLoS One. 2015;10:e0124776.
86. Storniolo JL, Chaulan M, Esposti R, Cavallari P. A single session of whole-body cryotherapy boosts maximal cycling performance and enhances vagal drive at rest. Exp Brain Res. 2023;241:383–93.

Multiple Sclerosis

12

Ewa Zielińska-Nowak and Elżbieta Miller

Introduction

Multiple sclerosis (MS) is a multifactorial autoimmune disease of the central nervous system (CNS) that is characterized by chronic inflammation, demyelination, oxidative stress, and axon and neuronal loss [1]. It is the most common nontraumatic disabling disease that predominantly affects young adults [2]. Over time, the incidence and prevalence of MS have been rising in both developed and developing countries, though the exact underlying cause remains unclear. MS is known to be a multifaceted condition, influenced by a combination of factors. Genetic factors play a role, with several genes contributing to a modest increase in disease susceptibility. Research indicates that oxidative/nitroxidative stress plays a significant role in the development, progression, and clinical manifestations of MS [3]. Additionally, specific environmental factors have been identified, including exposure to vitamin D or ultraviolet B light (UVB), infection with the Epstein-Barr virus (EBV), obesity, and smoking, which have been linked to the development and progression of MS [4]. Traditionally, MS has been found as a two-stage disease process. The initial stage is characterized by inflammation, which is primarily responsible for the relapsing-remitting course of the disease. In this stage, patients experience periods of neurological exacerbations followed by partial or complete recovery. The second stage involves delayed neurodegeneration, leading to a nonrelapsing progressive course, referred to as secondary and primary progressive MS, respectively. During this stage, patients may experience a gradual worsening of symptoms and disability, without experiencing distinct relapses and remissions [5].

E. Zielińska-Nowak · E. Miller (✉)
Department of Neurological Rehabilitation, Medical University of Lodz, Lodz, Poland
e-mail: ewa.zielinska@umed.lodz.pl; elzbieta.dorota.miller@umed.lodz.pl

P. Capodaglio (ed.), *Whole-Body Cryostimulation*,
https://doi.org/10.1007/978-3-031-18545-8_12

The clinical symptoms of MS may vary depending on the location of the demyelinating lesions. They can include motor, sensory, and cognitive impairment. The most prevalent symptoms are numbness, muscle spasms, ataxia, gait disturbances, bladder disfunctions, visual problems, fatigue, pain, depression, and MS-related dementia [6, 7].

The management of MS involves the treatment with immunomodulatory agents, which aim to modify the disease's course and symptomatic management, which focuses on alleviating specific symptoms experienced by MS patients. During acute relapses, corticosteroids, such as methylprednisolone, and adrenocorticotropic hormone (ACTH) are commonly used. These medications possess anti-inflammatory and immunomodulatory properties and are used to expedite recovery from acute relapses, hastening the return to a more stable neurological state [6].

The Role of WBC as Adjuvant Treatment of MS

Standard treatment of MS may not be fully effective for all patients. Some individuals may experience limited benefits or adverse effects, leading to a demand for alternative options. Some patients may benefit from a combination of conventional and alternative therapies. Integrating alternative approaches with standard treatments can be a way to optimize patient outcomes and address multiple aspects of the disease.

Ongoing research is aimed on discovering potential advantages of whole-body cryotherapy (WBC) on patients with MS. Several potential benefits have already been confirmed, indicating an expanding array of possible applications. In Table 12.1, there is a summary of existing research on the effect of WBC on individuals with MS (Table 12.1).

Table 12.1 Research on the influence of WBC on individuals with MS

Author, year	Number of participants	WBC protocol		Main outcomes
		Total WBC procedures/ WBC per week/number of weeks	Procedure	
Miller et al. (2010) [8]	MS WBC + kinesiotherapy = 16 MS WBC n = 16 Control n = 20	10/5/2	Time: 2–3 min Temp: Atrium = −60 °C Main chamber = First session: −110 °C Last session: −160 °C	Positive antioxidant effects Increase of TAS
Miller et al. (2011) [9]	MS D (depression) n = 12 MS non-D (nondepressive) n = 10	10/5/2	Time: 2–3 min Temp: Atrium = −60 °C Main chamber = First session: −110 °C Last session: −160 °C	Suppresses oxidative stress, especially in depressive MS patients
Miller et al. (2013) [10]	WBC (SPMS) = 22 Control n = 22	10/5/2	Time: 3 min Temp: Atrium = −60 °C Main chamber = −130 °C	Increase of uric acid blood level Improvement in functional status
Miller et al. (2016) [11]	WBC low fatigue (LF) = 24 WBC high fatigue (HF) = 24	10/5/2	Time: 2–3 min Temp: Atrium = −60 °C Main chamber = First session: −110 °C Last session: −160 °C	Improvement in the functional status and in the feeling of fatigue

(continued)

Table 12.1 (continued)

Author, year	Number of participants	WBC protocol		Main outcomes
		Total WBC procedures/ WBC per week/number of weeks	Procedure	
Bryczkowska et al. (2018) [12]	WBC $n = 30$	30	Time: 3 min Temp: Atrium = −60 °C Main chamber = −130 °C	Significant increase in SOD1 activity 2. No significant changes in total protein, albumin, uric acid, and glucose concentrations and lipid profile
Ptaszek et al. (2021) [13]	WBC-MS = 15 Control-MS = 20 Control-WBC = 15	20/5/4	Time: 1, 5–3 min Temp: Atrium = −60 °C Main chamber = −120 °C	Changes in the levels of RBC, HGB, HCT, elongation index, AMP, and proteins (including fibrinogen) No significant effect on changes in blood counts, rheology, and biochemistry
Ptaszek et al. (2022) [14]	WBC = 15 Control = 15	20/5/4	Time: 1, 5–3 min Temp: Atrium = −60 °C Main chamber = −120 °C After: cycloergometer 15 min	No significant effect on changes in iron status and neuroplasticity biomarkers (BDNF, NGF, PDGF, VEGF, and IGF-1) in either MS or healthy women Lower level of transferrin in MS

Author, year	Number of participants	WBC protocol		Main outcomes
		Total WBC procedures/ WBC per week/number of weeks	Procedure	
Lubkowska et al. (2019) [15]	WBC = 25	20/5/4	Time: 2–3 min Temp: −110 °C After: 30 min of individual physical rehabilitation	Improvement of thumb strength No statistically significant changes in global walking function
Pawik et al. (2019) [16]	WBC = 20 WBC + gym = 20 Gym = 20	10/5/2	Temp: First session: −110 °C Last session: −160 °C After: 60 min exercises for WBC + gym and gym group	Reduction of depressive symptoms; improved functional status
Radecka et al. (2021) [17]	WBC = 60 Control = 54	20/5/4	Time: 2–3 min Temp: −110 °C After: 15-min kinesiotherapy exercises conducted in groups of 5–6 people	In the rest electromyograms, an increase of extensor carpi radialis (ECR) and a decrease of flexor carpi radialis (FCR) amplitude; gait improvement; decrease of fatigue

Impact of WBC on Biochemical Markers

Oxidative Stress

Growing evidence indicates that oxidative stress significantly contributes to the development of various neurodegenerative diseases, including MS. Markers related to inflammation, myelination, and neuronal integrity have been areas of interest and advancement for years, but oxidative stress has remained an area of unrealized potential [18]. Studies have shown that there is a possibility of using antioxidant therapies as an additional treatment of MS. Given the involvement of oxidative damage in inflammatory and autoimmune-mediated tissue destruction, the modulation of oxygen-free radical production emerges as a promising new approach for the treatment of inflammatory and autoimmune diseases [19].

Studies exploring the effects of WBC on oxidative stress in patients with MS have shown promising results. The study by Miller et al. revealed positive antioxidant effects of WBC on MS patients; moreover, WBC caused statistically significant increase of total antioxidative status (TAS) in plasma of MS patients (from 0.3468 to 0.8126 mM) compared to non-WBC MS patients [8]. In another study the increase of TAS was also noted, whereas antioxidative enzymes superoxide dismutase (SOD) and catalase (CAT) activities in erythrocytes of MS patients were not changed in response to a series of ten WBC sessions. The change was more significant in a group of MS patients with depression compared to a group of nondepressive MS patients [9]. On the other hand, in a study Bryczkowska et al., where the effect of WBC on the systemic antioxidant potential in MS patients was investigated, a significant increase in the activity of two antioxidant enzymes, SOD and glutathione transferase (GST), was observed.

Uric acid, which is also associated with antioxidant and neuroprotective properties, has been the focus of research to explore its potential role in mitigating oxidative stress, protecting nerve cells, and modulating inflammation in various neurological conditions, including MS [20]. Higher levels of uric acid could help neutralize reactive oxygen species (ROS) and reduce oxidative stress, which contributes to the progression of MS. The effect of WBC on this parameter has also been a subject of interest. One study found that WBC led to an increase in uric acid (UA) concentration in patients' plasma not only immediately after ten WBC exposures but also 1 and 3 months later [10], whereas another investigation revealed no significant changes in UA concentration after 30 sessions of WBC in MS patients [12]. Due to the limited and conflicting evidence available, further investigations are needed to establish a clear understanding of the relationship between WBC and uric acid levels.

Other Blood Parameters

There are also studies assessing other blood parameters, not directly related to oxidative stress. Ptaszek et al. assessed the impact of 20 WBC sessions on the biochemical and rheological indices of blood in people with MS and noted statistically significant differences and changes after WBC in the levels of red blood cells (RBCs), hemoglobin (HGB), hematocrit (HCT), elongation index, total extend of aggregation (AMP), and proteins (including fibrinogen). There was no significant effect on changes in blood counts, rheology, and biochemistry in women with MS. The results confirmed that WBC constitutes a secure therapeutic approach for individuals with MS concerning the examined parameters. This conclusion is based on the fact that changes in blood rheology are not the determining factor behind the treatment's efficacy, and WBC does not exert any adverse effects on red blood cell deformability and aggregation [13]. In another study the effect of a series of 20 WBC sessions on iron levels and neuroplasticity biomarkers (BDNF, NGF, PDGF, VEGF, and IGF-1) in women with MS was analyzed and then compared with a group of healthy women. At the beginning of the study, there were no statistically significant differences between groups, and after 20 sessions, no statistically significant changes were observed in the level of neuroplasticity biomarkers, as well as iron status [14].

WBC as an Impairment-Based Approach

Physical therapy is mainly a symptom-based therapy (impairment-based approach) aimed at individual management tailored to the patient's current needs at a given moment of the disease. While the available literature is still limited, some studies have explored the potential benefits of WBC in MS patients. Although it is sometimes used as a complementary therapy for various conditions, including MS, its effectiveness in managing MS symptoms such as spasticity, fatigue, or depression is still a topic of debate and research. Several studies have explored the effects of WBC on various outcomes in patients with MS, including symptom management, quality of life, and physical performance. The summary of the influence of WBC on MS symptoms with potential future research areas is presented in Fig. 12.1.

Spasticity

Spasticity is a common symptom experienced by people with MS and it refers to muscle stiffness, involuntary muscle contractions, and difficulty with muscle control and coordination. It can cause pain, muscle spasms, and difficulties with movement and mobility.

In general, managing spasticity in MS often involves a multifaceted approach that may include physical therapy, complementary/alternative medicine interventions, oral medications, chemodenervation, implantation of an intrathecal baclofen pump medications, assistive devices, and lifestyle modifications [21]. Multiple sclerosis (MS) stands as the most prevalent autoimmune disease impacting the CNS, with spasticity emerging as one of its most debilitating symptoms. Occurring in over 80% of MS patients at some stage of the disease, spasticity significantly

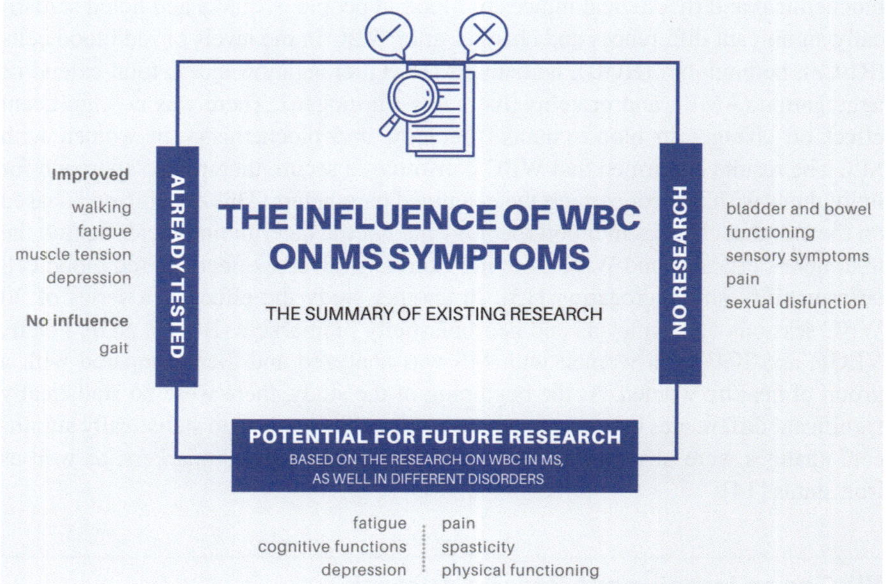

Fig. 12.1 The influence of WBC on MS symptoms and potential future research

impairs ambulation, induces pain, and contributes to development of contractures [22].

The available literature lacks data about the influence of WBC on muscle activity in patients with MS. Based on several studies, it is suggested that the beneficial impact of WBC on muscles could be linked to alterations in its bioelectric state due to reduced nerve conduction and decreased reactivity of peripheral sensory nerve endings [23, 24].

There is limited scientific evidence regarding the specific effects of WBC on spasticity in MS; however, there are studies confirming the positive impact of local cryotherapy on spasticity in different neurological conditions such as stroke [25]. There is only one study where MS patients underwent a series of 20 WBC treatments and in the rest electromyograms—an increase of extensor carpi radialis (ECR) and a decrease of flexor carpi radialis (FCR) amplitude were demonstrated (nonnormalized signal ECR $p = 0.0001$). It was also observed that significant differences in sEMG rest signals between ECR and FCR have decreased, and for voluntary contraction in both assessed antagonistic muscles, amplitude was significantly decreased, which may suggest a normalizing effect of the WBC treatment on muscle tension in MS patients [17].

Taking that into account, it is worth considering WBC as a potential factor supporting the treatment of spasticity also in MS; however, it is important to note that the existing research in this area is limited, and more rigorous studies are needed to draw definitive conclusions.

Fatigue

Fatigue syndrome occurs in approximately 75–95% of patients with MS [26–28] and may be unnoticed in physical examination and be misinterpreted as a symptom of depression. Symptoms of fatigue may affect both physically fit and severely disabled people, significantly reducing the ability to function in everyday life, perform professional work, and/or participate in social life [29, 30].

Fatigue can have a significant impact on various aspects of life, including quality of life, emotional well-being (depression and anxiety), motor function, and sleep patterns [26]. Despite ongoing research, the underlying mechanisms of fatigue in MS have not been fully elucidated, leading to challenges in effectively treating this symptom. Fatigue occurrence is associated with structural damage of white matter and gray matter and inflammation within or outside the CNS [27]. Furthermore, sleep disturbances, depression, heat, physical deconditioning, or side effects of medications can also exacerbate this symptom. The research on the effect of WBC on fatigue is limited; however, there are some studies indicating the potential of WBC in alleviating this troublesome symptom. In a group of 32 participants with chronic fatigue syndrome (CFS), a significant decrease in fatigue was noted in response to ten sessions of WBC and static stretching exercises. It was also observed that some domains of cognitive functioning also improved both in SCS and control groups [28]. There is also one study evaluating the influence of WBC on fatigue in MS, where 72 patients with fatigue were divided into two groups depending on the level of fatigue, high fatigue (HF) and low fatigue (LF). After ten sessions of WBC, fatigue was reduced in both of them; however, greater changes were observed in the HF group [11].

Functional Status

The way WBC affects functional status of MS patients has also been an area of interest.

A study published in 2016 investigated the effects of WBC on functional status in individuals with MS. The researchers observed improvements in all three Rivermead tests after a series of ten WBC sessions [11]. Furthermore, in the same study, patients showed a decrease in the disability score (Expanded Disability Status Scale [EDSS]). Pawik et al. noticed a statistically significant improvement in the functional status, measured with the Rivermead Mobility Index after 14 days of therapy with WBC [16].

On the contrary, no significant effect of 20 WBC treatments on improving the walking function, measured by the timed 25-foot walk (T25-FW) test, among people with MS was found; however, researchers stated that the T25-FW test, due to its low sensitivity, seems to be an inappropriate tool for assessing the effect of WBC on this parameter [15].

Psychological Well-Being

Psychological well-being and mental health are significant factors in the overall quality of life for individuals with MS, as the disease can have a substantial impact on emotional and cognitive status. Depression is a common concern among MS patients due to the challenges and uncertainties associated with managing a chronic condition. Certain research investigations have delved into the potential advantages of WBC in enhancing psychological well-being and mitigating symptoms of depression. The mechanism of WBC that can be likened to an "antidepressant" effect involves the activation of hypothalamic structures and the release of endogenous catecholamines, ACTH, cortisol, and beta-endorphins, as indicated by studies [29]. Few studies have confirmed the positive impact of WBC on depressive symptoms [30]. Pawik et al. tested whether WBC could complement standard pharmacological treatment particularly in MS, and the results indicated that the use of WBC reduced anxiety and depressive symptoms in the studied population, particularly when combined with physical exercise training [16].

Cognitive Functioning

Cognitive decline has been extensively reported in patients with MS, with deficits most commonly present in attention, processing speed, working memory, verbal fluency, and executive function. Some studies have shown that ten sessions of WBC might improve cognitive functions among population with mild cognitive impairments [31, 32]; however, none of them were performed among individuals with MS. The evidence regarding the effects of WBC on cognitive function is still evolving and may vary depending on the specific condition. Given the potential implications for individuals with MS, it would be valuable for future research to specifically focus on this population. Tailored studies involving individuals with MS could provide more targeted insights into the potential cognitive benefits of WBC and help establish its role in enhancing cognitive function within this specific context.

Pain

Cryogenic temperatures have proven to have analgesic effect in numerous studies [33–35], although studies examining pain relief through WBC have not been conducted exclusively among MS patients, thus hindering the ability to draw direct conclusions about its efficacy in this context. However, despite this limitation, it remains worthwhile to delve into this subject due to the significant potential it holds for enhancing the quality of life.

Conclusion

In summary, while there is some evidence suggesting potential positive effects of WBC on certain outcomes in patients with MS, the overall research is limited, and the results are not entirely consistent. It is important to consider that the studies in this area have used different protocols for WBC, including variations in temperature, duration, and frequency of sessions. This lack of standardization makes it challenging to draw definitive conclusions; however, available data already show some promising results. Considering the positive impact on overall patient well-being and the low risk of side effects, WBC has the potential to be significantly expanded as a part of symptom management in MS. Further well-designed studies with larger sample sizes and standardized protocols are needed to determine the specific effects of WBC on patients with MS and to establish its role as a complementary therapy for symptom management.

References

1. Compston A, Coles A. Multiple sclerosis. Lancet. 2008;372(9648):1502–17.
2. Kobelt G, Thompson A, Berg J, Gannedahl M, Eriksson J. New insights into the burden and costs of multiple sclerosis in Europe. Mult Scler. 2017;23(8):1123–36.
3. Tobore TO. Oxidative/Nitroxidative stress and multiple sclerosis. J Mol Neurosci. 2021;71(3):506–14.
4. Ascherio A. Environmental factors in multiple sclerosis. Expert Rev Neurother. 2013;13(12 Suppl):3–9.
5. Dobson R, Giovannoni G. Multiple sclerosis—a review. Eur J Neurol. 2019;26(1):27–40.
6. Garg N, Smith TW. An update on immunopathogenesis, diagnosis, and treatment of multiple sclerosis. Brain Behav. 2015;5(9):e00362.
7. Pegoretti V, Swanson KA, Bethea JR, Probert L, Eisel ULM, Fischer R. Inflammation and oxidative stress in multiple sclerosis: consequences for therapy development. Oxid Med Cell Longev. 2020;2020:7191080.
8. Miller E, Mrowicka M, Malinowska K, Zołyński K, Kedziora J. Effects of the whole-body cryotherapy on a total antioxidative status and activities of some antioxidative enzymes in blood of patients with multiple sclerosis-preliminary study. J Med Invest. 2010;57(1–2):168–73.
9. Miller E, Mrowicka M, Malinowska K, Mrowicki J, Saluk-Juszczak J, Kędziora J. Effects of whole-body cryotherapy on a total antioxidative status and activities of antioxidative enzymes in blood of depressive multiple sclerosis patients. World J Biol Psychiatry. 2011;12(3):223–7.
10. Miller E, Saluk J, Morel A, Wachowicz B. Long-term effects of whole body cryostimulation on uric acid concentration in plasma of secondary progressive multiple sclerosis patients. Scand J Clin Lab Invest. 2013;73(8):635–40.
11. Miller E, Kostka J, Włodarczyk T, Dugué B. Whole-body cryostimulation (cryotherapy) provides benefits for fatigue and functional status in multiple sclerosis patients. A case-control study. Acta Neurol Scand. 2016;134(6):420–6.
12. Bryczkowska I, Radecka A, Knyszyńska A, Łuczak J, Lubkowska A. Effect of whole body cryotherapy treatments on antioxidant enzyme activity and biochemical parameters in patients with multiple sclerosis. Fam Med Prim Care Rev. 2018;20:214–7.
13. Ptaszek B, Teległów A, Adamiak J, Głodzik J, Podsiadło S, Mucha D, et al. Effect of whole-body cryotherapy on morphological, rheological and biochemical indices of blood in people with multiple sclerosis. J Clin Med. 2021;10(13):2833.

14. Ptaszek B, Podsiadło S, Czerwińska-Ledwig O, Maciejczyk M, Teległów A. Effect of whole-body cryotherapy on iron status and biomarkers of neuroplasticity in multiple sclerosis women. Healthcare (Basel). 2022;10(9):1681.
15. Lubkowska A, Radecka A, Knyszyńska A, Łuczak J. Effect of whole-body cryotherapy treatments on the functional state of patients with MS (multiple sclerosis) in a timed 25-foot walk test and hand grip strength test. Pomeranian J Life Sci. 2019;65(4):46–9.
16. Pawik M, Kowalska J, Rymaszewska J. The effectiveness of whole-body cryotherapy and physical exercises on the psychological well-being of patients with multiple sclerosis: a comparative analysis. Adv Clin Exp Med. 2019;28(11):1477–83.
17. Radecka A, Knyszyńska A, Łuczak J, Lubkowska A. Adaptive changes in muscle activity after cryotherapy treatment: potential mechanism for improvement the functional state in patients with multiple sclerosis. NeuroRehabilitation. 2021;48(1):119–31.
18. Hollen C, Neilson LE, Barajas RF Jr, Greenhouse I, Spain RI. Oxidative stress in multiple sclerosis-emerging imaging techniques. Front Neurol. 2022;13:1025659.
19. Mirshafiey A, Mohsenzadegan M. Antioxidant therapy in multiple sclerosis. Immunopharmacol Immunotoxicol. 2009;31(1):13–29.
20. Spitsin S, Koprowski H. Role of uric acid in multiple sclerosis. Curr Top Microbiol Immunol. 2008;318:325–42.
21. Hughes C, Howard IM. Spasticity management in multiple sclerosis. Phys Med Rehabil Clin N Am. 2013;24(4):593–604.
22. Patejdl R, Zettl UK. Spasticity in multiple sclerosis: contribution of inflammation, autoimmune mediated neuronal damage and therapeutic interventions. Autoimmun Rev. 2017;16(9):925–36.
23. Ferreira-Junior JB, Vieira CA, Soares SR, Guedes R, Rocha Junior VA, Simoes HG, et al. Effects of a single whole body cryotherapy (−110°C) bout on neuromuscular performance of the elbow flexors during isokinetic exercise. Int J Sports Med. 2014;35(14):1179–83.
24. Giemza C, Matczak-Giemza M, Ostrowska B, Bieć E, Doliński M. Effect of cryotherapy on the lumbar spine in elderly men with back pain. Aging Male. 2014;17(3):183–8.
25. Garcia LC, Alcântara CC, Santos GL, Monção JVA, Russo TL. Cryotherapy reduces muscle spasticity but does not affect proprioception in ischemic stroke: a randomized sham-controlled crossover study. Am J Phys Med Rehabil. 2019;98(1):51–7.
26. Krupp LB, Serafin DJ, Christodoulou C. Multiple sclerosis-associated fatigue. Expert Rev Neurother. 2010;10(9):1437–47.
27. Manjaly ZM, Harrison NA, Critchley HD, Do CT, Stefanics G, Wenderoth N, et al. Pathophysiological and cognitive mechanisms of fatigue in multiple sclerosis. J Neurol Neurosurg Psychiatry. 2019;90(6):642–51.
28. Kujawski S, Słomko J, Godlewska BR, Cudnoch-Jędrzejewska A, Murovska M, Newton JL, et al. Combination of whole body cryotherapy with static stretching exercises reduces fatigue and improves functioning of the autonomic nervous system in chronic fatigue syndrome. J Transl Med. 2022;20(1):273.
29. Rymaszewska J, Tulczynski A, Zagrobelny Z, Kiejna A, Hadrys T. Influence of whole body cryotherapy on depressive symptoms—preliminary report. Acta Neuropsychiatr. 2003;15(3):122–8.
30. Krzystanek M, Romańczyk M, Surma S, Koźmin-Burzyńska A. Whole body cryotherapy and hyperbaric oxygen treatment: new biological treatment of depression? A systematic review. Pharmaceuticals (Basel). 2021;14(6):595.
31. Rymaszewska J, Lion KM, Stańczykiewicz B, Rymaszewska JE, Trypka E, Pawlik-Sobecka L, et al. The improvement of cognitive deficits after whole-body cryotherapy—a randomised controlled trial. Exp Gerontol. 2021;146:111237.
32. Rymaszewska J, Urbanska KM, Szczesniak D, Stanczykiewicz B, Trypka E, Zablocka A. The improvement of memory deficits after whole-body cryotherapy—the first report. Cryo Letters. 2018;39(3):190–5.
33. Salas-Fraire O, Rivera-Pérez JA, Guevara-Neri NP, Urrutia-García K, Martínez-Gutiérrez OA, Salas-Longoria K, et al. Efficacy of whole-body cryotherapy in the treatment of chronic low back pain: quasi-experimental study. J Orthop Sci. 2023;28(1):112–6.

34. Klemm P, Hoffmann J, Asendorf T, Aykara I, Frommer K, Dischereit G, et al. Whole-body cryotherapy for the treatment of rheumatoid arthritis: a monocentric, single-blinded, randomised controlled trial. Clin Exp Rheumatol. 2022;40(11):2133–40.
35. Chruściak T. Subjective evaluation of the effectiveness of whole-body cryotherapy in patients with osteoarthritis. Reumatologia. 2016;54(6):291–5.

Parkinson's Disease

13

Riccardo Cremascoli

Introduction

Parkinson's disease (PD) is a neurodegenerative disorder predominantly affecting the dopamine-producing ('dopaminergic') neurons in a specific area of the brain called substantia nigra [1]. The death of dopaminergic neurons is associated with α-synuclein (αSyn) containing inclusion bodies (Lewy pathology; LP) in the surviving neurons, according to a spreading pattern toward the central nervous system via the olfactory bulb and the vagus nerve [2]. Eventually, the aggregated α-Synuclein arrives at the substantia nigra [2]. In this view, clinical symptoms of PD are not only restricted to motor impairment (as a result of dopamine deficit), but they also include olfactory loss, constipation, mood disorder, cardiac sympathetic denervation, reduction in heart rate variability, orthostatic hypotension and rapid eye movement (REM) behaviour disorder [1]. Cognitive impairment is also a frequent event in the late stage of PD [3]. This chapter presents a summary of the potential effects of cryostimulation on Parkinson's disease, taking into account the evidence about cold exposure in this pathology.

Whole-Body Cryostimulation and Autonomic Dysfunction in Parkinson's Disease

Due to the link between LP deposition in brainstem and vagal nerve impairment in PD, the autonomic nervous system has been deeply investigated in PD patients both in pre-clinical and clinical settings. Autonomic dysfunction in PD covers a broad

R. Cremascoli (✉)
Neurology and Neurorehabilitation Unit, IRCCS Istituto Auxologico Italiano,
Piancavallo (Verbania), Italy
e-mail: r.cremascoli@auxologico.it

P. Capodaglio (ed.), *Whole-Body Cryostimulation*,
https://doi.org/10.1007/978-3-031-18545-8_13

spectrum that includes gastrointestinal, cardiovascular, sexual, urological and thermoregulatory dysfunctions [4]. Stated the purpose of this summary, we will focus the attention on cardiovascular and thermoregulatory dysfunctions.

Cardiovascular Dysfunction

Cardiovascular autonomic dysfunction in PD could be characterised by both preganglionic (baroreflex failure) and postganglionic (sympathetic denervation) lesions [5]. The association of these two factors leads to the development of neurogenic orthostatic hypotension (nOH), supine hypertension and postprandial hypotension [5]. Cardiac sympathetic denervation clearly is evident in PD [6] and can be visualised by both I123-meta-iodobenzylguanidine (I123-MIBG) imaging [7] and 18fluoro-dopamine PET imaging [8]. Cardiac denervation by itself, however, does not appear to be responsible for the blood pressure irregularities that characterise PD [5, 9, 10]. In fact, abnormal aggregation of α-synuclein is present in the autonomic parasympathetic system, in particular in the dorsal vagal motor nucleus (DMV) [2]. Recent studies indicate that cardiac parasympathetic dysfunction occurs in the early phase of PD, but not necessarily in parallel with cardiac sympathetic dysfunction [11]. These observations are in line with the fact that PD patients show more frequently parasympathetic dysfunction signs (such as reduction in heart rate variability) than sympathetic ones (such as orthostatic hypotension). It is also noteworthy that cardiac preganglionic parasympathetic neurons arise predominantly from the nucleus ambiguus rather than the DMV [12], and that a previous study has shown no evident neuronal loss in the nucleus ambiguus in PD, unlike what is observed in the DMV [13]. Further pathological studies are necessary, as the nucleus ambiguus is difficult to identify anatomically. In this view, there is only one study regarding pathological changes in the nucleus ambiguus in PD [13]. Whole-body cryostimulation has been indicated as a 'training method' for the autonomic nervous system [14]. In fact, cold activates afferent signals from the peripheral receptors that converge in the medial preoptic region of the hypothalamus, from which efferent signals cause reflex cutaneous vasoconstriction, leading to a shift in blood volume toward the core resulting in increased central pressure. This effect is responsible for reducing sympathetic nerve activity through baroreflex activation and shifting autonomic control of heart rate toward parasympathetic dominance [15]. Remote from cold stimulation, an increase in parasympathetic cardiac control occurs even overnight [16]. In an experiment of Louis and colleagues on healthy subjects, $-110\,^{\circ}\mathrm{C}$ cryostimulation proved to stimulate the sympathetic nervous system, marked by the rise in plasma norepinephrine [15]. After five daily exposures, a lower sympathetic response was recorded compared to day one, therefore suggesting the development of physiological habituation to whole-body cryostimulation (WBC). Conversely, heart rate variability increased from pre- to post-WBC sessions, but only in the $-110\,^{\circ}\mathrm{C}$ condition. Unfortunately, we have so far a lack of studies focusing on cryostimulation in PD, in particular concerning heart rate variability (HRV) changes.

Thermoregulatory Dysfunction

Although it has received poor attention in clinical literature, thermoregulatory dysfunction is quite common in PD, having a reported prevalence of 30–70% [17, 18]. Thermoregulatory dysfunction is associated with abnormalities both in the central nervous system and in the peripheral nervous system. In fact, LP and αSyn deposition has been confirmed in hypothalamus [19], in preganglionic neurons in the intermediolateral cell column of the spinal cord and in the sympathetic ganglia [20, 21]. Furthermore, small fibre peripheral neuropathy, with reduced innervation of blood vessels, sweat glands and erector pili muscles, is a common finding in PD, although its aetiology remains uncertain [17]. Interestingly, thermoregulatory dysfunction in PD could result in both heat and cold intolerance, and both hyperhidrosis and hypohidrosis [4]. Few studies have investigated the effect of cold exposure in PD. Kolev and colleagues evaluated basal skin microcirculatory blood flow and its change in response to a cold caloric stimulus (cold water, 5 °C, exposure of one foot for 30 s) in a group of PD patients compared to healthy controls [22]. PD patients showed no detectable change in the red cell flux (RCF) on cold water exposure, evidencing that the cold caloric reflex was attenuated or absent, although there was no difference in the basal microcirculatory blood flow compared to normal subjects [22]. Similar findings are reported from Purup and colleagues, who found that PD patients exhibited significant reduction in thermal recovery rate compared to healthy controls [23]. In a preclinical model of PD, Tsai and coworkers investigated the effects of 4 °C cold exposure after exercise on exercise-induced thermal responses and neuroprotection in an MPTP (1-methyl-4-phenyl-1,2,3,6-tetrahydropyridine)-induced Parkinsonian mouse model [24]. They found that 4 °C exposure for 2 h after exercise impeded the neuroprotective effects of exercise on thermoregulation and UCP4 expression in MPTP-treated mice.

Metabolism

Irisin is an myokine induced by physical exercise and cold exposure [25]. It is expressed as a bioactive peptide in multiple tissues and organs, including the brain [25]. Irisin plays an important protective role in the nervous system, especially the central nervous system [26], and can induce neurogenesis and neural differentiation of mouse embryonic stem cells [27]. Researchers have demonstrated that increased concentration of irisin in blood can lead to the overexpression of brain-derived neurotrophic factor (BDNF) in both blood and brain [28]. Furthermore, molecules such as PGC-1α induced by endurance exercise can stimulate the expression of irisin precursor *FNDC5* gene in nerve cells, and the overexpression of *FNDC5* can upregulate the expression of BDNF by fourfold. Irisin can promote the degradation of fat and reduce the accumulation of fat [29], thereby reducing neuronal damage caused by chronic inflammatory infiltration. In addition, mitochondrial dysfunction is one of the pathogenic mechanisms of PD [30]. PGC-1α is a key regulator involved in mitochondrial respiration and insulin resistance, and plays a vital role in the pathogenesis of neuronal degeneration in patients with PD [31]. Moreover, as the downstream protein regulated by PGC-1α, irisin exerts a protective effect on mitochondrial function by inhibiting excessive mitochondrial division, promoting mitochondrial biosynthesis and reducing oxidative stress [32–34]. In summary, targeting irisin is a novel direction for the prevention, control and treatment of PD, and cryostimulation could act on this pathway. Although there are no studies evaluating irisin level in PD under cryostimulation, Dulian and coworkers investigated the influence of the whole-body cryostimulation on irisin in a group of middle-aged obese men [35]. Patients were exposed to a series of ten sessions in a cryogenic chamber (once a day at 9:30 a.m., for 3 min, at temperature −110 °C). Prior to treatment body composition and fitness level were determined. Patients were divided in "active" and "nonactive" according to fitness levels. It also reduced the high-sensitivity C-reactive protein (hsCRP) and hepcidin (Hpc) concentration confirming its anti-inflammatory effect. Finally, irisin values recorded 24 h after the last cryosession correlated significantly with the fat tissue, yet inversely with the skeletal muscle mass. Therefore, authors concluded the subcutaneous fat tissue to be the main source of irisin in response to cold exposures [35].

Motor Dysfunction

Exposure to cold induces several physiological changes in muscle, nerve and circulatory functioning. In particular, cooling results in reduced nerve conduction velocity, reduction of core muscle temperature, vasoconstriction and lowering of skeletal muscle tension [36]. It also decreases both the extensibility of soft tissue and muscle strength [37, 38]. Cooling, therefore, has been used therapeutically with orthopaedic patients to reduce muscle spasm [36, 37]. In contrast to cold, heat results in faster nerve conduction, vasodilatation, increased extensibility or reduced resistance of soft tissue, and improved mobility of joints [37, 38]. Therapeutically, heat is used to reduce muscle spasms in chronic cases, whereas cold is used in the acute stage. In the orthopaedic setting, heat and cold are applied to control pain and to prime musculoskeletal tissue for exercises. Both heat and cold are thought to promote relaxation of underlying muscle indirectly through nerve stimulation [36]. Several studies have explored the effect of temperature on motor performance, in particular on tremor. Lakie and colleagues studied the effect of cooling and heating on target shooting performance in normal subjects [39]. They found that cooling the limb resulted in a reduction in the amplitude of physiologic tremor and better target shooting performance, whereas warming the limb led to an increase in the amplitude of physiologic tremor [39]. Comparable results are found by Arblaster and coworkers; cooling one forearm immersed in water at 10–15 °C for 4 min resulted in a 50% reduction in physiologic tremor for at least 1 h [40]. Both Lakie and Arblaster studied the effect of cooling on patients with essential tremor (ET) [40, 41]. Essential tremor is the most common movement disorder seen clinically [42–44]. Its cause is unknown [44]. It is characterised by postural and action (intention) tremors without other associated features. Following cooling, in both studies, the subjects with ET demonstrated a 'striking' decrease in tremor, with improvement in writing performance lasting for 36 up to 150 min [41]. In the study of Lakie and colleagues, following heating of the same extremity, tremor increased in amplitude up to threefold [41]. In three subjects, the tremor became visible after heating. The increase in tremor amplitude following heating was of shorter duration than was the decrease following cooling. Authors hypothesised that an oscillation in a peripheral feedback circuit leads to tremor in ET patients, and the oscillation rate is determined by the delay in that circuit [41]. They hypothesised that temperature change of the circuit's muscles and neural components modified the delay and thereby changed the tremor frequency and amplitude. Literature is scarce on the effect of limb temperature in PD. It is not uncommon though, to hear from PD patients subjectively that their rigidity, bradykinesia and walking are worse during winter, and better during summer. Cooper and colleagues exposed 20 PD patients' arm to cold water (15 °C = 59 °F) or warm water (44 °C = 111.2 °F) for 5 min [45]. No statistically significant differences were noted between treatments or from baseline except the score for small common objects, which was improved following exposure to warm water than at baseline [45].

Conclusion

Parkinson's disease is a complex disease, evolving over time in a neurodegenerative way. However, the application of WBC in PD patients is a promising field in both therapeutic and rehabilitative settings. In fact, pre-clinical and clinical data on cooling in PD pave the way for its application on autonomic dysfunction, motor symptoms, fat and muscle metabolism and neuroprotection. Furthermore, in healthy subjects and in patients with other neurological disorders such as multiple sclerosis and cognitive impairment, WBC proved to have beneficial effects also on sleep quality, restless leg syndrome and cognitive performance [46, 47]. In this view, it could become a precious 'rehabilitation booster' in Parkinson's disease [14].

References

1. Postuma RB, et al. MDS clinical diagnostic criteria for Parkinson's disease. Mov Disord. 2015;30(12):1591–601. https://doi.org/10.1002/mds.26424.
2. Braak H, Del Tredici K, Rüb U, de Vos RAI, Steur ENHJ, Braak E. Staging of brain pathology related to sporadic Parkinson's disease. Neurobiol Aging. 2003;24:197–211. https://doi.org/10.1016/S0197-4580(02)00065-9.
3. Emre M, et al. Clinical diagnostic criteria for dementia associated with Parkinson's disease. Mov Disord. 2007;22(12):1689–707; quiz 1837. https://doi.org/10.1002/mds.21507.
4. Pfeiffer RF. Autonomic dysfunction in Parkinson's disease. Neurotherapeutics. 2020;17:1464–79. https://doi.org/10.1007/s13311-020-00897-4.
5. Goldstein DS. Dysautonomia in Parkinson's disease: neurocardiological abnormalities. Lancet Neurol. 2003;2(11):669–76.
6. Amino T, Orimo S, Itoh Y, Takahashi A, Uchihara T, Mizusawa H. Profound cardiac sympathetic denervation occurs in Parkinson disease. Brain Pathol. 2005;15(1):29–34.

7. Rascol O, Schelosky L. 123I-Metaiodobenzylguanidine scintigraphy in Parkinson's disease and related disorders. Mov Disord. 2009;24(Suppl 2):S732–41.
8. Goldstein DS, Holmes C, Bentho O, et al. Biomarkers to detect central dopamine deficiency and distinguish Parkinson disease from multiple system atrophy. Parkinsonism Relat Disord. 2008;14(8):600–7.
9. Haensch CA, Lerch H, Jörg J, Isenmann S. Cardiac denervation occurs independent of orthostatic hypotension and impaired heart rate variability in Parkinson's disease. Parkinsonism Relat Disord. 2009;15(2):134–7.
10. Katagiri A, Asahina M, Araki N, et al. Myocardial (123)I-MIBG uptake and cardiovascular autonomic function in Parkinson's disease. Parkinsons Dis. 2015;2015:805351.
11. Suzuki M, et al. Cardiac parasympathetic dysfunction in the early phase of Parkinson's disease. J Neurol. 2017;264(2):333–40. https://doi.org/10.1007/s00415-016-8348-0. Epub 2016 Nov 29.
12. Greene JG. Causes and consequences of degeneration of the dorsal motor nucleus of the vagus nerve in Parkinson's disease. Antioxid Redox Signal. 2014;21(4):649–67. https://doi.org/10.1089/ars.2014.5859.
13. Eadie MJ. The pathology of certain medullary nuclei in Parkinsonism. Brain J Neurol. 1963;86:781–92.
14. Capodaglio P, Cremascoli R, Piterà P, Fontana JM. Whole-body cryostimulation. A rehabilitation booster. J Rehabil Med Clin Commun. 2022;5:2810. https://doi.org/10.2340/jrmcc.v5.2810. eCollection 2022.
15. Louis J, Theurot D, Filliard JR, Volondat M, Dugué B, Dupuy O. The use of whole-body cryotherapy: time- and dose-response investigation on circulating blood catecholamines and heart rate variability. Eur J Appl Physiol. 2020;120(8):1733–43.
16. Douzi W, Dupuy O, Tanneau M, Boucard G, Bouzigon R, Dugué B. 3-min whole body cryotherapy/cryostimulation after training in the evening improves sleep quality in physically active men. Eur J Sport Sci. 2019;19(6):860–7.
17. Coon EA, Low PA. Thermoregulation in Parkinson disease. Handb Clin Neurol. 2018;157:715–25.
18. Skorvanek M, Bhatia KP. The skin and Parkinson's disease: review of clinical, diagnostic, and therapeutic issues. Mov Disord Clin Pract. 2016;4(1):21–31.
19. Langston JW, Forno LS. The hypothalamus in Parkinson disease. Ann Neurol. 1978;3(2):129–33.
20. Beach TG, Adler CH, Sue LI, et al.; Arizona Parkinson's Disease Consortium. Multi-organ distribution of phosphorylated alphasynuclein histopathology in subjects with Lewy body disorders. Acta Neuropathol. 2010;119(6):689–702.
21. Gelpi E, Navarro-Otano J, Tolosa E, et al. Multiple organ involvement by alpha-synuclein pathology in Lewy body disorders. Mov Disord. 2014;29(8):1010–8.
22. Kolev OI, et al. Cold caloric microcirculatory reflex disturbance in patients with Parkinson's disease. Clin Auton Res. 1997;7(2):81–3. https://doi.org/10.1007/BF02267751.
23. Purup MM, et al. Skin temperature in Parkinson's disease measured by infrared thermography. Parkinsons Dis. 2020;2020:2349469. https://doi.org/10.1155/2020/2349469.
24. Tsai YJ, et al. Cold exposure after exercise impedes the neuroprotective effects of exercise on thermoregulation and UCP4 expression in an MPTP-induced Parkinsonian mouse model. Neuroscience. 2020;14:573509. https://doi.org/10.3389/fnins.2020.573509.
25. Zhang H, et al. Irisin, an exercise-induced bioactive peptide beneficial for health promotion during aging process. Ageing Res Rev. 2022;80:101680. https://doi.org/10.1016/j.arr.2022.101680.
26. Novelle MG, Contreras C, Romero-Picó A, López M, Diéguez C. Irisin, two years later. Int J Endocrinol. 2013;2013:746281. https://doi.org/10.1155/2013/746281.
27. Grygiel-Górniak B, Puszczewicz M. A review on irisin, a new protagonist that mediates muscle-adipose-bone-neuron connectivity. Eur Rev Med Pharm Sci. 2017;21(20):4687–93.
28. Chao MV, Rajagopal R, Lee FS. Neurotrophin signalling in health and disease. Clin Sci. 2006;110(2):167–73. https://doi.org/10.1042/cs20050163.

29. Boström P, Wu J, Jedrychowski MP, Korde A, Ye L, Lo JC, Rasbach KA, Boström EA, Choi JH, Long JZ, Kajimura S, Zingaretti MC, Vind BF, Tu H, Cinti S, Højlund K, Gygi SP, Spiegelman BM. A PGC1- α-dependent myokine that drives brown-fat-like development of white fat and thermogenesis. Nature. 2012;481(7382):463–8. https://doi.org/10.1038/nature10777.
30. Westbroek W, Gustafson AM, Sidransky E. Exploring the link between glucocerebrosidase mutations and parkinsonism. Trends Mol Med. 2011;17(9):485–93. https://doi.org/10.1016/j.molmed.2011.05.003.
31. Aviles-Olmos I, Limousin P, Lees A, Foltynie T. Parkinson's disease, insulin resistance and novel agents of neuroprotection. Brain. 2013;136(2):374–84. https://doi.org/10.1093/brain/aws009.
32. Bi J, Zhang J, Ren Y, Du Z, Li Q, Wang Y, Wei S, Yang L, Zhang J, Liu C, Lv Y, Wu R. Irisin alleviates liver ischemia-reperfusion injury by inhibiting excessive mitochondrial fission, promoting mitochondrial biogenesis and decreasing oxidative stress. Redox Biol. 2019;20:296–306. https://doi.org/10.1016/j.redox.2018.10.019.
33. Chen K, Xu Z, Liu Y, Wang Z, Li Y, Xu X, Chen C, Xia T, Liao Q, Yao Y, Zeng C, He D, Yang Y, Tan T, Yi J, Zhou J, Zhu H, Ma J, Zeng C. Irisin protects mitochondria function during pulmonary ischemia/reperfusion injury. Sci Transl Med. 2017;9(418):eaao6298. https://doi.org/10.1126/scitranslmed.aao6298.
34. Wang FS, Kuo CW, Ko JY, Chen YS, Wang SY, Ke HJ, Kuo PC, Lee CH, Wu JC, Lu WB, Tai MH, Jahr H, Lian WS. Irisin mitigates oxidative stress, chondrocyte dysfunction and osteoarthritis development through regulating mitochondrial integrity and autophagy. Antioxidants. 2020;9(9):810. https://doi.org/10.3390/antiox9090810.
35. Dulian K, et al. The whole body cryostimulation modifies irisin concentration and reduces inflammation in middle aged, obese men. Cryobiology. 2015;71(3):398–404. https://doi.org/10.1016/j.cryobiol.2015.10.143.
36. Griffin JE, Karselis TC. Physical agents for physical therapists. 2nd ed. Springfield: Charles C Thomas. Pain; 1982. pp. 3–18.
37. Mullins PAT. Use of therapeutic modalities in upper extremity rehabilitation. In: Hunte JM, Mackin EJ, Callahan AD, editors. Rehabilitation of the hand: surgery and therapy. 4th ed. St. Louis: Mosby-Year Book; 1995. p. 1495–519.
38. Powell SG, Burke AL. Surgical and therapeutic management of tennis elbow: an update. J Hand Ther. 1991;4(2):64–8.
39. Lakie M, Villagra F, Bowman I, Wilby R. Shooting performance is related to forearm temperature and hand tremor size. J Sports Sci. 1995;13:313–20.
40. Arblaster LA, Lakie M, Roberts RC. Localized cooling can reduce essential tremor in man. J Physiol. 1992;452:26P.
41. Lakie M, Walsh EG, Arblaster LA, Villagra F, Roberts SC. Limb temperature and human tremors. J Neurol Neurosurg Psychiatry. 1994;57:35–42.
42. Anouti A, Koller WE. Tremor disorders and diagnosis management. West J Med. 1995;162:510–3.
43. Britton TC. Essential tremor and its variants. Curr Opin Neurol. 1995;8:314–9.
44. Findley LJ. Classification of tremors. J Clin Neurophysiol. 1996;13(2):122–32.
45. Cooper C, et al. The effect of temperature on hand function in patients with tremor. J Hand Ther. 2000;2000(13):276–88.
46. Happe S, Evers S, Thiedemann C, Bunten S, Siegert R. Whole body and local cryotherapy in restless legs syndrome: a randomized, single-blind, controlled parallel group pilot study. J Neurol Sci. 2016;370:7–12. https://doi.org/10.1016/j.jns.2016.09.006.
47. Rymaszewska J, Lion KM, Stańczykiewicz B, Rymaszewska JE, Trypka E, Pawlik-Sobecka L, et al. The improvement of cognitive deficits after whole-body cryotherapy—A randomised controlled trial. Exp Gerontol. 2021;146:111237. https://doi.org/10.1016/j.exger.2021.111237.

Post-COVID-19 Condition

14

Paolo Piterà, Federica Verme, Jacopo Maria Fontana,
Stefania Cattaldo, Stefania Mai, and Paolo Capodaglio

Post-COVID Condition (PCC): Overview and Clinical Manifestations

Coronavirus disease 2019 (COVID-19), caused by the severe acute respiratory syndrome coronavirus 2 (SARS-CoV-2) virus, is an infectious disease with over 750 million confirmed cases worldwide as of January 2023 [1]. While pulmonary issues are the most common, COVID-19 also presents various extrapulmonary symptoms affecting the psychosocial, cardiovascular, hematologic, renal, gastrointestinal, and central nervous systems, along with postintensive care syndrome. The presence of a pro-inflammatory cytokine storm during COVID-19, which can persist in the subacute phase, may lead to muscular complications like critical illness

P. Piterà (✉) · F. Verme · J. M. Fontana
Research Laboratory in Biomechanics, Rehabilitation and Ergonomics, IRCCS Istituto
Auxologico Italiano, Piancavallo (Verbania), Italy
e-mail: p.pitera@auxologico.it; f.verme@auxologico.it; j.fontana@auxologico.it

S. Cattaldo
Laboratory of Clinical Neurobiology, IRCCS Istituto Auxologico Italiano,
Piancavallo (Verbania), Italy
e-mail: s.cattaldo@auxologico.it

S. Mai
Laboratory of Metabolic Research, IRCCS Istituto Auxologico Italiano,
Piancavallo (Verbania), Italy
e-mail: s.mai@auxologico.it

P. Capodaglio
Research Laboratory in Biomechanics, Rehabilitation and Ergonomics,
IRCCS Istituto Auxologico Italiano, Piancavallo (Verbania), Italy

Physical Medicine and Rehabilitation, Department of Surgical Sciences,
University of Torino, Torino, Italy
e-mail: p.capodaglio@auxologico.it; paolo.capodaglio@unito.it

P. Capodaglio (ed.), *Whole-Body Cryostimulation*,
https://doi.org/10.1007/978-3-031-18545-8_14

myopathy (CIM) [2] and acute sarcopenia [3]. The long-term consequences of the "post-COVID-19 condition" (PCC) [4], characterized by persistent symptoms occurring at least 3 months after initial onset in individuals with confirmed or probable SARS-CoV-2 infection, lasting for a minimum of 2 months, and without an alternative diagnosis, still require further exploration [5–8]. The most commonly reported symptoms include musculoskeletal discomfort (fatigue and muscle pain) and psychological issues (impaired concentration and memory, depression, and anxiety), as well as dyspnea, persistent cough, fever, and loss of smell or taste [4, 5, 7, 9].

More than 30% of individuals impacted by COVID-19, including those without symptoms, and approximately 80% of hospitalized COVID-19 patients show symptoms of PCC [5, 10]. PCC patients require comprehensive multidisciplinary rehabilitation programs that aim to restore their ability to perform basic daily activities independently [11]. Unlike temporary symptoms such as anosmia [12], fatigue and cognitive impairment tend to persist or even worsen in susceptible individuals [13]. The World Health Organization has released rehabilitation guidelines for PCC patients, while Cochrane Rehabilitation has launched REH-COVER, and ongoing updates on rehabilitation best practices for these patients are available within the scientific community [10, 14, 15]. An integrated approach combining physiotherapy, resistance training, and nutritional interventions and addressing the inflammatory state is crucial for PCC patients to regain their independence. An extensive range of clinical manifestations associated with PCC, which impact activity ability and overall quality of life, have attracted significant attention. Patients with severe illness or those receiving intensive care unit treatment are particularly vulnerable to experiencing long COVID symptoms, including reduced activity ability, cognitive difficulties, and psychological impairment, similar to postintensive care syndrome (PICS). A surprising number of extrapulmonary manifestations of severe acute respiratory SARS-CoV-2 infection have been described with a review of imaging [16], shedding some light on a range of musculoskeletal, nerve, joint, and bone involvement, and leading to the manifestation of prolonged symptoms. These individuals require medical rehabilitation services to mitigate disability [17], and an intensive and multidisciplinary rehabilitation approach becomes imperative to optimize functional recovery and facilitate the return to the individual's preillness state, especially considering that fatigue and cognitive impairment may persist or even worsen in susceptible individuals [13].

Preliminary Evidence

Our research group conducted preliminary investigations on the clinical, metabolic, and functional effects of whole-body cryostimulation (WBC) on PCC patients. To our knowledge, no previous studies on this particular topics are present in the literature. During the first COVID pandemic wave in Italy, we studied an elderly patient after discharge from the intensive care unit. He was in a severe health condition and underwent a cycle of 15 WBC sessions, leading to remarkable functional and clinical improvements [18]. Encouraged by these novel, promising findings, we proceeded to study seven PCC patients [19]. Again, we observed rapid and significant functional benefits, in line with the findings of our previous case report. We then expanded the sample of PCC patients comparing the outcomes of this group with a control group of PCC patients undergoing the same rehabilitation program without WBC [20]. The results we obtained showed clinically significant improvements in health and function in all patients who underwent a WBC cycle. Specifically, improvements were observed in pain relief, dyspnea, fatigue, sleep, mood, and physical performance. Biochemical analyses revealed a significant decrease in high-density lipoprotein (HDL), low-density lipoprotein (LDL), total cholesterol, and triglycerides. Glucose and HBA1c% also decreased significantly in both WBC and control groups at discharge. Systolic blood pressure (PAS) and heart rate (HR) significantly decreased, but diastolic pressure (PAD) did not show a significant change. Improvements were also present in the 6-min walking test (6-MWT) distance and timed up and go (TUG), though not statistically significant. The rapid anti-inflammatory action of WBC may be responsible for the quick benefits observed, making it a suitable addition to rehabilitation programs for patients with typical PCC symptoms like pain, inflammation, and fatigue. We have therefore shown that introduction of WBC sessions had a positive impact on subjective and objective improvements in health and function, and the improvements in physical performance, hematological and metabolic parameters, sleep, mood, and pain suggest that WBC may represent an effective adjunct for functional recovery in PCC patients.

In conclusion, our research provides preliminary but promising evidence of WBC's potential as an effective and safe adjuvant in the recovery from PCC symptoms within a multidisciplinary rehabilitation program. The observed improvements in various parameters support its use as a booster in rehabilitation, but further research on larger samples is needed to establish its full utility and mechanisms of action.

Conclusive Remarks

The rationale for prescribing WBC in post-COVID symptoms appears in line with the existing evidence of clinical and functional benefits following WBC documented in other musculoskeletal, neurological, and psychiatric conditions (Fig. 14.1). Pain, fatigue, and alleviation of inflammatory symptoms after WBC, as also shown in this report, appear to be related to reduced nerve conduction and acetylcholine formation and lower levels of oxidative stress and inflammation [21], but a full understanding of the underlying mechanisms is yet to be fully disclosed. Importantly, the benefits of WBC seem to appear rapidly (1 week). WBC seems to trigger rapid anti-inflammatory actions, which could explain our encouraging results and support its use as a booster for rehabilitation programs, as the improvement in physical performance in each case described was noteworthy. In support of this suggestion, findings by Lubkowska and collaborators [21] highlighted that WBC leads to a rapid decrease in the concentration of the pro-inflammatory cytokine interleukin 1a

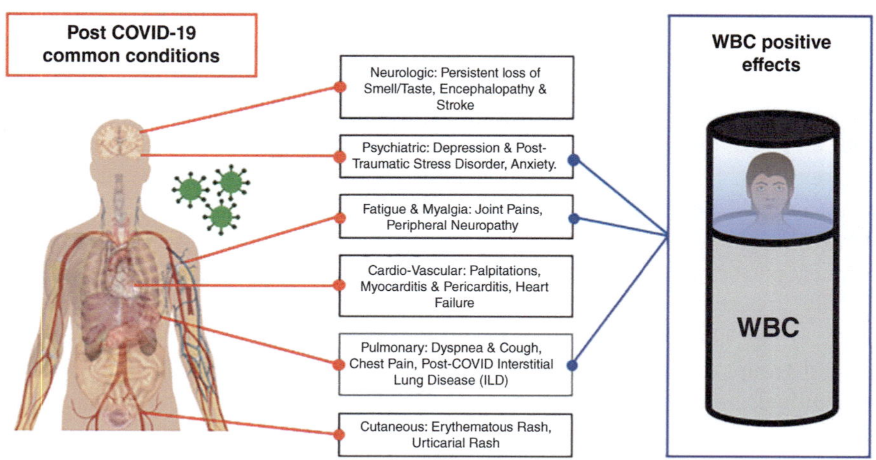

Fig. 14.1 WBC as a rehabilitation booster that can improve symptoms and accelerate the achievement of functional outcomes in patients recovering from PCC

(IL-1a), and a rapid increase in the anti-inflammatory cytokine interleukin 10 (IL-10). In addition, the use of cryostimulation prior to training or competition has been shown to exert beneficial effects through a multifactorial hypothesis, such as hormonal changes, peripheral vasoconstriction with improved muscle oxygenation, reduced fatigue and pain, an anti-inflammatory effect, and subsequent psychological well-being [22].

WBC can act as a "training method" for the autonomic nervous system on top of the well-known anti-inflammatory and antioxidant effects. It is in fact widely used as a postexercise recovery technique in elite athletes [23], and the positive effects of 10 serial sessions of WBC have been previously reported on patients with PCC [18, 19].

Given these known rapid effects, WBC sessions were performed early in the day with the goal of improving patients' overall physical performance and improving patients' adherence and motivation to the rehabilitation program [19]. Because we provided a variety of interventions, including nutritional and psychological support along with physical exercise, it was not possible to determine to what extent WBC may per se have accounted for observed clinical and functional improvements, and randomized control trials with sham WBC sessions are needed for that purpose. Moreover, the reduction in the inflammatory status encountered cannot be attributed merely to WBC treatment. In fact, it is known that weight loss results in a reduction in pro-inflammatory markers, suggesting that the anti-inflammatory effect could be a synergic result of WBC and weight loss interventions [24]. Another present limitation of this report, and, in general, in current WBC studies shows that no blinding of participants has been used, which could have influenced the outcomes.

Considering the current severity and prevalence of PCC in the general population, the identification of adjuvants that can act as a booster for rehabilitation programs appears to be of paramount importance. Independent research must proceed with caution in gathering data and evidence from larger studies on the benefits of WBC to avoid dangerous scientific shortcuts. We are aware of commercial and nonmedical use of cryostimulation as some sort of panacea, but scientific evidence of its clinical utility in several specific conditions is growing rapidly. Our preliminary results indicate that integrating WBC into a multidisciplinary rehabilitation approach may provide benefits for individuals recovering from PCC [25]. Given the evidence of effectiveness of WBC on a range of symptoms common in PCC, we believe that our published papers, written according to the CARE checklist, provide some inputs to promote further research on the use of WBC in boosting the recovery from PCC within a multidisciplinary rehabilitation program. Sturdy evidence that WBC has beneficial effects in various musculoskeletal and neurological conditions indeed exists, but larger and controlled studies on PCC patients are needed to generalize our preliminary suggestions.

References

1. CSR COVID-19 situation updates for week 4 (22–28 January 2023). In: World Health Organization - Regional Office for the Eastern Mediterranean. http://www.emro.who.int/pandemic-epidemic-diseases/covid-19/covid-19-situation-updates-for-week-4-2228-january-2023.html. Accessed 5 Feb 2024.
2. Bagnato S, Boccagni C, Marino G, Prestandrea C, D'Agostino T, Rubino F. Critical illness myopathy after COVID-19. Int J Infect Dis. 2020;99:276–8.
3. Gobbi M, Bezzoli E, Ismelli F, et al. Skeletal muscle Mass, Sarcopenia and rehabilitation outcomes in post-acute COVID-19 patients. J Clin Med. 2021;10:5623.
4. Coronavirus disease (COVID-19): Post COVID-19 condition. https://www.who.int/newsroom/questions-andanswers/item/coronavirus-disease-(covid-19)-post-covid-19-condition. Accessed 30 Nov 2022.
5. Ceban F, Ling S, Lui LMW, et al. Fatigue and cognitive impairment in Post-COVID-19 Syndrome: A systematic review and meta-analysis. Brain Behav Immun. 2022;101:93–135.
6. Dani M, Dirksen A, Taraborrelli P, Torocastro M, Panagopoulos D, Sutton R, Lim PB. Autonomic dysfunction in 'long COVID': rationale, physiology and management strategies. Clin Med J R Coll Physicians Lond. 2021;21:E63–7.
7. Gupta A, Madhavan MV, Sehgal K, et al. Extrapulmonary manifestations of COVID-19. Nat Med. 2020;26:1017–32.
8. Higgins V, Sohaei D, Diamandis EP, Prassas I. COVID-19: from an acute to chronic disease? Potential long-term health consequences. Crit Rev Clin Lab Sci. 2021;58:297–310.
9. Ferioli M, Prediletto I, Bensai S, et al. Spontaneous evolution of COVID-19 lung sequelae: results from a double-step follow-up. Respir Int Rev Thorac Dis. 2022;101:381–93.
10. Tenforde MW, Kim SS, Lindsell CJ, et al. Symptom duration and risk factors for delayed return to usual health among outpatients with COVID-19 in a multistate health care systems network - United States, March-June 2020. MMWR Morb Mortal Wkly Rep. 2020;69:993–8.
11. Lam MH, Wing YK, Yu MW, Leung CM, Ma RC, Kong AP, So WY, Fong SY, Lam SP. Mental morbidities and chronic fatigue in severe acute respiratory syndrome survivors. 2021
12. Lopez M, Bell K, Annaswamy T, Juengst S, Ifejika N. COVID-19 guide for the rehabilitation clinician: a review of nonpulmonary manifestations and complications. Am J Phys Med Rehabil. 2020;99:669–76.

13. Hopkins C, Surda P, Whitehead E, Kumar BN. Early recovery following new onset anosmia during the COVID-19 pandemic—An observational cohort study. J Otolaryngol Head Neck Surg. 2020;49:1–6.
14. Vitacca M, Lazzeri M, Guffanti E, et al. Italian suggestions for pulmonary rehabilitation in COVID-19 patients recovering from acute respiratory failure: results of a Delphi process. Monaldi Arch Chest Dis. 2020; https://doi.org/10.4081/monaldi.2020.1444.
15. Zhao H-M, Xie Y-X, Wang C. Recommendations for respiratory rehabilitation in adults with coronavirus disease 2019. Chin Med J (Engl). 2020;133:1595–602.
16. Ramani C, Davis EM, Kim JS, Provencio JJ, Enfield KB, Kadl A. Post-ICU COVID-19 outcomes: a case series. Chest. 2021;159:215–8.
17. Zhang H, Cao B. Post-infection rehabilitation of COVID-19 patients: Findings and prospects. Lancet Reg Health Eur. 2022;22:100496.
18. Gobbi M, Trotti G, Tanzi M, Kasap F, Piterà P, Capodaglio P. Post-covid symptoms and whole-body cryotheraphy: a case report. J Rehabil Med Clin Commun. 2022;5:1000075.
19. Piterà P, Gobbi M, Fontana JM, Cattaldo S, Massucci M, Capodaglio P. Whole-body cryostimulation: a rehabilitation booster in post-COVID patients? A case series. Appl Sci. 2022;12:4830.
20. Fontana JM, Alito A, Piterà P, Verme F, Cattaldo S, Cornacchia M, Mai S, Brunani A, Capodaglio P. Whole-body cryostimulation in post-COVID rehabilitation for patients with obesity: a multidisciplinary feasibility study. Biomedicines. 2023;11:3092. https://doi.org/10.3390/biomedicines11113092.
21. Lubkowska A, Szyguła Z, Chlubek D, Banfi G. The effect of prolonged whole-body cryostimulation treatment with different amounts of sessions on chosen pro- and anti-inflammatory cytokines levels in healthy men. Scand J Clin Lab Invest. 2011;71:419–25.
22. Bouzigon R, Dupuy O, Tiemessen I, De Nardi M, Bernard J-P, Mihailovic T, Theurot D, Miller ED, Lombardi G, Dugué BM. Cryostimulation for post-exercise recovery in athletes: a consensus and position paper. Front Sports Act Living. 2021;3:302.
23. Rose C, Edwards KM, Siegler J, Graham K, Caillaud C. Whole-body cryotherapy as a recovery technique after exercise: a review of the literature. Int J Sports Med. 2017;38:1049–60.
24. Bianchi VE. Weight loss is a critical factor to reduce inflammation. Clin Nutr ESPEN. 2018;28:21–35.
25. Capodaglio P, Cremascoli R, Piterà P, Fontana JM. Whole-body cryostimulation: a rehabilitation booster. J Rehabil Med Clin Commun. 2022;5:2810.

Cryostimulation as a Nonpharmacological Intervention for the Promotion of Mental Health: A Focus on Depressive and Anxiety Disorders

15

Fabien D. Legrand

Definition, Prevalence, and Incidence of Depressive and Anxiety Disorders

Major depressive disorder is defined as having five or more symptoms, which cause significant distress or impairment during the same 2-week period, and at least one of these should be a depressed mood or loss of interest or pleasure. Other symptoms can include change in weight, sleep disturbances, psychomotor agitation or retardation, fatigue or loss of energy, guilt, impaired concentration, and thoughts of death (Diagnostic and Statistical Manual of Mental Disorders, Fifth Edition [DSM-V], American Psychiatric Association) [1].

Anxiety disorders have been redefined from the DSM-IV to the DSM-V. In the DSM-IV [2], anxiety disorders included panic disorder, phobia (social phobia, specific phobia, and agoraphobia), posttraumatic stress disorder, acute stress disorder, generalized anxiety disorder, and obsessive-compulsive disorder. Anxiety disorders in the DSM-V have been narrowed with posttraumatic stress disorder and acute stress disorder being moved into a category entitled "stress-related disorders," and obsessive-compulsive disorder placed in a category entitled "obsessive-compulsive and related disorders."

Current psychiatric epidemiological studies are primarily based on DSM-IV definitions of depressive and anxiety disorders. Prevalence and incidence studies have been conducted using representative community household surveys and generally consisted of structured interviews (most of these interviews were based on the Composite International Diagnostic Interview, CIDI [3]).

F. D. Legrand (✉)
Cognition Santé Société, Département de Psychologie, University of Reims Champagne Ardennes, Reims, France
e-mail: fabien.legrand@univ-reims.fr

P. Capodaglio (ed.), *Whole-Body Cryostimulation*,
https://doi.org/10.1007/978-3-031-18545-8_15

The prevalence of major depressive disorder (MDD) varies widely cross-nationally. For example, the 1-year prevalence ranges from 0.3% in Vietnam to 10.2% in Iran. Similarly there is a broad range of lifetime prevalence rates from 3.2% in Nigeria to 20.4% in France. The median lifetime prevalence is estimated at 9.9% ($n = 39$ studies, see Table 15.1). It appears that MDD has an early age of onset with a median age of approximately 28 years.

Table 15.1 Twelve-month and lifetime prevalence rates and age of onset of major depressive episodes and anxiety disorders from selected countries worldwide

Country	Major depression			Anxiety disorders		
	1 year	Lifetime	Onset	1 year	Lifetime	Onset
Australia	4.8	12.8		11.8	20.0	
Belgium	5.2	14.1	29.4	8.4	13.1	22.8
Brazil	10.1	18.0	24.3	19.9	28.1	20.3
Bulgaria	3.0	6.7		5.6		
Canada	4.8	12.2		4.7		
Chile	5.7	9.2		9.9	16.2	
China	2.0	3.8	30.3	3.0	4.8	28.1
Colombia	5.3	11.8	23.5	14.4	25.3	22.8
Czech Republic	2.0	7.8				
Finland	7.4					
France	5.6	20.4	28.4	13.7	22.3	25.5
Germany	3.1	10.3	27.6	8.3	14.6	27.1
Guatemala	0.8	3.2		2.3	5.2	
India	4.5	9.0	31.9			
Iran	10.2			15.6		
Iraq	3.9	7.2	46.0	10.4	13.8	39.6
Israel	5.9	9.8	25.5	3.6	5.2	22.0
Italy	2.9	9.7	27.7	6.5	11.0	26.9
Japan	2.4	6.8	30.1	4.2	6.9	28.2
Lebanon	4.9	10.3	23.8	12.2	16.7	25.0
Mexico	3.7	7.6	23.5	8.4	14.3	24.1
Netherlands	4.9	18.0	27.2	8.9	15.9	27.0
New Zealand	5.7	15.8	24.2	15.0	24.6	21.4
Nigeria	1.1	3.2	29.2	4.2	6.5	20.7
Northern Ireland	8.8	17.7		12.3		
Norway	7.3	17.8				
Peru	2.7	6.4	38.0	7.9	14.9	29.9
Poland	1.6	3.8				
Portugal	7.0	17.4		13.7		
Romania	1.5	2.9		4.2		
Singapore	2.2	5.8	26.0	0.4	0.9	27.6
South Africa	4.9	10.4	22.3	8.2	15.8	24.2
South Korea	3.1	6.7		6.8	8.7	
Spain	3.8	10.6	30.0	6.6	9.9	26.6
Thailand		19.9			10.2	
Turkey	3.5	6.3		5.8	7.4	
United States	8.3	19.2	22.7	19.0	31.0	20.8
Ukraine	8.4	14.6	27.8	6.8	8.9	24.9
Vietnam	0.3			0.4		

The Netherlands Mental Health Survey and Incidence Study (NEMESIS) [4] revealed several risk factors associated with the incidence of MDD: female gender, having a negative life event in the past 12 months, ongoing difficulties in the past 12 months, high neuroticism, and sleep problems [5].

Global Burden of Disease and Societal Cost

Major depression results in 34.4 mean days out of role per year [6], which is similar to values seen in patients with cancer (31.9). The number of mean days out is highest in lower-income countries (i.e., 35.8) compared to medium-income countries (34.8) and higher-income countries (33.7). MDD is not the psychiatric disorder with the most days out of role; bipolar disorder (41.2), panic disorder (42.9), posttraumatic stress disorder (42.7), social phobia (39.8), or still generalized anxiety disorder (39.8) all have higher days out of role. Approximately half of the negative impact of MDD on role functioning is mediated by problems with cognition and by feelings of embarrassment and shame [7].

The global burden of disease generally uses two measures of disability. Disability-adjusted life years (DALY) is a measure of overall disease burden expressed as the number of years lost due to ill-health, disability, or early death. Years lived with disability (YLD) is another disability measure defined as years of healthy life lost as a result of disability [8]. Broadly speaking, mental disorders account for a significant amount of the burden of disease: 7.1% DALY and 21.2% YLD [9]. Depressive disorders (MDD + dysthymia) alone account for 36.4% DALY and 38.3% YLD caused by mental disorders. Overall, depressive disorders are the 11th ranked disorder contributing to DALY, while it is the second highest ranked for YLD (see Table 15.2). The available data regarding anxiety disorders are much more limited, but it appears that anxiety disorders rank ninth among diseases contributing to YLD; and among persons aged 15–49 years, anxiety disorders are the fifth leading cause of YLD (see Table 15.2). One of the reasons for the higher rate of DALY and YLD in developed countries for depressive and anxiety disorders compared to developing countries is that diarrheal diseases, malaria, HIV, and preterm birth complications are all disorders that result in early mortality or life years lost in developing countries, whereas mental disorders result in relatively few deaths.

Table 15.2 Percentage and ranking of DALY and YLD accounted by MDD and anxiety disorders out of 301 diseases and injuries by gender, country development status, and age group

		Males		Females		Developed		Developing	
		%	Rank	%	Rank	%	Rank	%	Rank
		Major depressive disorder							
DALY	All ages	1.48	17	2.85	6	2.58	8	2.02	13
	5–14	2.20	10	3.65	5	5.08	4	2.72	8
	15–49	2.88	7	5.53	2	4.96	3	3.92	3
	50–69	1.24	20	2.85	7	2.12	11	1.87	10
	≥70	0.59	47	1.26	17	0.97	23	0.91	20
YLD	All ages	5.51	2	7.92	2	5.76	2	7.09	2
	5–14	4.46	3	7.09	3	6.08	4	5.67	2
	15–49	7.40	2	10.18	1	8.20	2	9.01	2
	50–69	4.44	6	6.85	3	5.13	5	5.94	4
	≥70	2.50	11	4.01	9	2.86	11	3.77	7
		Anxiety disorders							
DALY	All ages	0.62	51	1.43	19	1.48	18	0.90	38
	5–14	1.31	16	2.76	7	5.49	3	1.73	13
	15–49	1.25	21	2.87	7	2.96	7	1.82	14
	50–69	0.43	57	1.19	24	1.10	29	0.68	32
	≥70	0.17	194	0.42	60	0.39	116	0.24	179
YLD	All ages	2.32	9	3.97	7	3.31	9	3.16	9
	5–14	4.46	6	7.09	3	6.08	3	5.67	5
	15–49	3.20	6	5.28	5	4.89	5	4.18	5
	50–69	1.55	16	2.88	10	2.67	11	2.08	11
	≥70	0.70	44	1.34	17	1.16	19	1.00	19

Source: Institute for Health Metrics and Evaluation (IHME). GBD Compare. Seattle, WA: IHME, University of Washington, 2015. Available from http://vizhub.healthdata.org/gbd-compare

Treatment Gap

Most people with depressive or anxiety disorders are often seen for the first time at the primary health care level (i.e., general practitioner). However, these disorders are not always managed appropriately. When depression, in particular, is not treated properly or in a timely manner, it often leads to recurrent symptoms or becomes chronic, resulting in severe disability, death by suicide, or the prolonged suffering of the patient and his/her family. One reason behind the failure by general practitioners (GPs) to provide depressed people with appropriate medical/psychiatric help is that depression can be masked by physical symptoms or diverse complaints, leading to repeated and unproductive consultations among physicians that do not improve the patient's condition and increase the cost of medical care. As a result of these factors and other patient's related barriers such as believing the problems will resolve on their own or one can resolve the problem themselves, having no time to seek treatment, or lack of confidence in the health care system, a wide treatment gap has emerged for both depression and anxiety disorders that needs to be bridged.

The concept of "treatment gap" can be defined as the absolute difference between the true prevalence of a disorder and the treated proportion of individuals affected by the disorder [10]. Over the last two decades, the treatment gap for MDD has been estimated to be 56% worldwide, with huge disparities between countries. In Africa and the Arab countries, the treatment gap for MDD is estimated to peak at around 70%, while in Europe and the USA, it stands at 43–45% [11]. The treatment gap for anxiety disorders is even higher than for MDD. For instance, among European countries, the treatment gap for anxiety disorders has been estimated to be 74% [12].

In the United States, treatment lag (i.e., the delay between onset of disorder and obtaining treatment) may be as high as 4 years, with only 35% of patients receiving treatment in the first year following diagnosis of MDD or anxiety disorder [13]. The median duration of delay is shorter in some European countries, China, and Japan (approximately 1 year), and the longest median delay is 14 years in Mexico. Earlier onset of disorder, older age, and male gender are associated with greater delay in treatment.

The World Health Organization [14] has outlined 10 recommendations to address the treatment gap for MDD as well as other mental disorders. These recommendations can be implemented at both the national and community levels: make mental health treatment accessible in primary care; make psychotropic drugs readily available; shift care away from institutions toward community; educate the public; involve family; establish national mental health programs; increase and improve training of mental health professionals; increase links with other governmental and nongovernmental institutions; provide monitoring of the mental health system with quality indicators; and support more research actions.

Treating Depression or Anxiety with Repeated Cold Exposure: An Immune Perspective

The literature has evidenced a strong association between noncommunicable diseases such as cardiovascular, diabetes, cancer, or respiratory illness (the ones with the highest worldwide rate of mortality) and emotional disorders [15]. There is much evidence showing that the immune system is the molecular connection linking these conditions. Inflammation is a protective and coordinated response to cellular stress that results from the communication among different types of immune cells. Acute inflammation is an early (almost immediate) tissue response to injury. It is nonspecific and of short duration. At this stage, the main objective is to remove the cellular stress (injury, injurious agents, and foreign bodies) or resolve hypersensitivity reactions. On the other hand, chronic inflammation is not part of the natural healing process, and in the long run, it will cause organ damage, including mental illness, since the body is not prepared to cope with persistent unfocused immune activity.

Cytokines are immunomodulatory molecules produced by immune cells that coordinate the inflammatory response. The functions of the various existing cytokines are very complex and depend on the context and concentration of cytokines in relation to one another. However, cytokines such as interleukin-6 (IL-6), tumor necrosis factor-α (TNF-α), interleukin-1α, and interleukin-1β (IL-1β) are considered to have profound pro-inflammatory functions [16]. On the contrary, cytokines such as interleukin-4 (IL-4) and interleukin-10 (IL-10) are regarded as anti-inflammatory [16]. The idea that afferent pathways communicate the inflammatory status of peripheral tissues to the brain dates back to the beginning of the twentieth century, with observations by Wagner-Jauregg (Nobel Prize, 1927) that activation of the immune system by an infectious agent (malaria inoculation) could affect psychiatric symptoms and cognitive functions.

Studies showing that increased pro-inflammatory cytokines plasma concentrations correlated with the severity of illness in patients with MDD were the basis for proposing the cytokines-induced model of depression [17, 18].

Whole-body cryostimulation (WBC) is a promising intervention for the prevention and treatment of various diseases characterized by chronic inflammation, including mental and neurological disorders. Many experimental studies have shown that 5 to 20 sessions of WBC can result in statistically and clinically significant increases in IL-10 levels (anti-inflammatory cytokines) as well as decreases in IL-1β (pro-inflammatory cytokines) that are still visible 2 weeks after participation [19].

The impact of the immune system activation on mental health—and particularly on depression and anxiety—has been extensively studied over the last decade [20, 21]. In response to WBC, the cascade in cytokines release differs from the classical response to infections. For instance, it has been demonstrated that a four- to fivefold decrease in TNF-α could be achieved in obese men with poor cardiovascular fitness after ten WBC sessions [22]. It has also been reported that blood IL-10 levels considerably increased after 5, 10, or 20 WBC sessions in healthy men [19]. Increased anti-inflammatory IL-10 levels in the circulation can cause suppression of the pro-inflammatory cytokines IL-1α, IL-1β, and TNF-α at the central nervous system level [16]. This cascade of effects is schematically illustrated in Fig. 15.1.

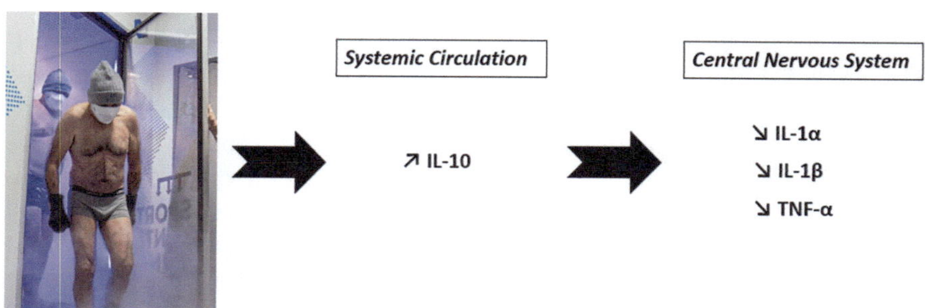

Fig. 15.1 Increased secretion of IL-10 in the systemic circulation reduces the brain levels of inflammatory cytokines IL-1α, IL-1β, and TNF-α. (Photo provided by CRYOTERA Bezannes, France. Copyright free)

Can Cryostimulation Programs Prevent or Treat Clinical Depression or Anxiety?

There are hardly seven studies published on the effects of cold therapy on mental health to date. In addition, only small samples were used; as a result, the participants used might not be representative of the general population. Of these studies, four included participants with MDD or anxiety diagnosis [23–26], two of which had no control group [23, 25]. Since the absence of a proper control group poses several threats to the internal validity of research using pre- and postintervention measures, we decided to discard them as it may be difficult to determine the "true" effect of WBC.

In their 2008 study, Rymaszewska and Ramsey [24] recruited 60 participants (53 females, mean age: 45 years) with diagnosis of MDD or anxiety disorder. They were randomized into two groups. The study group ($n = 26$) received 15 WBC sessions over a 3-week period (Monday to Friday, 3 weeks in a row). Each session was performed in a standard cryogenic chamber and lasted 2–3 min at a temperature of -110 °C to -160 °C (during the final sessions). Participants in the control group ($n = 34$) did not receive the WBC program. The Hamilton Depression Rating Scale (HDRS) and the Hamilton Anxiety Rating Scale (HARS) were used to evaluate depression and anxiety symptoms pre- and post-study for each participant. The HDRS is a 17-item clinician-rated instrument allowing a comprehensive evaluation of depressive symptomatology (e.g., guilt feelings, retardation, suicide ideation, and weight loss). Items are scored from 0 to 4, and the higher the total score the more severe the depression. The HARS is a clinician-rated instrument too. It aims at evaluating the various symptoms of anxiety (e.g., fears, insomnia, and respiratory symptoms). It includes 13 items, each being rated on a 5-point scale. The five scores are none (0), mild (1), moderate (2), severe (3), and very severe (4). Regarding the HDRS, all symptoms except gastrointestinal symptoms and weight loss significantly improved pre- to post-study among participants who received the WBC intervention compared to those in the control group. Likewise, comparing the two groups over the 3-week-long intervention, there were more favorable changes in HARS scores for participants in the study group, except for gastrointestinal and genitourinary symptoms. However, this study, despite having a control group, is limited by the lack of a procedure randomly assigning participants into the study groups.

This limitation was addressed in a recent randomized controlled trial published by the same research group [26]. A prospective, randomized, double-blind sham-controlled research design was used. The study involved 56 adults (mean age: 47 years, 40 females) with a diagnosis of an MDD who completed all evaluations. Thirty of them (study group) received ten WBC sessions over 2 weeks (five sessions per week, Monday to Friday) at a temperature of -110 °C to -160 °C (during the final sessions). The remaining participants (control group, $n = 26$) received a "sham" intervention, which consisted of WBC sessions at less extreme temperatures (-50 °C, the control group). The Hamilton Depression Rating Scale (HDRS) and the Beck Depression Inventory (BDI-II) were completed at baseline (T1), beginning of the second week of intervention (T2), end of intervention (T3), and 2 weeks after the end of intervention (T4). The BDI-II is a self-assessed measure of depression consisting of 21 items scored between 0 (lack of symptoms) and 3 (the highest severity of the described symptom). Scores between 0 and 13 indicate the lack of depressive symptoms, 14–19 indicate mild depressive symptoms, 20–29 indicate depressive symptoms of moderate intensity, and 30–63 reflect symptoms of severe intensity. The main findings revealed early decreases in self-reported depression (BDI-II scores), which appeared as soon as the first week of treatment, after five WBC sessions (T2). Similarly, evidence was found for a more significant decrease of clinically rated depressive symptoms (HDRS) at T4 (2 weeks after study completion) in participants who received the "true" WBC intervention compared to those received the «sham» treatment. It is worth mentioning that no adverse event was reported, leading the authors to state that WBC might be an effective and safe intervention for adults with MDD. One disconcerting result of this study was that—despite significant improved clinical outcomes—authors did not observe any significant change in the levels of IL-6 and IL-10 from T1 to T3 (no measures had been taken at T2 or T4). One potential explanation for this paradox could be that all participants were under antidepressant treatment at the time of study initiation. In a recent meta-analysis [27], it has appeared that antidepressant drugs inhibit cytokines production on a long-term basis, especially IL-4, IL-6, and IL-10.

Alternatively, this uncoupling between clinical symptoms of depression and inflammatory biomarkers may suggest that other mechanisms could be responsible for the effects of WBC on mental health. Solid evidence exists that WBC can lead to increased sleep quality [28], as well as increased energy/reduced fatigue [29]. Since poor sleep and lack of energy are two of the signature symptoms of MDD, it is obvious that such improvements will have a positive impact on mental health and alleviate depressive symptoms.

Finally, the last three studies reviewed in this section did not directly evaluate the effects of WBC on MDD or anxiety disorders. They are summarized shortly here however, as they are still relevant to the broader topic of mental health.

In 2021, Rymaszewska et al. [30] published a randomized controlled trial, which involved 62 participants diagnosed with a mild neurocognitive disorder (mean age: 66 years, 40 females). After randomization into a study group ($n = 33$) or a control group ($n = 29$), those in the study group received ten WBC sessions (-110 °C to -135 °C) over 2 weeks (one session per day from Monday to Friday). Participants in the control group received a "sham" treatment using WBC with similar parameters except room temperature, which was set at -50 °C. Significant differences in general cognitive functioning and orientation ability were found between groups immediately after the 2 weeks of intervention in favor of the study group.

In the study by Happe and colleagues [31], 35 participants (mean age: 61 years, 28 females) with a diagnosis of sleep-wake disorder (restless legs syndrome, RLS) were randomized to either 14 sessions (one daily session over 2 weeks) of WBC at -60 °C ($n = 12$), 14 sessions of WBC at -10 °C ("sham" treatment, $n = 12$), or 14 sessions of local cryotherapy (on the affected legs) at -17 °C (control group, $n = 11$). Several questionnaires evaluating the severity of RLS symptoms and sleep quality were administered immediately before and after completion of the 14 sessions, and 4 weeks after the end of intervention. In addition, the number of periodic leg movements (PLM) was assessed via surface electrodes over the anterior tibial muscle of each leg before and after completion of the 14 sessions, and in the last 2 weeks of follow-up. Both the number of periodic leg movements and the severity of RLS symptoms significantly decreased following intervention in participants who received WBC at −60 °C. All this translated into a substantial and significant increase in total sleep time. These benefits were still present at the 4-week follow-up. No change was found for these variables among participants who received sham WBC or local cryotherapy.

Using a single-case experimental (A-B-A) design involving one patient diagnosed with restless legs syndrome, Kasmi and colleagues [32] extended on these findings by demonstrating that WBC (ten sessions over 2 weeks; room temperature: −90 °C) can also result in significantly decreased daytime sleepiness. Excessive daytime sleepiness has been documented to cause negative behavioral, physiological, and cognitive effects, which limit people's actions and quality of life [33].

Conclusion and Perspectives

Major depression and anxiety are common mental health disorders that can have serious effects. More often than not, decision for psychiatric treatments—which are time-consuming and costly—is made after a long delay. In addition, side effects of pharmacological interventions may include fatigue, cardiovascular complications, and possible addiction. Thus, nonpharmacological interventions may be a desirable alternative or adjunct treatment.

Published research has so far principally involved participants with depression. Overall, the literature supports some clinically significant benefits of WBC on alleviating depressive symptoms in people diagnosed as having mild-to-moderate depression. However, the number of published studies on this topic is still very limited to date, and all follow-up periods were short-lived (<1 month).

Burgeoning evidence also suggests that WBC programs may contribute to reduction in severity and symptoms of mild neurocognitive disorders and sleep-wake disorders (which are among the most common types of mental health disorders worldwide). However, sleep-wake disorders are a group of conditions including more than a dozen specific problems, and published studies have exclusively focused on restless legs syndrome to date.

Overall, an important issue is that serious questions remain about the potential for bias in most of the studies reviewed in this chapter.

Consequently, for now, clinicians and health professionals can be recommended to consider promoting WBC as a treatment option for MDD, anxiety, mild neurocognitive disorders, and sleep-wake disorders, but should be mindful of the methodological concerns raised and be aware that current evidence points toward WBC being effective only in the shorter term.

Future research is strongly needed to (a) determine whether benefits can be obtained through the use of WBC programs in participants with true anxiety disorders (not only above-average anxiety); (b) identify the specific parameters of WBC duration, frequency, and intensity that should be used for optimizing positive effects; and (c) understand the mechanisms—especially the neurobiological mechanisms—whereby WBC promotes mental health.

References

1. American Psychiatric Association. Diagnostic and statistical manual of mental disorders. 5th ed. Arlington, VA: American Psychiatric Association; 2013.
2. American Psychiatric Association. Diagnostic and statistical manual of mental disorders, 4th edition, text revised. Washington, DC: American Psychiatric Association; 2000.
3. Robins LN, Wing J, Wittchen HU, Helzer JE, Babor TF, Burke J, et al. The Composite International Diagnostic Interview. An epidemiologic instrument suitable for use in conjunction with different diagnostic systems and in different cultures. Arch Gen Psychiatry. 1988;45:1069–77.
4. Bijl RV, de Graaf R, Ravelli A, Smit F, Vollebergh WAM. Gender and age-specific first incidence of DSM-III R psychiatric disorders in the general population: Results from The Netherlands Mental Health Survey and Incidence Study (NEMESIS). Soc Psychiatry Psychiatr Epidemiol. 2002;37:372–9.
5. de Graaf R, Bijl RV, Ravelli A, Smit F, Vollebergh WAM. Predictors of first incidence of DSM III R psychiatric disorders in the general population: Findings from The Netherlands Mental Health Survey and Incidence Study. Acta Psychiatr Scand. 2002;106:303–13.
6. Alonso J, Petukhova M, Vilagut G, Chatterji S, Heeringa S, Ustun TB, et al. Days out of role due to common physical and mental conditions: Results from the WHO World Mental Health surveys. Mol Psychiatry. 2011;16:1234–46.
7. Buist-Bouwman MA, Ormel J, de Graaf R, de Jonge P, van Sonderen E, Alonso J. Mediators of the association between depression and role functioning. Acta Psychiatr Scand. 2008;118:451–8.
8. Murray CJL, Lopez AD. The global burden of disease: A comprehensive assessment of mortality and disability from diseases, injuries, and risk factors in 1990 and projected to 2020. Cambridge, MA: Harvard University Press; 1996.
9. Institute for Health Metrics and Evaluation (IHME). GBD compare. Seattle, WA: University of Washington; 2015. http://vizhub.healthdata.org/gbd-compare
10. Kohn R, Saxena S, Levav I, Saraceno B. The treatment gap in mental health care. Bull World Health Organ. 2004;82:858–66.
11. Kohn R. Treatment gap in the Americas. Washington, DC: Pan American Health Organization; 2013.
12. Alonso J, Angermeyer MC, Bernert S, Bruffaerts R, Brugha TS, Brysin H, et al. Use of mental health services in Europe: Results from the European Study of the Epidemiology of Mental Disorders (ESEMeD) project. Acta Psychiatr Scand. 2004;420:47–54.
13. Wang PS, Berglund P, Olfson M, Pincus AH, Wells KB, Kessler RC. Failure and delay in initial treatment contact after first onset of mental disorders in the National Comorbidity Survey replication. Arch Gen Psychiatry. 2005;62:603–13.
14. World Health Organization. The World Health Report 2001 Mental Health: New understanding, new hope. Geneva: WHO; 2001.
15. Huang W, Aune D, Ferrari G, Zhang L, Lan Y, Nie J, et al. Psychological distress and all-cause, cardiovascular disease, cancer mortality among adults with and without diabetes. Clin Epidemiol. 2021;13:555–65.
16. Svensson M, Lexell J, Deierborg T. Effects of physical activity on neuroinflammation, neuroplasticity, neurodegeneration, and behavior: What we learn from animal models in clinical settings. Neurorehabil Neural Repair. 2015;29:577–89.

17. Dantzer R, O'Connor JC, Freund GG, Johnson RW, Kelley KW. From inflammation to sickness and depression: When the immune system subjugates the brain. Nat Rev Neurosci. 2008;9:46–57.
18. Raison CL, Capuron L, Miller AH. Cytokines sing the blues: Inflammation and the pathogenesis of depression. Trends Immunol. 2006;27:24–31.
19. Lubkowska A, Szygula Z, Chlubek D, Banfi G. The effect of prolonged whole-body cryostimulation treatment with different amounts of sessions on chosen pro- and anti-inflammatory cytokines levels in healthy men. Scand J Clin Lab Investig. 2011;71:419–25.
20. Moons WG, Shields GS. Anxiety, not anger, induces inflammatory activity: an avoidance/approach model of immune system activation. Emotion. 2015;15:463–76.
21. Sorensen NV, Benros ME. The immune system and depression: From epidemiological to clinical evidence. Curr Top Behav Neurosci. 2023;61:15–34.
22. Ziemann E, Olek RA, Grzywacz T, Antosziewicz J, Kujach S, Luszczyk M, et al. Whole-body cryostimulation as an effective method of reducing low-grade inflammation in obese men. J Physiol Sci. 2013;63:333–43.
23. Rymaszewska J, Tulczynski A, Zagrobelny Z, Kiejna A, Hadrys T. Influence of whole body cryotherapy on depressive symptoms—preliminary report. Acta Neuropsychiatr. 2003;15:122–8.
24. Rymaszewska J, Ramsey D. Whole body cryotherapy as a novel adjuvant therapy for depression and anxiety. Arch Immunol Ther Exp. 2008;10:49–57.
25. Rymaszewska J, Urbanska K, Szczesniak D, Pawłowski T, Pieniawska K, Kokot I, et al. Whole-body cryotherapy: Promising add-on treatment of depressive disorders. Psychiatr Pol. 2019;53:1053–67.
26. Rymaszewska J, Lion KM, Pawlik-Sobecka L, Pawłowski T, Szczesniak D, Trypka E, et al. Efficacy of the whole-body cryotherapy as add-on therapy to pharmacological treatment of depression: a randomized controlled trial. Front Psych. 2020;11:522.
27. Wiedlocha M, Marcinowicz P, Krupa R, Janoska-Jazdzic M, Janus M, Debowska W, et al. Effect of antidepressant treatment on peripheral inflammation markers—A meta-analysis. Prog Neuro-Psychopharmacol Biol Psychiatry. 2018;80:217–26.
28. Douzi W, Dupuy O, Tanneau M, Boucard G, Bouzigon R, Dugué B. 3-min whole body cryotherapy/cryostimulation after training in the evening improves sleep quality in physically active men. Eur J Sport Sci. 2019;19:860–7.
29. Kujawski S, Zalewski P, Godlewska BR, Cudnoch-Jedrzejewska A, Murowska M, Newton JL, et al. Effects of whole-body cryotherapy and static stretching are maintained 4 weeks after treatment in most patients with chronic fatigue syndrome. Cryobiology. 2023;112:104546.
30. Rymaszewska J, Lion KM, Stanczykiewicz B, Rymaszewska JE, Trypka E, Pawlik-Sobecka L, et al. The improvement of cognitive deficits after whole-body cryotherapy: a randomised controlled trial. Exp Gerontol. 2021;146:111237.
31. Happe S, Evers S, Thiedemann C, Bunten S, Siegert R. Whole body and local cryotherapy in restless legs syndrome: a randomized, single-blind, controlled parallel group pilot study. J Neurol Sci. 2016;370:7–12.
32. Kasmi S, Filliard JR, Polidori G, Bouchet B, Blancheteau Y, Legrand FD. Effects of Whole-Body Cryostimulation (−90°C) on somnolence and psychological well-being in an older patient with restless legs syndrome. Appl Psychol Health Well-Being. 2020;12:259–67.
33. Liu X, Liu ZZ, Wang ZY, Yang Y, Liu BP, Xia CX. Daytime sleepiness predicts future suicidal behavior: a longitudinal study of adolescents. Sleep. 2019;42:zsy225.

Sleep Disorders

16

Elisa Perger, Laura Calvillo, and Riccardo Cremascoli

Introduction

Sleep involves roughly one-third of human lives and prolonged sleep deprivation is fatal in animals [1]. Sleep is a complex and precise body process with an essential role in physical restoration, learning and memory, neurocognitive performance, and for the immune system. One mechanism by which sleep is proposed to provide a survival advantage is in terms of supporting a neurally integrated immune system that might anticipate injury and infectious threats. Sleep disturbances, such as sleep apnea or restless legs syndrome, have negative consequences on the neural and cardiovascular system and can contribute to the dysregulation of inflammatory and antiviral responses. Thus, sleep deprivation is associated with increases in inflammatory molecules such as cytokines, interleukin-6, and C-reactive protein, exposing subjects with sleep disorders to cardiovascular disease, immunological disorders, and chronic diseases [2]. Within the sleep period, lowering the minimum body temperature has been suggested to increase slow wave sleep and to positively affect sleep quality [3]. Several results suggest that the evening lowering body temperature is mediated by endogenous melatonin [4, 5]. In this view, experimental data have shown that the hypothermic effects of exogenous therapeutic melatonin

E. Perger (✉)
Sleep Disorders Center, IRCCS Istituto Auxologico Italiano, Milan, Italy
e-mail: e.perger@auxologico.it

L. Calvillo
Sleep Disorders Center, Department of Cardiovascular, Neural and Metabolic Sciences, IRCCS Istituto Auxologico Italiano, Milan, Italy

R. Cremascoli
Sleep Medicine Unit, IRCCS Istituto Auxologico Italiano, Piancavallo (Verbania), Italy

may mediate its hypnotic effects [6, 7]. Several cooling protocols have been proposed in scientific literature, which effects range from transient skin temperature drop to several degrees of hypothermia (from mild degree when the human body temperature reaches 32–34°C to severe hypothermia for a temperature of 28°C or lower) [8]. Although hypothermia could induce torpor and be associated with sleep changes [8, 9], this chapter will focus only on cryostimulation and its effect on sleep.

Whole-body cryostimulation (WBC) or partial-body cryostimulation (PBC) is a physical treatment that exposes the body to cryogenic temperatures (−110°C to −140°C) for a short period (2–3 min), producing in first instance a transient drop in skin temperature.

The extreme cold of body cryostimulation (BC) has become an emerging tool, demonstrating changes in inflammatory response [10], reduction in pain [11], improved muscle strength recovery [12], and benefits to range of motion [13]. Cooling therapies are often used in sports medicine and in athletes after training and competitions to reduce inflammation, oxidative stress and to enhance sleep quality. Although cryostimulation has a recognized effect on the human body [14–16], its possible role in influencing sleep and sleep-related disorders is still largely unknown.

Effect of BC on Sleep Quality

With BC having a recognized effect especially for sports and exercise recovery [17], literature available up to now explores sleep during muscle recovery or during training studies. Douzi and colleagues found that WBC on physically active human males could improve the quality of sleep [18]. Three-minute exposure to a temperature of −40 °C under a wind speed of 2.3 m/s was compared to passive recovery in 22 healthy participants [18]. Each night after regular training, subjective sleep quality was assessed using Spiegel's questionnaire and perceived pain was evaluated, thanks to a visual analogue scale. Movements during sleep were evaluated with a wrist actigraph. While the time spent in bed was similar between WBC treatment and regular recovery, Spiegel's total questionnaire score was significantly higher after WBC exposure than after passive recovery (WBC: 20.9 ± 3.5 vs control: 23.1 ± 2.5, $p < 0.05$), which indicated improved subjective sleep quality. The number of movements during the night following WBC was significantly reduced ($p < 0.05$), together with a perception of pain relief [18]. Qu and colleagues evaluated cryostimulation on subjective sleep quality in Chinese middle- and long-distance runners after muscle damage protocol [19]. Pittsburgh Sleep Quality Index scores indicated that the cryostimulation protocol had improved sleep quality compared with the control and cold water immersion conditions ($p < 0.05$) [19]. The results from this study suggest that cryostimulation improves subjective sleep quality and reduces muscle damage and inflammatory responses.

Conversely, in a postexercise study on healthy subjects, while WBC was more effective than cold water immersions for muscle strength postexercise recovery, this treatment did not improve sleep [12]. However, in this study, sleep quality was evaluated with wrist watches (Fitbit Inspire, California) instead of a validated actigraph and sleep quality was expressed with a self-reported scale from 1 to 5 and not with more accurate questionnaires [12]. An analogous sleep quality scale applied to off-season athletes failed to show acute sleep improvement after a single evening partial body cryostimulation (approximately −180 °C in a specially designed cabin for 3 min) [20].

Regarding high-performance athletes, only partial preliminary results on sleep quality emerged in ten elite synchronized female swimmers after WBC and intense training [21]. In 27 professional basketball players during tournaments for the European championship, a 3-min exposure between −110 °C and −150 °C was performed after a training or a match session. Sleep was assessed with a perceptual 1–5 scale adapted from Spiegel's questionnaire and showed an amelioration after WBC [22]. In soccer players, Douze and coauthors evaluated a partial body cryostimulation (the all body excluding the head and the neck) after a training session [23]. Each player experienced different exposure durations at −180 °C in a partial-body chamber (Cryotechno®, Castelnau le Lez, France) in a random order (no cryostimulation, 180-s exposure, twice 90-s exposure separated by a 5-min rest at room temperature, and 90-s exposure). The sleep quality was evaluated using Spiegel's sleep quality perception questionnaire, and movements during sleep were recorded with an actigraph. The number of accelerations detected during the night following the exposure was significantly lower after the 180-s exposure than in the control and in other tested conditions. Sleep efficiency and the subjective sleep quality were similar in all the tested conditions. Similarly, a 12-week partial-body cryostimulation intervention (2 min at a temperature of −120°C in a cryosauna *CryoPod*, Cumbria, UK) showed no effects on the sleep quality questionnaire in Elite Rugby Union Players During the Competitive Phase of the Season [24].

While actigraphy is able to detect indirectly sleep quality by analyzing the time spent in bed, lights, and movement during sleep, the correct evaluation of sleep architecture and respiratory quality needs nocturnal polysomnography with electro-encephalograms. In our knowledge, polysomnography after WBC was performed in only one study on 19 professional rugby players by Aloulou and coauthors [25]. After a 3-min exposure of an extreme cold temperature at −110 °C 2 h before bedtime, no differences in sleep quality were observed. Unfortunately, no data regarding sleep stages or sleep respiratory parameters were presented.

Outside the sport field, literature is still lacking in terms of cryotherapy for sleep evaluation in nonhealthy subjects. Only one study applied whole-body cryotherapy in patients hospitalized for coronavirus disease 2019 (COVID-19). Long COVID-19 syndrome is a disease that follows acute COVID-19 and it is known to affect sleep quality [26]. In a case series, seven patients suffering post-COVID-19 condition underwent a WBC cycle of 10–15 sessions at −110 °C in the morning in a cryochamber, before physical exercise classes and physiotherapy [27]. After treatment, the most frequently reported improvements were related with quality of life, sleep, and mood, together with a reduced fatigue, dyspnea, and pain.

The efficacy of WBC as add-on treatment to pharmacotherapy in patients affected by depression was explored by Rymaszewska et al. [28]. While whole-body cryotherapy was effective in decreasing depressive symptoms, self-assessed mood, and in increased self-perception of life quality, no improvements were noted in sleep quality explored with a visual analogue scales (VAS) questionnaire. Finally, recently, Verme and colleagues described a positive effect on sleep quality of 10 whole-body cryotherapy sessions (twice a day, the first at 9 a.m. and the second at 12 p.m. inside a cryochamber Artic, CryoScience, Rome, at −110 °C for 2 min) on a 74-year-old woman suffering from active rheumatic polymyalgia [29]. Also in this study, sleep quality was assessed using the Pittsburgh sleep quality index (PSQI) clinical scale.

Effect of BC on Sleep-Related Diseases

Sleep might also be disrupted by respiratory disorders such as apneas or hypopneas or by leg movement. Restless legs syndrome (RLS) is a neurological sleep disorder that causes an uncomfortable feeling and the urge to move the legs. RLS is highly related to insomnia, sleep deprivation, and fragmentation [30], with a consequent increase in systemic inflammation and somnolence.

Nevertheless, few studies were performed relating to medical application of whole-body cryotherapy, where sleep quality was considered.

In a randomized, single-blind, controlled parallel group pilot study [31], 35 patients with idiopathic RLS were randomized into three groups for 3 min over 2 weeks: cold air chamber at −60 °C; cold air chamber at −10 °C, and local cryotherapy at −17 °C. The severity of symptoms was documented weekly by using the RLS Severity Scale, as well as daily completion of the VAS for rating the feelings/perceptions. The Epworth Sleepiness Scale (ESS) as evaluation of sleepiness was also conducted. Significant improvements of RLS symptoms and quality of life were observed only in the −60 °C group as compared to baseline. Local cryotherapy led to improvement in quality of life and sleep quality but not in RLS relief and in somnolence as detected by the ESS. In the −10 °C group, the only significant effect was shortening the number of wake phases per night [31].

Kasmi and colleagues exposed a patient affected by RLS who experienced somnolence to whole-body cryotherapy at −90 °C for 2 weeks daily [32]. Reported levels of sleepiness decreased immediately following the beginning of the treatment phase. Whole-body cryotherapy was well tolerated and self-reported well-being significantly increased during cold exposure.

The most common sleep disordered breathing is obstructive sleep apnea (OSA) that is responsible for systemic inflammation, sympathetic overactivity, free radicals' formations due to intermittent hypoxia, sleep fragmentation, and cognitive impairment. As exposure to cold (e.g., winter swimming, cold-water immersion, and WBC) has been shown to reduce inflammation, oxidative stress and to improve sleep quality, it has been hypothesized that whole-body cryotherapy might also have a beneficial effect in the alleviation of OSA consequences [33]. However, to our knowledge, up to now, no studies have investigated the role of WBC as an adjunct to OSA therapy. Only recently has a randomized controlled trial (RCT) been proposed from researchers of Sohag University to evaluate the role of cryotherapy in

OSA patients (NCT05206916). Twenty-five OSA patients aged between 25 and 65 years and a body mass index between 28 and 40 kg/m^2 will be exposed to local cryotherapy at sites of vibration as origin of snoring and site of collapse.

Conclusion

Although cryostimulation is known to improve sleep quality following intense physical activity, its application in patients with sleep disorders is almost unexplored to date. Sleep perception assessed by questionnaires and sleep quality in terms of movements during sleep have been evaluated in healthy subjects, but there is a lack of studies that have carefully examined changes in sleep stages with polysomnography and the effect of cryotherapy on sleep breathing disorders. Theoretically, cryostimulation can improve sleep quality, but to date literature is still immature in this field. In particular, there is a need of neurophysiological investigations on the effects of cryostimulation on both the homeostatic and circadian processes of sleep, with a particular focus on core body temperature and melatonin alterations. New, more accurate studies regarding sleep and its pathologies are needed to explore the possible role of cryotherapy.

References

1. Samson ZA, Montserrat D-A, Emerson MW, Steven MS. The functions of sleep. AIMS Neuroscience. 2015;2(3):155–71.
2. Irwin MR. Sleep and inflammation: partners in sickness and in health. Nat Rev Immunol. 2019;19(11):702–15.
3. Togo F, Aizawa S, Arai J, et al. Influence on human sleep patterns of lowering and delaying the minimum core body temperature by slow changes in the thermal environment. Sleep. 2007;30(6):797–802.
4. Badia P, Myers B, Murphy PI. Melatonin and thermoregulation. 1994.
5. Dawson D, Encel N. Melatonin and sleep in humans. J Pineal Res. 1993;15(1):1–12.
6. Attenburrow ME, Cowen PJ, Sharpley AL. Low dose melatonin improves sleep in healthy middle-aged subjects. Psychopharmacology. 1996;126(2):179–81.
7. Zhdanova IV, Wurtman RJ, Lynch HJ, et al. Sleep-inducing effects of low doses of melatonin ingested in the evening. Clin Pharmacol Ther. 1995;57(5):552–8.
8. Lee CC. Is human hibernation possible? Annu Rev Med. 2008;59:177–86.
9. Glees P, Blumer WFC, Cole J. A study of monkeys subjected to hypothermia. Minim Invasive Neurosurg. 1963;6(03):108–16.
10. Pournot H, Bieuzen F, Louis J, Fillard J-R, Barbiche E, Hausswirth C. Time-course of changes in inflammatory response after whole-body cryotherapy multi exposures following severe exercise. PLoS One. 2011;6(7):e22748.
11. Hausswirth C, Louis J, Bieuzen F, et al. Effects of whole-body cryotherapy vs. far-infrared vs. passive modalities on recovery from exercise-induced muscle damage in highly-trained runners. PLoS One. 2011;6(12):e27749.
12. Haq A, Ribbans WJ, Hohenauer E, Baross AW. The comparative effect of different timings of whole body cryotherapy treatment with cold water immersion for post-exercise recovery. Front Sports Act Living. 2022;4:940516.

13. De Nardi M, La Torre A, Benis R, Sarabon N, Fonda B. Acute effects of whole-body cryotherapy on sit-and-reach amplitude in women and men. Cryobiology. 2015;71(3):511–3.
14. Bleakley CM, Bieuzen F, Davison GW, Costello JT. Whole-body cryotherapy: empirical evidence and theoretical perspectives. Open Access J Sports Med. 2014;5:25–36.
15. Bouzigon R, Grappe F, Ravier G, Dugue B. Whole- and partial-body cryostimulation/cryotherapy: current technologies and practical applications. J Therm Biol. 2016;61:67–81.
16. Kujawski S, Newton JL, Morten KJ, Zalewski P. Whole-body cryostimulation application with age: a review. J Therm Biol. 2021;96:102861.
17. Lombardi G, Ziemann E, Banfi G. Whole-body cryotherapy in athletes: from therapy to stimulation. An updated review of the literature. Front Physiol. 2017;8:258.
18. Douzi W, Dupuy O, Tanneau M, Boucard G, Bouzigon R, Dugué B. 3-min whole body cryotherapy/cryostimulation after training in the evening improves sleep quality in physically active men. Eur J Sport Sci. 2019;19(6):860–7.
19. Qu C, Wu Z, Xu M, et al. Cryotherapy on subjective sleep quality, muscle, and inflammatory response in Chinese middle- and long-distance runners after muscle damage. J Strength Cond Res. 2021;36:2883–90.
20. Hoshikawa M, Dohi M, Nakamura M. Effects of evening partial body cryostimulation on the skin and core temperatures. J Therm Biol. 2019;79:144–8.
21. Schaal K, Le Meur Y, Louis J, et al. Whole-body cryostimulation limits overreaching in elite synchronized swimmers. Med Sci Sports Exerc. 2015;47(7):1416–25.
22. Bouzigon R, Ravier G, Dugue B, Grappe F. The use of whole-body cryostimulation to improve the quality of sleep in athletes during high level standard competitions. Br J Sports Med. 2014;48(7):572.
23. Douzi W, Dupuy O, Theurot D, Boucard G, Dugué B. Partial-body cryostimulation after training improves sleep quality in professional soccer players. BMC Res Notes. 2019;12(1):1–5.
24. Grainger A, Comfort P, Heffernan S. No effect of partial-body cryotherapy on restoration of countermovement-jump or well-being performance in elite Rugby union players during the competitive phase of the season. Int J Sports Physiol Perform. 2019;15:1–23.
25. Aloulou A, Leduc C, Duforez F, et al. Effect of an innovative mattress and cryotherapy on sleep after an elite Rugby match. Med Sci Sports Exerc. 2020;52(12):2655–62.
26. Giuliano M, Tiple D, Agostoni P, et al. Italian good practice recommendations on management of persons with long-COVID. Front Public Health. 2023;11:1122141.
27. Piterà P, Gobbi M, Fontana JM, Cattaldo S, Massucci M, Capodaglio P. Whole-body cryostimulation: a rehabilitation booster in post-COVID patients? A case series. Appl Sci. 2022;12(10):4830.
28. Rymaszewska J, Lion KM, Pawlik-Sobecka L, et al. Efficacy of the whole-body cryotherapy as add-on therapy to pharmacological treatment of depression-a randomized controlled trial. Front Psych. 2020;11:522.
29. Verme F, Scarpa A, Varallo G, Piterà P, Capodaglio P, Fontana JM. Effects of whole-body cryostimulation on pain management and disease activity in active rheumatic polymyalgia: a case-report. Biomedicine. 2023;11(6):1594.
30. Vlasie A, Trifu SC, Lupuleac C, Kohn B, Cristea MB. Restless legs syndrome: an overview of pathophysiology, comorbidities and therapeutic approaches (review). Exp Ther Med. 2022;23(2):185.
31. Happe S, Evers S, Thiedemann C, Bunten S, Siegert R. Whole body and local cryotherapy in restless legs syndrome: a randomized, single-blind, controlled parallel group pilot study. J Neurol Sci. 2016;370:7–12.
32. Kasmi S, Filliard JR, Polidori G, Bouchet B, Blancheteau Y, Legrand FD. Effects of whole-body cryostimulation (−90°C) on somnolence and psychological Well-being in an older patient with restless legs syndrome. Appl Psychol Health Well Being. 2020;12(2):259–67.
33. Douzi W, De Bisschop C, Dugué B. Regular short exposures to cold environment as an adjunct therapy for patients with sleep apnea syndrome (SAS). Med Hypotheses. 2022;161:110795.

Risks 17

Fabien D. Legrand, Benoit Dugué, Elzbieta Miller,
Guillaume Polidori, Giovanni Lombardi,
Jacopo Maria Fontana, Paolo Capodaglio,
and the Whole-Body Cryostimulation Working
Group of the International Institute
of Refrigeration

the Whole-Body Cryostimulation Working Group of the International Institute of
Refrigeration

F. D. Legrand
Cognition Santé Société, Department of Psychology, University of Reims Champagne
Ardennes, Reims, France
e-mail: fabien.legrand@univ-reims.fr

B. Dugué
Laboratory Mobilité, Vieillissement, Exercice (MOVE), Faculty of Sports Sciences,
University of Poitiers, Poitiers, France
e-mail: benoit.dugue@univ-poitiers.fr

E. Miller
Neurological Rehabilitation Department, Medical University of Lodz, Lodz, Poland
e-mail: elzbieta.dorota.miller@umed.lodz.pl

G. Polidori
University of Reims Champagne Ardennes, "MATIM", Reims, France
e-mail: guillaume.polidori@univ-reims.fr

G. Lombardi
Laboratory of Experimental Biochemistry and Molecular Biology, IRCCS Istituto Ortopedico
Galeazzi, Milan, Italy

Department of Athletics, Strength and Conditioning, Poznań University of Physical
Education, Poznań, Poland
e-mail: giovanni.lombardi@grupposandonato.it; lombardi@awf.poznan.pl

J. M. Fontana
Research Laboratory in Biomechanics, Rehabilitation and Ergonomics, IRCCS Istituto
Auxologico Italiano, Piancavallo (Verbania), Italy
e-mail: j.fontana@auxologico.it

P. Capodaglio (✉)
Research Laboratory in Biomechanics, Rehabilitation and Ergonomics, IRCCS Istituto
Auxologico Italiano, Piancavallo (Verbania), Italy

Physical and Rehabilitation Medicine, Department of Surgical Sciences,
University of Torino, Torino, Italy
e-mail: p.capodaglio@auxologico.it; paolo.capodaglio@unito.it

P. Capodaglio (ed.), *Whole-Body Cryostimulation*,
https://doi.org/10.1007/978-3-031-18545-8_17

Evaluating the effectiveness of an intervention is inseparable from assessing its safety. Thus, it is crucial to put the expected benefits of whole-body cryotherapy (WBC) into perspective with the potential harms and risks it may impose on those who will receive it. There is historical evidence that traditional cold-based therapies, such as cold water immersion and ice pack application, are safe and can result in significantly decreased body temperature that will trigger a range of beneficial effects. WBC is often regarded as a superior and more comfortable mode of cooling; however, there is no conclusive evidence that it offers distinct advantages over traditional methods of cryotherapy [1]. In a randomized controlled trial, Hirvonen et al. [2] reported that WBC (-110 °C) seems to relieve pain more effectively than other types of cryostimulation (WBC -60 °C, local cold air -30 °C, cold water immersion, and cold packs) in participants with rheumatoid arthritis. Similarly, Costello et al. [3, 4] showed that WBC was able to elicit a greater decrease in skin temperature as compared to cold water immersion for 4 min at 8 °C. Average and minimum skin temperatures were lower immediately after WBC (19.0 ± 0.9 °C) compared to cold water immersion (20.5 ± 0.6 °C). However, during the assessments conducted after the end of cold exposure (10–60 min post-interventions), the average, minimum, and maximum skin temperatures were lower for participants who had been immersed in cold water. The authors also concluded that none of the tested protocols had decreased skin temperature to the supposedly required level for achieving an analgesic effect or stimulating systemic anti-inflammatory processes (i.e., <13 °C). Future studies are needed to compare the clinical benefits that can be obtained from different types of cryostimulation, and their cost-effectiveness, and shed further light on the target of skin temperature to be achieved for obtaining those benefits. This chapter only focuses on contraindications, risks, and reported adverse events related to WBC.

Consensus on Contraindications

The use of WBC has grown exponentially worldwide. According to the French Society of Whole-Body Cryotherapy, over one million WBC sessions were delivered for the year 2019 in France. In Poland, where WBC is covered under the national health fund, the number of reimbursed WBC sessions was estimated to be around 650,000 sessions per year over the last decade. The high number of exposures may result in an increased number of complications, but, surprisingly, only a few cases of complications have been reported in the literature to date. Part of the reason for this are, on one side, the precautionary measures taken for safety and security (see list of absolute contraindications jointly released and implemented by the Bad Voslau [5] and the International Institute of Refrigeration consensus [6]) (Tables 17.1 and 17.2) and, on the other, the absence of a clear register of adverse events and a lack of reporting.

Medical assessments determining participants' ability to receive WBC treatment are still poorly defined and vary from one country to another. For instance,

Table 17.1 Bad Voslau absolute contraindications to WBC

Whole-body cryostimulation contraindications	
• Untreated high blood pressure • Heart attack within the past 6 months • Decompensated diseases of the cardiovascular and respiratory system • Unstable angina • Pacemaker • Peripheral artery occlusive disease (Fontaine's stages III and IV) • History of deep vein thrombosis	• Acute febrile diseases of the respiratory tract • Acute renal and urinary disorders • Severe anemia • Signs or symptoms of cold allergy • Severe wasting diseases • Seizure disorder • Large-area bacterial and viral skin infections, wound-healing problems • Alcohol and drug influence

Table 17.2 International Institute of Refrigeration Medical contraindications

• Serious hypertension • Serious cardiopathies • Cold allergy • Raynaud syndrome • Sickle cell anemia • Cryoglobulinemia • Claustrophobia • Skin problems • Frostbites • Severe hypothyroid diseases

blood pressure monitoring is mandatory for the routine diagnosis of hypertension (serious hypertension is one of the main contraindications to WBC), but there is no agreement on the cut-off values for allowing subjects' access to WBC. In Poland, the cut-off value is rather strict and subjects with systolic blood pressure over 130 mmHg are not allowed to be exposed. Protocols still need to be universally defined and validated in order to limit the risks of health issues during and after cold exposure.

Documented WBC-Related Adverse Events

The lack of evidence on adverse events is thought to be underestimated due to either underreporting or a lack of uniform reporting standards. In response to calls by several experts for further investigations on WBC safety [7], a panel of experts critically analyzed each reported case of WBC-induced adverse events using well-established reporting standards [8]. To do so, the Common Terminology Criteria for Adverse Events grading system [9] was used for assessing the seriousness of any adverse event, which allowed to distinguish between «minor» (Grade 1 or Grade 2) and "serious" (Grade 3, Grade 4, or Grade 5) adverse events in the present review. Adverse events classified into the Grade 3 (or more) category define severe complications requiring at least hospitalization or invasive healing therapy,

Table 17.3 Grades to classify the severity of adverse events (common terminology criteria for adverse events)

Grades to classify the severity of harms (common terminology criteria for adverse events)	
Grade 1—Mild	Asymptomatic or minor symptoms Clinical or diagnostic observations only No intervention needed
Grade 2—Moderate	Minimal, local, or noninvasive intervention indicated
Grade 3—Severe	Medically significant but not immediately life-threatening Hospitalization or prolongation of hospitalization indicated Disabling
Grade 4—Life-threatening	Life-threatening consequences (i.e., immediate risk of death) Urgent intervention indicated
Grade 5—Death	Death related to adverse events

while Grade 1 and Grade 2 adverse events require no or noninvasive interventional procedures (Table 17.3). As the weight of scientific evidence for a causal relationship in each of the cases to be presented differs somewhat, a judgment has been made at the end of each section. This assigned associations to one of four categories: (1) convincing evidence for a causal relationship, (2) probable evidence, (3) possible evidence, and (4) insufficient evidence. "Convincing" and "probable" evidence for a causal disease/exposure relationship should result in policy recommendations, while "possible" and "insufficient" evidence indicates the need for more research.

This panel of experts recently produced a preprint paper [8], in which a literature search was performed in the PubMed, Scopus, Cochrane, and Web of Science electronic databases using the following keywords and Boolean operators "adverse OR side OR negative AND effects OR complications AND whole-body cryotherapy OR extreme cold exposure OR cryostimulation." Studies published in languages other than English and French were excluded. No temporal restriction was performed. A combined search for these keywords returned 19 records, published up to February 2023. In the second step, literature screening was done based on a set of inclusion and exclusion criteria to identify the papers to be read in detail. Eight papers were found to be duplicates, and another three records were excluded as they used cryosauna interventions (despite having indicated whole-body cryotherapy in the title). One master's thesis was also excluded. In total, seven articles were reviewed. Six were written in English and one in French. Our search strategy located seven articles reporting a total of 16 documented adverse events (Table 17.1). Five of these seven articles were case reports studies [10–14], and the remaining two papers were randomized controlled trials (RCT), which mentioned safety data in their results section [2, 15]. Reported cases were mostly middle-aged to aged individuals treated for benign, self-limiting conditions such as back pain, joint pain (rheumatism/arthritis), or sleep disturbances. There was no clear over-representation of one sex over another. In most reported cases, patients fully recovered in less than 1 month.

Dermatological

Cold Panniculitis

Greenwald et al. [11] reported a case of cold panniculitis in a 47-year-old man who received eight WBC sessions over the 2 weeks preceding symptom onset. After a diagnosis of panniculitis was made, cessation of cold exposure was the only treatment received and the patient's condition improved spontaneously within a couple of weeks. Greenwald concluded that reported symptoms were most consistent with cold panniculitis. However, an overlooked information is that this patient had a history of autoimmune neutropenia, which is a disease known to increase the risk for cutaneous bacterial infections [15, 16]. Therefore, what can be concluded is only "possible evidence" for a causal relationship between WBC and panniculitis.

Urticaria

Hirvonen et al. [2] published a randomized controlled trial (RCT) in which 40 patients with rheumatoid arthritis received three daily 3-min-long sessions of WBC at −60 °C ($n = 20$) or −110 °C ($n = 20$) over 1 week. One patient in the WBC at −110 °C group reported urticaria. No further information is given on how and when it appeared, whether it was medically confirmed, and what treatments were prescribed (if any). As a general and indiscriminate account of adverse events in their RCT, Hirvonen et al. concluded that no serious or permanent adverse events occurred and that all except one participant felt WBC acceptable or tolerable. Urticaria is a common condition with a lifetime prevalence of approximately 15% and females being more affected than males. Many trigger factors have been identified such as specific food proteins, pollen, or drugs and also specific medical conditions, hormonal imbalances, or physical stress (heat, cold, pressure, sunlight) [17]. There is evidence that the risk for cold urticaria is increased in patients with cold-dependent antibodies such as cryoglobulins or cold agglutinins [18]. Given that no other reason for urticaria was reported in this study, it seems logical to conclude that there is convincing evidence for a causal relationship between WBC participation and urticaria.

Neurological

Transient Global Amnesia

A 63-year-old male presented with transient global amnesia after undertaking a WBC session [10]. The patient did not have any other symptoms. This WBC session was the second one in his life, and the first went without any problems. The amnesia covered a period starting 30 min before the WBC session and ending 3 h after it. Brain magnetic resonance angiography revealed no sign of ischemic or hemorrhagic lesions and no stenosis of the arteries perfusing the brain. Blood analyses showed a somewhat elevated glycemia, which persisted on the following day, vitamin D and B_{12} deficits, and dyslipidemia. In addition, an electrocardiogram (ECG) and transthoracic echocardiogram were performed, revealing a normal cardiac rhythm pattern and heart morphology. The patient received intensive hospital-based monitoring for 24 h and completely recovered in 24 h. The authors concluded that WBC can potentially result in transient global amnesia. It is true that cold exposure can trigger transient amnesia attacks, but this is also true for other precipitating events such as vigorous exercise or stressful events [19]. By his own admission, the patient was experiencing a lot of stress at work at the time his amnesia occurred [10]. In addition, there is growing concern over proton pump inhibitors (PPIs) neurological side effects, including memory impairments [20]. It happens that the patient in this case study was on omeprazole (a medication in the category of PPIs) for 2 years at the time the event was recorded [10]. All that can be said from this report is that WBC had a "possible" causal relation to the patient's transient amnesia.

Intracerebral Hemorrhage

Intracerebral hemorrhage is a life-threatening complication [21]. The first case of intracerebral hemorrhage during a WBC session was reported by French authors [13]. A 61-year-old woman during her first WBC session, as she moved from the pre-chamber (−60 °C) to the main chamber (−110 °C), suddenly complained of severe headache and nausea, accompanied by left-sided hemiparesis. The next day, the MRI images revealed a $36 \times 22 \times 10$ mm-sized edema in the right superior frontoparietal region. Complementary brain activity measures and cerebrospinal fluid analyses revealed no other lesions or signs of disease. She was treated with nimodipine (180 mg per day) and regained the use of her left leg and arm in a few weeks. Considering that no alternative explanation could be found for this subject's intracerebral hemorrhage, the authors proposed that WBC was the precipitating cause. Nevertheless, this woman had a long history of ocular migraine at the time she engaged in her first WBC session, a condition which has been found to increase the risk of hemorrhagic stroke by 50% [22]. The role of WBC (more particularly of the hypertensive pike resulting from extreme cold exposure) in relation to the onset of cerebral bleeding in this patient cannot be dismissed. However, this complication is at least partly attributable to the well-established underlying vascular vulnerability of individuals prone to migraine.

Vascular

Moyamoya Angiopathy

Chen et al. [12] recently described a manifestation of moyamoya syndrome, a progressive stenosis of the intracranial carotid arteries, following WBC at −90 °C in a

32-year-old woman with no medical history. She felt unwell after an unusually long (>4 min) WBC session. The main reported symptoms were inability to speak and a sudden decrease of strength in her right arm. A computed tomography angiogram showed a near-occlusion of the left internal carotid artery as well as a severe narrowing of the left posterior cerebral artery. Her clinical condition rapidly improved in the emergency room and she was discharged receiving no treatment except aspirin (325 mg). At 1-month follow-up, the patient showed no sign of neurological deficits. The authors concluded that WBC may induce cerebral vasoconstriction and suggested that cold-induced hyperventilation could trigger this side effect. There is probable evidence for a cause-and-effect association between cold exposure and the onset of symptoms in this patient. However, the performed session (first-ever WBC session, healthy but nonathlete woman) was too long compared to the recommendations from the Bad Voslau consensus. If recommendations are followed, the risk of angiopathy might actually be minimal.

Abdominal Aortic Dissection

A case of a 56-year-old male with sudden abdominal pain accompanied by dyspnea and lightheadedness 1 week after he had completed a 15-session long WBC program (3 min per session, −150 to −160 °C) was published [14]. A chest CT angiogram revealed no evidence of any abnormalities of the major arteries and all laboratory findings were within the reference interval. The patient was discharged 2 days later with no abdominal pain. Nine days later, he was admitted again, with identical abdominal pain. The abdominal CT angiogram showed an anterior aortic dissection of 36 mm that ended 13 mm before the iliac bifurcation. An endovascular prosthesis was placed. During the 2 following months, the patient experienced episodes of abdominal pain, most of which were associated with cold exposure. After receiving clonidine (0.5 mg per day) and avoiding cold temperatures, the patient improved. Based on these elements, the authors suggested that the implication of WBC in the occurrence of aortic dissection was at least probable. However, the patient had a documented history of hypertension and hypercholesterolemia and described himself to be an "avid runner." Arterial hypertension is one of the 14 absolute contraindications to WBC defined by the Bad Voslau consortium [5] and excessive exercise is one of the risk factors for abdominal aortic aneurysms [23].

Other Complications

All other WBC-induced adverse events reported in the literature ($n = 10$) were of mild severity. They were not described in detail on a case-by-case basis and were simply mentioned in the Results section from the published articles by Happe et al. [12] and Hirvonen et al. [2]. In total, there were three cases of cold-induced headache, four cases of discomfort/dizziness, one case of reactive hypertension, and two cases of long-lasting shivering. None of these events resulted in the discontinuation of the study protocol and none required medical investigation, surveillance, or treatment.

Kelly et al. [24] recently recruited via email 457 collegiate athletes to participate in a retrospective survey about adverse events during and after WBC. In this sample, negative adverse effects of WBC were mild-to-moderate, mainly including skin burns and itching in the first hour following WBC. No life-threatening or severe adverse effects were reported. There were fewer reports of adverse effects afterward (i.e., beyond the first 60 min following intervention). Because cold-induced skin reactions are quite common, strict adherence to preparation guidelines is recommended (e.g., WBC cannot be completed with any moisture present, no thick lotion on skin or hair within 1-h prior WBC). However, due to the study being a retrospective survey, recall bias potentially impacted the results, leading to over- or underestimation of the number and types of adverse events.

Concluding Remarks

A definitive conclusion on possible safety risks associated with WBC should be reached once large-scale studies are available. Most of the studies conducted so far have neglected the monitoring of adverse events during and after WBC. Some institutions have expressed concerns regarding WBC safety over the last decade. The American Academy of Dermatology warns that "extreme cold can injure your skin" and that "there is very little evidence about WBC safety or effectiveness in treating the conditions for which it is being promoted." In 2016, the US Food and Drug Administration (FDA) released a consumer update warning that "WBC is a trend that lacks evidence and poses potential health risks" [25]. The report stated that the FDA "does not have evidence that WBC effectively treats diseases or conditions like Alzheimer's, fibromyalgia, migraines, rheumatoid arthritis, multiple sclerosis, stress, anxiety or chronic pain" and that no WBC devices have been cleared or approved by the FDA. Potential hazards include "frostbite, burns, and eye injuries from the extreme temperatures and asphyxiation when liquid nitrogen is used for cooling. Asphyxiation could occur because nitrogen vapors lower the amount of oxygen in the room, resulting in oxygen deficiency and loss of consciousness." No more recent reports are available from the FDA since then. On the contrary, in Poland, where WBC has been consistently used for 40 years as a therapy reimbursed by the national health system, no official safety concerns have been raised. In Italy, the Ministry of Health has recently (May 2023) released indications for the clinical use of WBC in the following conditions: fibromyalgia, obesity, mood disorders, and rheumatological conditions [26]. The American analysis and conclusions are flawed in one critical way: partial-body (body in a cryosauna but head remaining outside, direct injection of liquid nitrogen mist inside the cabin) and whole-body (entire body exposure in a cryochamber filled with breathable air) technologies have been amalgamated under the alleged banner "whole-body cryotherapy." As an illustration of this point, Ben Kheder et al.'s analysis of WBC safety [27] is based on four studies, one of which used cryosauna cooling equipment [28]. Another example is the case study by O'Connor and colleagues [29] regularly cited as scientific evidence in support of the dangerousness of WBC. It actually describes a cold burn injury in a 71-year-old man who accidentally had his back burned by liquid nitrogen while standing in a cryosauna (i.e., partial-body cryotherapy). Indisputably, special care must be taken when using cryosauna as there are inherently high risks of cold burns and anoxia due to the direct injection of vaporized nitrogen gas. The data discussed in the present chapter suggest that WBC is associated with relatively infrequent, and mostly minor and transient adverse effects. Evidence of its adverse effects is strongest for vascular/neurological complications: intracerebral hemorrhage, moyamoya angiopathy, and abdominal aortic dissection. However, careful examination of each of these reported serious adverse events allowed to notice significant patient's related risk factors, or inappropriate WBC exposure parameters in terms of session length or ambient temperature.

In conclusion, looking back on the past four decades, adverse events appear to be rare in relation to the extent to which WBC has grown worldwide. The level of scientific evidence of serious adverse events related to the use of WBC is still low to date, limited to published case reports. Some of the adverse reactions reported here could have been possibly prevented with a better understanding or better application of Bad Voslau's list of contraindications. At present, it is difficult to reach a definitive conclusion on possible risks associated with WBC, as studies have not undertaken active surveillance of predefined adverse events. We reaffirm the importance of considering medical contraindications before involving any subject in a WBC program. In this regard, we propose to upgrade Bad Voslau's list by including migraine due to the documented association with increased risk of hemorrhagic stroke. Also, a special concern regarding lipid disorders should be raised, as one case of abdominal aortic aneurysm has been observed. The International Institute of Refrigeration Working Group on Whole Body Cryotherapy/Cryostimulation is actively working on the development and update of safe guidelines using evidence-based information to overcome recommendations for WBC parameters based on anecdote [30].

References

1. Bleakley CM, Bieuzen F, Davison GW, Costello JT. Whole-body cryotherapy: empirical evidence and theoretical perspectives. Open Access J Sports Med. 2014;5:25–36.
2. Hirvonen HE, Mikkelsson MK, Kautiainen H, Pohjolainen TH, Leirisalo-Repo M. Effectiveness of different cryotherapies on pain and disease activity in active rheumatoid arthritis. A randomised single blinded controlled trial. Clin Exp Rheumatol. 2006;24:295–301.
3. Costello JT, Culligan K, Selfe J, Donnelly AE. Muscle, skin and core temperature after −110°C cold air and 8°C water treatment. PLoS One. 2012;7:e48190.
4. Costello JT, Donnelly AE, Karki A, Selfe J. Effects of whole body cryotherapy and cold water immersion on knee skin temperature. Int J Sports Med. 2014;35:35–40.
5. Zimmer Medizin System. Consensus declaration on whole-body cryotherapy (WBCT). Austria: Bad Vöslau; 2006.

6. Dugué B, Bernard J-P, Bouzigon Romain, De Nardi M, Douzi W, Ferreira JJ, Guilpart J, Lombardi G, Miller E, Tiemessen I. Whole body cryotherapy/cryostimulation, 39th Informatory Note on Refrigeration Technologies. 2020. https://doi.org/10.18462/iif.NItec39.09.2020.

7. Costello JT, Baker PRA, Minett GM, Bieuzen F, Stewart IB, Bleakley C. Whole-body cryotherapy (extreme cold air exposure) for preventing and treating muscle soreness after exercise in adults. Cochrane Database Syst Rev. 2015:CD010789.

8. Legrand FD, Dugué B, Costello J, et al. Evaluating safety risks of whole-body cryotherapy/cryostimulation (WBC): a scoping review from an international consortium. 2023. https://doi.org/10.21203/rs.3.Rs-2879229/v1.

9. Qureshi R, Mayo-Wilson E, Li T. Harms in systematic reviews paper 1: an introduction to research on harms. J Clin Epidemiol. 2022;143:186–96.

10. Carrard J, Lambert AC, Genné D. Transient global amnesia following a whole-body cryotherapy session. BMJ Case Rep. 2017;2017:bcr2017221431.

11. Greenwald E, Christman M, Penn L, Brinster N, Liebman TN. Cold panniculitis: adverse cutaneous effect of whole-body cryotherapy. JAAD Case Rep. 2018;4:344–5.

12. Chen PM, Chen MM, Chiang C-C, Olson S, Bolar DS, Agrawal K. Moyamoya presenting after whole body cryotherapy. Acta Neurol Taiwanica. 2020;29(2):64–6.

13. Cronier R, Fardellone P, Goëb V. Cerebral bleeding during a cryotherapy session: a case report. Rev Med Interne. 2020;41:843–5.

14. Camara-Lemarroy CR, Azpiri-Lopez JR, Vasquez-Diaz LA, Galarza-Delgado DA. Abdominal aortic dissection and cold-intolerance after whole-body cryotherapy: a case report. Clin J Sport Med. 2017;27(5):e67–8.

15. Quesada-Cortés A, Campos-Muñoz L, Díaz-Díaz RM, Casado-Jiménez M. Cold panniculitis. Dermatol Clin. 2008;26(485–489):vii.

16. Autrel-Moignet A, Lamy T. Autoimmune neutropenia. Presse Medicale Paris Fr. 2014;1983(43):e105–18.

17. Deacock SJ. An approach to the patient with urticaria. Clin Exp Immunol. 2008;153:151–61.

18. Gorevic PD. Cryopathies: cryoglobulins and cryofibrinogenemia. In: Samter M, Talmage DW, Frank MM, Austen KF, Claman HN, et al., editors. Immunological diseases, 1988:1;687–713. https://www.wolterskluwer.com/en/solutions/ovid/samters-immunologic-diseases-841. Accessed 28 Aug 2023.

19. Hodges JR, Warlow CP. Syndromes of transient amnesia: towards a classification. A study of 153 cases. J Neurol Neurosurg Psychiatry. 1990;53:834–43.

20. Makunts T, Alpatty S, Lee KC, Atayee RS, Abagyan R. Proton-pump inhibitor use is associated with a broad spectrum of neurological adverse events including impaired hearing, vision, and memory. Sci Rep. 2019;9:17280.

21. Caceres JA, Goldstein JN. Intracranial haemorrhage. Emerg Med Clin North Am. 2012;30:771–94.

22. Sacco S, Ornello R, Ripa P, Pistoia F, Carolei A. Migraine and hemorrhagic stroke: a meta-analysis. Stroke. 2013;44:3032–8.

23. Franklin BA, Thompson PD, Al-Zaiti SS, et al. Exercise-related acute cardiovascular events and potential deleterious adaptations following long-term exercise training: placing the risks into perspective-an update: a scientific statement from the American Heart Association. Circulation. 2020;141:e705–36.

24. Kelly EA, Forootan NS, Checketts JX, Frank A, Tangen CL. Retrospective analysis of whole-body cryotherapy adverse effects in division I collegiate athletes. J Osteopath Med. 2023;123:249–57.

25. Commissioner O of the. Whole body cryotherapy (WBC): a "cool" trend that lacks evidence, poses risks. FDA; 2020.

26. Ministero della Salute. Comitato tecnico sanitario—Sezione per i dispositivi medici. sezione f)—dispositivi medici "Crioterapia whole-body e partial-body". May 2023.

27. Ben Khedher Balbolia S, Barry C, Hassler C, Falissard B. Evaluation de l'efficacité et de la sécurité de la cryothérapie corps entier à visée thérapeutique. 2019. https://iifiir.org/en/fri-

doc/assessing-the-efficiency-and-safety-of-whole-body-cryotherapy-for-4829. Accessed 28 Aug 2023.

28. Bourrain JL, Raison-Peyron N, Du Thanh A, Dereure O. Urticaire chronique au froid survenue au décours d'une cryothérapie corps entier. Ann Dermatol Vénéréol. 2014;141:S425.

29. O'Connor M, Wang JV, Gaspari AA. Cold burn injury after treatment at whole-body cryotherapy facility. JAAD Case Rep. 2019;5:29–30.

30. New IIR Informatory Note on Whole Body Cryotherapy/Cryostimulation, 2020. https://iifiir.org/en/news/new-iir-informatory-note-on-whole-body-cryotherapy-cryostimulation. Accessed 28 Aug 2023.

Toward Personalized Protocols: A Scoping Review

18

Guillaume Polidori, Fabien Beaumont, Fabien Bogard, and Sébastien Murer

Introduction

Whole-body cryotherapy (WBC) is an innovative therapeutic approach involving the exposure of the human body to extremely low temperatures, typically 3 min at $-110\ °C$. This technique has recently gained popularity as a modality for recovery, enhancing athletic performance, and treating various medical conditions. WBC is performed in specialized chambers, known as cryotherapy chambers, which are designed to generate and regulate the required cold temperatures while ensuring the safety and well-being of users.

The effects of WBC on the body are manifold and complex. Exposure to extreme cold leads to peripheral vasoconstriction, resulting in reduced blood flow to the extremities and redistribution of blood toward the heart and vital organs. This can have beneficial effects, such as reducing inflammation [1, 2], enhancing muscle recovery [3, 4], alleviating pain [5], and stimulating the immune system [6]. In the realm of sports, research has shown that WBC can reduce muscle soreness [3], improve physical performance, and enhance exercise tolerance [7]. Additionally, WBC may promote the release of endorphins [8], which can induce a sense of well-being and alleviate anxiety and depression. Studies have also examined the effectiveness of WBC as a therapeutic approach for a number of conditions, such as arthritis, dermatological disorders, autoimmune diseases, sleep disorders, and mood disorders. It should be noted that WBC requires appropriate supervision to avoid any risk [9]. Indeed, precautions must be taken to prevent frostbite and potential

G. Polidori (✉) · F. Beaumont · F. Bogard · S. Murer
MATIM Faculty of Exact and Natural Sciences, Université de Reims Champagne-Ardenne, Reims, France
e-mail: guillaume.polidori@univ-reims.fr; fabien.beaumont@univ-reims.fr; fabien.bogard@univ-reims.fr; sebastien.murer@univ-reims.fr

P. Capodaglio (ed.), *Whole-Body Cryostimulation*, https://doi.org/10.1007/978-3-031-18545-8_18

209 "

medical complications associated with extreme cold exposure. Therefore, it is essential that WBC is administered by trained professionals and in safe facilities.

The process of skin cooling is a fundamental concept that delineates the efficacy of whole-body cryostimulation (WBC) in its endeavor to target localized attainment of analgesic thresholds and avoid adverse effects [10]. Recent updates to guidelines in 2010, as published by the Association of Chartered Physiotherapists in Sports and Exercise Medicine (ACPSM) and endorsed by the Chartered Society of Physiotherapists (London), underline that the presently acknowledged threshold for inducing effective local analgesia occurs when the absolute skin temperature is decreased to below 13 °C. This threshold value closely approximates the measurement defined by Bugaj [11], previously regarded as the benchmark standard, which was established at 13.6 °C.

The attainment of these target values of skin temperature corresponding to analgesic thresholds does not adhere to the use of a universal protocol, but rather is inherent to the conjunction of several combined parameters, encompassing both thermo-aerodynamic aspects related to WBC chambers and physiological as well as anthropometric aspects related to users. Indeed, an optimized benefit of the dose/response ratio is linked to the optimized coupling of an exposure temperature and an exposure duration for a given category of individuals. The exposure temperature, representing the actual temperature to which the body is exposed, is a variable that is currently challenging to ascertain precisely. It is customary in the literature to associate it with the set temperature of the refrigeration machine. But what is the actual scenario? Elfahem [12] demonstrated that due to the opening and closing of cryotherapy chamber doors during client passages, a drop of approximately 16% in the actual temperature within a dual chamber could occur. It is imperative that research efforts be directed toward this aspect in the near future. Regarding the optimization of exposure durations, it is contingent upon both the exposure temperatures and the anthropometric characteristics of patients (body mass index, fat mass).

The most effective regimen for whole-body cryotherapy (WBC) treatment in terms of duration, temperature, frequency, and timing is a topic of ongoing debate, a viewpoint that is echoed by various researchers [13–15]. The specific protocol that would result in the utmost physiological and biochemical advantages, optimal muscle recovery, and enhanced sports performance remains a point of uncertainty [16].

The objective of this article is to review the current state of literature that can provide insights into the optimization of WBC protocols. Firstly, initial milestones are established to propose equivalences between different pairs of temperature/exposure duration parameters, given the wide array of WBC devices available with varying set temperatures. Subsequently, we delve into an aspect that has drawn our attention and remains unaddressed. To minimize operational costs, operators often tend to accommodate multiple individuals in the chambers simultaneously. We aim to ascertain whether this practice leads to alterations in exposure temperature values. Lastly, we will substantiate the hypothesis that there is no justification for offering the same cryotherapy protocol to individuals of diverse characteristics such as gender, body composition, age, and physique.

All the aforementioned elements are part of the questions also raised by the "Whole Body Cryotherapy/Cryostimulation" working group of the International

Institute of Refrigeration in its 39th Informatory Note [17]. The frequency of sessions that can be offered to patients in the context of specific treatments will not be discussed here.

Overview of Cryostimulation Chambers

Whole-body cryotherapy (WBC) chambers are devices used to expose the human body to extremely low temperatures for short periods. Each different type of chamber utilizes specific technologies to generate the necessary cold. The most common one is based on cooled air, to reach temperatures generally ranging from −60 °C to −110 °C, according to the number of chambers (single or multiple) and their dimensions. The standardization of exposure protocols is primarily contingent upon the characteristics of individuals and the anticipated effects. However, it also relies on the cold environment, specifically the intensity of cold within the chambers.

The raised question is, for instance: at equal exposure duration, what is the influence of the set temperature on the average skin temperature of individuals? A review of the literature reveals limited findings regarding averaged skin temperature data across the entire body surface. In this context, the set temperature is considered, as currently, there are no studies demonstrating the relationship between the actual temperature within the chamber and the setpoint temperature.

To exemplify our assertion, Table 18.1 presents the variations in averaged skin temperatures over the whole exposed body surface in an environment with a wide temperature range. The current analysis is confined to male subjects undergoing standard 3-min cryosessions. The collected data include raw, extrapolated, and, in one instance, even unrelated to cryostimulation. The latter aids in determining whether a general trend can be discerned.

These data are plotted in Fig. 18.1. Surprisingly, a strong correlation is observed between the skin and setpoint temperatures, with a Pearson correlation coefficient $r = 0.975$. Let us compare two setpoint temperatures frequently used in

Table 18.1 Room and skin temperature, pre- and post-cryosession

Authors	Sample	Ambient		Cryostimulation session	
		T room	T skin	T chamber	T skin
[18]	$N = 40$	24 °C	32.0 ± 0.5 °C	−110 °C −60 °C −10 °C	−42% (18.6 °C)[a] −27% (23.4 °C)[a] −12% (28.2 °C)[a]
[19]	$N = 8$	21 °C	32.1 ± 0.6 °C	−110 °C	19.0 ± 1.7 °C
[20]	$N = 10$	26 °C	33.5 ± 0.5 °C	−110 °C	22.1 ± 2.2 °C
[21]	$N = 15$	24 °C	31.9 °C	−110 °C	18.2 °C
[12]	$N = 8$	22 °C	32.9 ± 0.5 °C	−76 °C	25.6 ± 1.3 °C
[22]	$N = 18$	21.6 °C	32.2 ± 0.8 °C	−110 °C	22.0 ± 2.1 °C
[23][b]	$N = 10$	40 °C	34.2 ± 0.9 °C		

[a] Data extrapolated from the article
[b] Article not related to cryostimulation chambers

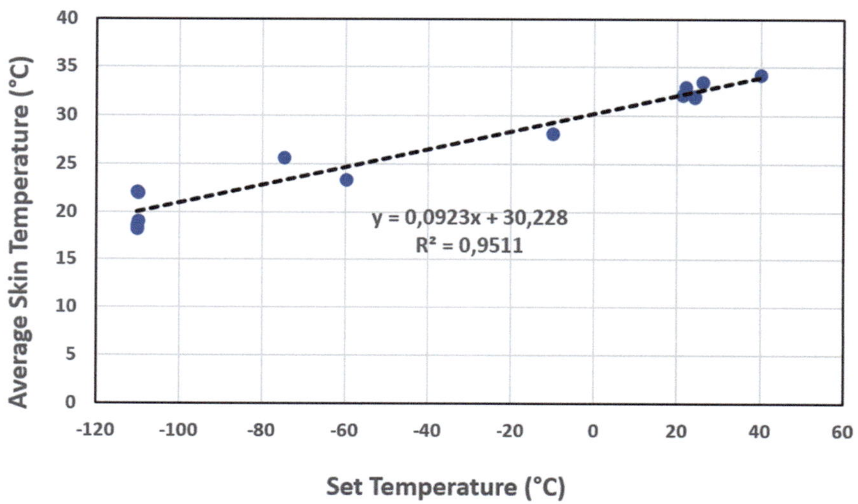

Fig. 18.1 Average skin temperature vs. setpoint temperature, from Table 18.1

cryostimulation devices, e.g., −85 °C and −110 °C. The linear regression equation deduced from Fig. 18.1 is $|\Delta T_{skin}| = 0.0923\ |\Delta T_{setup}|$. Subsequently, considering for males an equal exposure period of 3 min, the average skin temperature is 2.31 °C lower in a −110 °C chamber than in a −85 °C chamber, for a difference of 25 °C between the two types of exposures.

The question that arises is: how much longer should be an exposure at −85 °C to achieve the same dose/response as a −110 °C session? Based on Polidori et al. [19], the cutaneous behavior of the human body obeys negative exponential cooling in the first seconds, followed by a linear evolution over time. The latter should therefore be used as the basis for the calculation of an exposure duration. It is mentioned that the thermal gradient over time is −0.0467 °C/s for males. Considering the average skin temperature as the key parameter and an identical dose/response as the objective, the following equivalence can be proposed:

$$3\,\text{min at}-110°C \cong 3\,\text{min}\,50\,\text{s at}-85°C \tag{18.1}$$

Despite the reservations that can be made about this approach, this semi-analytical analysis allows us to identify a very interesting trend and displays consistency with the common empirical practice where sessions of 4 min are typically recommended for a temperature of −85 °C. This represents a deviation of 4.1% from the analytically determined duration.

More generally, considering the example of exposure to −110 °C, which is the most common, one can determine the exposure duration t_{exp} at a new temperature T_{setup} using the formula:

$$t_{exp} \approx 180\,\text{s} - 2\left(-110°C - T_{setup}\right) \tag{18.2}$$

While this correlation Cannot be universally extrapolated without additional research, It underscores the pivotal role of the environment in refining treatment protocols. An analogous examination could be conducted among female subjects, contingent upon the availability of supplementary data within existing literature.

Overview of Common Practices

Another aspect that appears fundamental in estimating exposure durations to achieve an equivalent dose/response effect pertains to the practices of the operators. A common scenario, when the chamber size permits, consists in performing a cryo-session on several people together, in order to reduce the overall energetic cost. However, it is legitimate to question the consequences that this practice has on the temperature fields within the chamber, as each individual, in a very cold environment, behaves as a heat source. As shown in the preceding paragraph, any change in temperature within the chamber leads to a modification in skin temperature. Consequently, it appears important to account for this practice in the duration of the protocols.

Extreme atmospheres constitute obstacles, even barriers, to any experimental endeavor, as the electronics and optics of the equipment are unable to withstand such low temperatures. Furthermore, employing a semi-analytical modeling approach and/or computational fluid dynamics (CFD) can help overcome this significant limitation and provide crucial insights for operators to refine protocol durations.

In a recent study, Elfahem et al. [24] employed both CFD and experimental approaches. The intricate numerical simulation relies in part on the development of a convective-radiative model, and the convective phase is not, contrary to common assumptions, purely natural convection, but rather mixed convection. In fact, in this type of geometry and technology, the thermal plume naturally created by the heat source represented by the human body is impeded by mechanical ventilation carrying the cold. The apparatus employed in this study consisted of a dual whole-body cryotherapy (WBC) chamber (Mecotec, BitterfeldWolfen, Germany, dimensions: $2.10 \times 1.84 \times 2.15$ m^3) supplied with cold air through a closed-circuit cascade refrigeration system. Cold air was introduced into the chamber via perforated grids on the ceiling, comprising a total of 3132 holes with a diameter of 13 mm. The extraction of cold air occurred through a slotted extraction plate (110 slotted holes, dimensions: 105×20 mm^2) situated at the lower part of one of the walls, with a flow rate of 1500 m^3/h. In the setup, a total of 15 thermocouples (type K 430-2000-2-1) were positioned throughout the volume, as shown in Fig. 18.2. These thermocouples were simultaneously connected to a data acquisition system for the purpose of recording local temperature variations. Additionally, the thermocouples facilitated volume mapping reconstruction using Abaqus software in conjunction with finite element interpolation.

The prescribed input temperature in the simulation was set to -80 °C, a value selected within a range to prevent potential breakdown of experimental equipment due to extremely low temperatures. Utilizing simplified adiabatic wall conditions to model the vacant chamber unveiled a three-dimensional primary curvilinear flow pattern, extending from the inlet to the outlet. This flow pattern was characterized

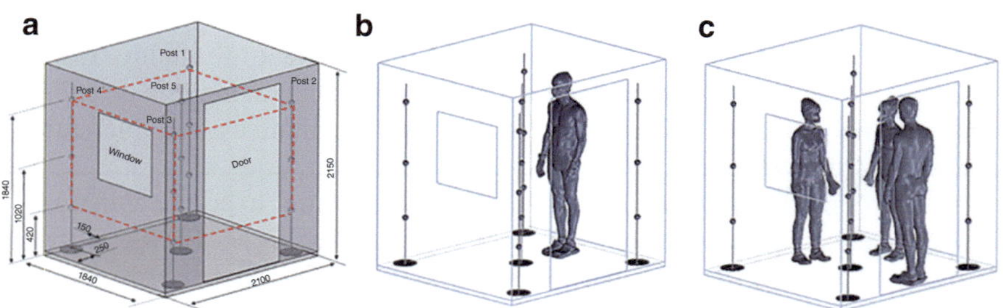

Fig. 18.2 Experimental WBC chamber: (**a**) empty; (**b**) with one person inside; (**c**) with three persons. From [24]

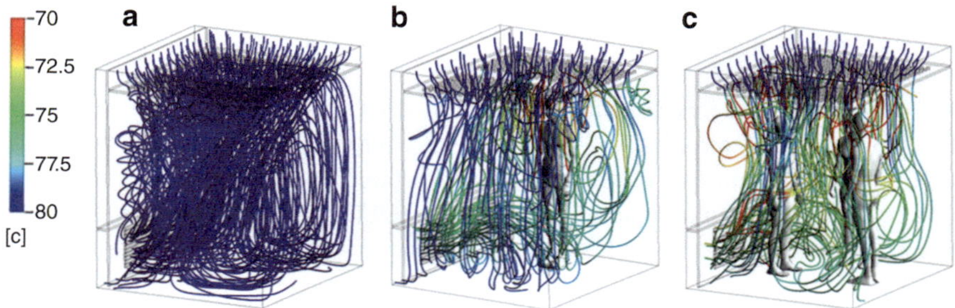

Fig. 18.3 Temperature color-coded 3D streamlines: (**a**) empty chamber; (**b**) chamber with one person inside; chamber with three persons inside (**c**). Inlet temperature −80 °C; average body skin temperature 27 °C. From [24]

by a substantial primary vortex cell and secondary spiral-like vortices situated at the upper and lateral edges of the chamber (see Fig. 18.3). To illustrate both flow dynamics and convective effects, the computational fluid dynamics (CFD) results demonstrate the propagation of heat emitted by an individual (with a mean skin temperature of 27 °C) positioned at the room's center to the exhaust vents. The resulting intricate three-dimensional convective flow generates localized temperature disparities, potentially giving rise to thermal stratification and nonhomogeneous mixing phenomena, warranting experimental confirmation.

Figure 18.4 illustrates the temporal evolution of temperature distribution within the cryochamber for three distinct scenarios, involving both participant presence and absence, during a standard 3-min cryotherapy session. The empty prism shapes represent an approximate depiction of each participant's location. The findings underscore the substantial influence exerted by the presence of multiple occupants on the thermal patterns within the cryochamber. Notably, the warmer convective plumes undergo displacement toward the outlet, positioned at the lower section of the rear wall. The practice of accommodating multiple individuals simultaneously within the cryochamber, motivated by economic considerations, necessitates meticulous scrutiny in terms of achieving a balanced response and dose. In essence, the protocol's duration should be correspondingly extended in accordance with the number of occupants present.

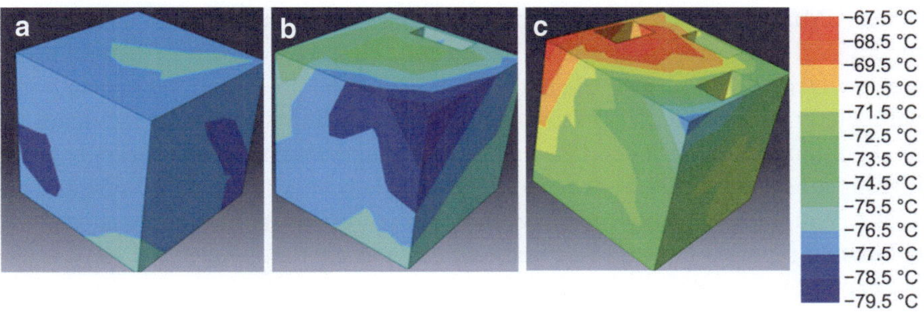

Fig. 18.4 Three-dimensional temperature fields inside the measurement volume after 3 min: (**a**) empty chamber, (**b**) chamber with one person, (**c**) chamber with three persons

Table 18.2 Increase in the cryotherapy protocol duration vs. number of persons inside the chamber, compared to an empty chamber. Percentages are calculated based on a 3-min session

	Male	Female
1 person	+ 4 s (2.2%)	+ 2.8 s (1.6%)
3 persons	+ 13.2 s (7.4%)	+ 9.5 s (5.3%)

In identical conditions, it is shown in [12] that the presence of a single person inside the chamber increases the average temperature by 2 °C, compared to the reference case of an empty chamber. For three persons inside, the computed increase is 6.7 °C. Using the relationship between skin temperature and setpoint temperature (Fig. 18.1), as well as the cooling ratios calculated for males and females [19], the additional duration required to achieve identical cooling compared to an empty chamber may be calculated. Results are summarized in Table 18.2 for a setpoint temperature of −80 °C taken as an example to illustrate this point.

After elucidating the specific attention cryotherapists must direct toward both the type of chamber employed, yielding varying exposure temperatures, and the repercussions of administering concurrent sessions for multiple individuals, our focus now shifts to the physiological and anthropometric data of patients. In substantiating our argument regarding the impact of body mass index (BMI) and fat mass on the optimization of WBC protocols, we confine this literature review to studies encompassing male and female populations. Ongoing research endeavors are presently investigating this theme concerning elderly individuals, obese subjects, athletes, and more. However, these investigations have yet to be disseminated through scientific literature publications.

Gender Influence on Body Thermal Resistance

Genetically predisposed for reproduction, women statistically exhibit a higher volume of adipose tissue compared to men. In cold environments, this adipose tissue assumes the role of thermal insulation. This tissue is directly linked to physiological parameters such as the percentage of body fat and, consequently, the body mass index (BMI). These two physiological parameters can be summarized using a thermophysical parameter employed in Engineering Sciences, known as thermal resistance, which plays a pivotal role in the heat dissipation process of the human body, particularly in extreme cold atmospheres. Understanding its behavior facilitates its incorporation into biophysical, mathematical, or numerical models, especially when investigating the kinetics of skin cooling during exposure to extreme cold environments. Within the existing literature, the thermal resistance of the human body is commonly reported to exhibit a consistent value of approximately 0.03 K/W, without explicit reference to anatomical sexual dimorphic variations between male and female individuals [25]. Polidori et al. [26] studied the temporal evolution of body thermal resistance between genders during the recovery phase following a WBC session and demonstrated its significance as a crucial factor in WBC protocols. Given the limited research on gender-based effects in WBC protocols, it was postulated that adiposity-related tissue characteristics, such as fat mass percentage, emerge as pivotal factors in body thermal resistance. These factors warrant consideration in devising appropriate protocols for both males and females.

At rest, in the absence of conduction and evaporation (as is likely during WBC sessions), it is postulated that the equilibrium of heat is upheld when the rate of heat production φ_{met} (metabolism) equals the heat dissipated through radiation φ_{rad}, convection φ_{conv}, and respiration φ_{resp}, with the assumption that storage effects are negligible, which is reasonable for minimal fluctuations in core (rectal) temperature. Considering the human body as a mildly transient thermal system, the preservation of thermal rate is adhered to, resulting in the subsequent system of equations:

$$\{\varphi_{\mathrm{met}}\left(t\right)=\varphi_{\mathrm{conv}}\left(t\right)+\varphi_{\mathrm{rad}}\left(t\right)+\varphi_{\mathrm{resp}}\left(t\right) \quad \varphi_{\mathrm{met}}\left(t\right)=\frac{T_c\left(t\right)-T_{\mathrm{Sk}}\left(t\right)}{\left[\mathrm{BSA}\right]R_b\left(t\right)} \tag{18.3}$$

where R_b represents the thermal resistance of the body, T_c denotes the core temperature, T_{Sk} signifies the skin temperature, BSA stands for body surface area, and φ_{resp} represents the cumulative effect of latent heat loss through respiration as well as dry heat loss through respiration. Integrating both Antoine's equation and the equation for the total respiratory heat loss as provided by the American Society of Heating, Refrigerating, and Air-Conditioning Engineers [27], establishes the connection between heat production and respiration losses:

$$\varphi_{\mathrm{resp}}\left(t\right)=10.5\%\varphi_{\mathrm{met}}\left(t\right) \tag{18.4}$$

Incorporating the principles of Newton's law of convection and Boltzmann's law of radiation heat loss into the equations of bio-heat transfer modeling culminates in the ultimate formulation of the intrinsic thermal resistance. This intrinsic thermal resistance stands as the principal parameter governing the assessment of individuals' insulative reactions in the context of whole-body cryotherapy:

$$R_b\left(t\right)=\frac{0.895\left(T\left(t\right)_c-T\left(t\right)_{\mathrm{Sk}}\right)}{\left[\mathrm{BSA}\right]\left[h_c\left(t\right)\left(T\left(t\right)_{\mathrm{Sk}}-T_a\right)+\left(T\left(t\right)_{\mathrm{Sk}}^4-T_a^4\right)\right]} \tag{18.5}$$

The temporal variation of the convective heat transfer coefficient is also contingent upon the skin temperature and can be reliably determined through empirical relationships applicable to both laminar and turbulent flows featuring uniform heat flux density as the thermal condition. The equation for the convective heat transfer coefficient h_c over time can be expressed as follows:

$$h_c(t) = \frac{0.0257}{H_b}\left[0.825 + 7.08\left(T(t)_{\text{Sk}} - T_a\right)^{\frac{1}{6}} H_b^{\frac{1}{2}}\right]^2 \tag{18.6}$$

where H_b represents the body height. The computation of the body surface area (BSA) is derived using the subsequent correlations established for both male and female subjects [27]:

$$[\text{BSA}]_m = 0.000579479\,W^{0.38}H_b^{1.24} \tag{18.7}$$

$$[\text{BSA}]_f = 0.000975482\,W^{0.46}H_b^{1.08} \tag{18.8}$$

where W is the body mass.

To illustrate the development of this bio-heat transfer model, Polidori et al. [26] employed the experimental findings of Cuttel et al. [20], which pertained to the investigation of the warming phase experienced by a group of young males and females following a 3-min session of WBC at -110 °C. Figure 18.5 presents a graphical representation depicting the temporal progression of the thermal resistance and the dynamic alterations in skin temperature for both male and female subjects. It is evident that irrespective of gender, these two parameters (T_{Sk} and R_b) exhibit an inversely proportional relationship. The decrease in thermal resistance corresponds to an elevation in skin temperature, underscoring the fact that, akin to thermal systems in general, thermal resistance acts in opposition to the internal dispersion of heat from the core to the periphery.

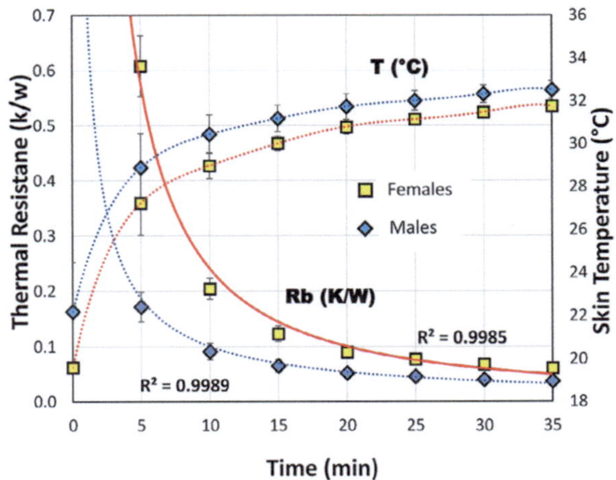

Fig. 18.5 Time-evolution of the thermal resistance R_b (left scale) and skin temperature T_{Sk} (right scale) for males and females in the rewarming after -110 °C (3 min) WBC, from [26]

This analysis enabled the authors to establish the asymptotic limits of the evolution of body thermal resistance at rest in both men and women, namely:

$$\{(R_b)_{\text{male}} = 0.027\,\text{K}\,/\,\text{W} \quad (R_b)_{\text{female}} = 0.037\,\text{K}\,/\,\text{W} \tag{18.9}$$

The comparison of the key thermal resistance parameter between males and females indicates a 37% disparity at rest. The findings of this study suggest that the adiposity of tissues, inherent in the percentage of fat mass, emerges as a pivotal factor affecting the body's thermal resistance, which necessitates consideration when formulating appropriate protocols for both genders. In other words, this study demonstrates that to achieve equivalent effects on skin temperature and, consequently, to uniformly cool tissues, the duration of cryotherapy protocols should be adjusted based on gender, with differences observed between females and males.

Influence of Gender on the Duration of Protocols

To further extend the conclusions drawn from the results of the previous study, Polidori et al. [19] undertook an analytical approach to demonstrate that the durations of WBC protocols should differ based on whether the patients are males or females, under the same exposure temperature and for the same amplitude of cutaneous cooling. Also targeting a young and healthy population, they focused on the cooling phase, which pertains to the evolution of skin behavior during exposure to extreme cold. The proposed analysis was systemic but also more localized, targeting more specific regions of interest.

In order to project the necessary duration of whole-body cryostimulation at $-110\,^{\circ}\text{C}$ for males and females to achieve an equivalent cold-induced dose-response effect, a mathematical model capturing the kinetics of skin cooling was formulated to accommodate experimental data. This model has the capability to deduce and extrapolate anticipated skin temperatures at any given point in time by fitting experimental observations. Assuming a negative power law due to the pronounced phenomenon of substantial vasoconstriction arising from abrupt exposure to extreme cold during the initial transient phase within the interval $t \in [0; 30]$, succeeded by a linear trend during the latter portion of the transient phase within the interval $t \in [30; \beta]$, they proposed an analytical formulation for the resultant skin temperature throughout the cooling process:

$$T_{\text{sk}}(t) = \left[T_{\text{sk}0} \left(\frac{T_{\text{sk}0}}{T\text{sk}_1 + C_0(30 - \beta)} \right)^{-\left(\frac{t}{30}\right)^n} \right]_{0 \to 30} + \left[C_0 t + (T_{\text{sk}1} - C_0 \beta) \right]_{30 \to \beta} \tag{18.10}$$

where $T_{\text{sk}0}$ denotes the initial baseline skin temperature, $T\text{sk}_1$ represents the skin temperature at the conclusion of the session, and C_0 signifies the cooling rate. The parameter β is indicative of the session's termination point. Figure 18.6 depicts the

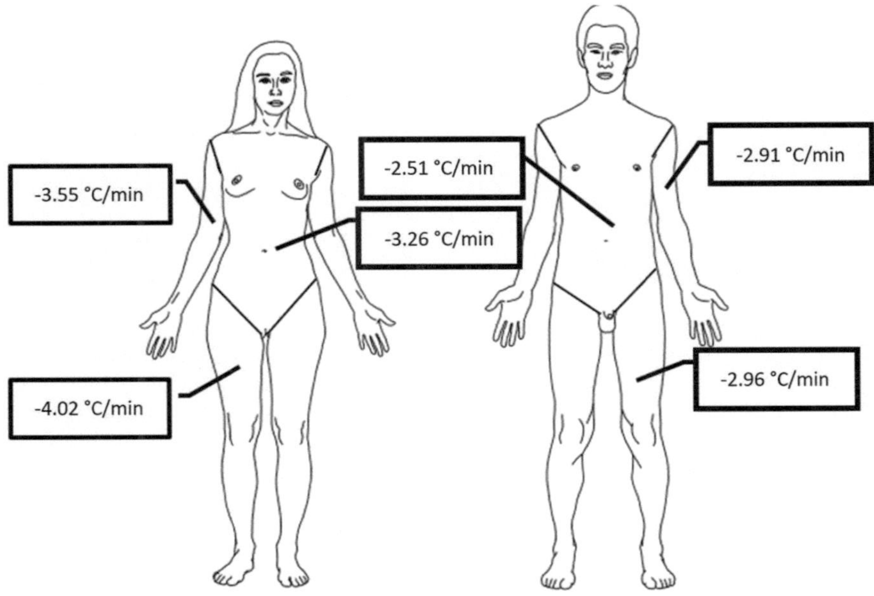

Fig. 18.6 Thermal gradient C_0 (converted in °C/min) during the linear cooling phase $t > 30$ s— Thermal gradients are built on the average of both front and back views

progression of the linear cooling phase, which occurs beyond the initial 30 s, characterized by rapid vasoconstriction. It is evident that, on the one hand, the cooling kinetics for females are faster than those for males, and on the other hand, this cutaneous cooling is contingent upon specific regions of the body.

All these findings suggest that males and females adapt differently to extreme cold air exposure, with females being more sensitive to environmental thermal conditions, depending on their body surface areas. This raises questions about the current clinical practices in WBC centers, which often employ identical cryostimulation protocols for both males and females. The magnitude of cutaneous variation, represented by $\Delta T = T_{sk} - T_{sk0}$, can be considered a key parameter for evaluating the impact of sex in cryostimulation. The analytical formulation of cutaneous thermal behavior (Eq. (18.10)) facilitates the prediction of protocol durations required to attain this target. Figure 18.7 provides a summary of numerically calculated durations within a range of cooling gradients ΔT, spanning from -8 °C to -20 °C, for various body regions examined in our investigation. It becomes evident that, in order to induce an equivalent thermal skin response, protocol durations for males need to exceed those for females. For instance, to achieve a cooling magnitude of -12 °C in the trunk region, the protocol duration must be extended by 36% for males compared to females. This discrepancy can reach 54% and even 62% for the upper and lower limbs, respectively.

Estimation of cryo-session protocol duration (s)

Cooling gradient	Trunk			Upper limbs			Lower limbs		
	Female	Male	E(%)	Female	Male	E(%)	Female	Male	E(%)
-8°C	55	78	42	24	58	141	27	59	120
-10°C	90	124	38	58	99	72	57	100	76
-12°C	125	170	36	91	140	54	87	140	62
-14°C	160	215	34	125	182	46	116	181	55
-16°C	195	261	-	158	223	41	146	222	51
-18°C	230	307	-	192	264	-	176	262	-
-20°C	265	352	-	225	305	-	206	303	-

Fig. 18.7 Analytical evaluation of the protocol durations (in seconds) based on gender and body surface areas. The shaded boxes represent an extrapolation for a cold exposure time of more than 3 min and less than 4 min. The blackened boxes refer to exposure times longer than 4 min, which are mentioned but should not be taken into account as they may compromise the health of patients. From [19]

Conclusion

Whole-body cryotherapy (WBC) is a therapeutic methodology that entails exposing the human body to extremely low temperatures within specialized cryotherapy chambers. The potential advantages of WBC are extensive, encompassing aspects like sports recovery and addressing various medical conditions. Nonetheless, further investigation is imperative to gain a comprehensive understanding of the underlying mechanisms and to establish optimized treatment protocols that can thoroughly evaluate the effectiveness of this technique. Of particular significance is the consideration of personalized protocols. Can it be assumed that what proves beneficial for one individual under a similar temperature-to-exposure duration ratio would yield the same benefits for another? Are we all equally responsive to cold stimuli?

Although based on a literature that is deficient in its coverage of this topic, the present review demonstrates that it is mathematically feasible, with the aim of minimizing time-consuming and costly experiments, to partially address these questions related to protocol personalization. Only a distinction between men and women has been the subject of investigatory efforts. Based on the values of the body's thermal resistance, it is analytically proven that men and women cannot physiologically achieve the same cutaneous response for an identical WBC protocol. Additionally, it is distinctly shown that, in order to attain a given cooling threshold, the exposure time for men must surpass that of women. A mathematical model is employed to compute these exposure durations. This personalization, hitherto restricted to populations of young men and women with standard BMI, can be extended to other targeted groups (elderly individuals, obese individuals, etc.) following the same principle. Ongoing research in this direction is poised to provide insights into protocol personalization on broader scales, encompassing both systemic analysis and specific body regions of minimal surface area such as joints.

References

1. Patel K, Bakshi N, Freehill MT, Awan TM. Whole-body cryotherapy in sports medicine. Curr Sports Med Rep. 2019;18(4):136–40.
2. Stanek A, Wielkoszyński T, Bartuś S, Cholewka A. Whole-body cryostimulation improves inflammatory endothelium parameters and decreases oxidative stress in healthy subjects. Antioxidants. 2020;9(12):1–11.
3. Rose C, Edwards KM, Siegler J, Graham K, Caillaud C. Whole-body cryotherapy as a recovery technique after exercise: a review of the literature. Int J Sports Med. 2017;38(14):1049–60. http://www.thieme-connect.de/products/ejournals/html/10.1055/s-0043-114861
4. Costello JT, Baker PRA, Minett GM, Bieuzen F, Stewart IB, Bleakley C. Whole-body cryotherapy (extreme cold air exposure) for preventing and treating muscle soreness after exercise in adults. Cochrane Database Syst Rev. 2015;2015:CD010789.
5. Lange U, Uhlemann C, Müller-Ladner U. Serielle ganzkörperkältetherapie im criostream bei entzündlich-rheumatischen erkrankungen. Eine pilotstudie Med Klin. 2008;103(6):383–8.
6. Banfi G, Melegati G, Barassi A, Dogliotti G, Melzi d'Eril G, Dugué B, et al. Effects of whole-body cryotherapy on serum mediators of inflammation and serum muscle enzymes in athletes. J Therm Biol. 2009;34(2):55–9.
7. Lombardi G, Ziemann E, Banfi G. Whole-body cryotherapy in athletes: from therapy to stimulation. An updated review of the literature. Front Physiol. 2017;8:258. /pmc/articles/PMC5411446/
8. Barłowska-Trybulec M, Zawojska K, Szklarczyk J, Góralska M. Effect of whole body cryotherapy on low back pain and release of endorphins and stress hormones in patients with lumbar spine osteoarthritis. Reumatologia. 2022;60(4):247–51.
9. Legrand FD, Dugué B, Costello J, Bleakley C, Miller E, Broatch JR, et al. Evaluating safety risks of wholebody cryotherapy/cryostimulation (WBC): a scoping review from an international consortium. European Journal of Medical Research. 2023;28(1):387, https://doi.org/10.1186/s40001-023-01385-z.
10. Costello JT, McInerney CD, Bleakley CM, Selfe J, Donnelly AE. The use of thermal imaging in assessing skin temperature following cryotherapy: a review. J Therm Biol. 2012;37(2):103–10.
11. Bugaj R. The cooling, analgesic, and rewarming effects of ice massage on localized skin. Phys Ther. 1975;55(1):11–9. https://pubmed.ncbi.nlm.nih.gov/1088989/
12. Elfahem R. Modélisation numérique CFD du comportement thermique cutané humain en Cryothérapie Corps Entier à −110°C. Université de Reims Champagne-Ardenne; 2023.
13. Bleakley CM, Hopkins JT. Is it possible to achieve optimal levels of tissue cooling in cryotherapy? Phys Therapy Rev. 2013;15(4):344–50. https://doi.org/10.1179/174328810X12786297204873.
14. Costello JT, Culligan K, Selfe J, Donnelly AE. Muscle, skin and core temperature after -110°c cold air and 8°c water treatment. PLoS One. 2012;7(11):e48190. https://doi.org/10.1371/journal.pone.0048190.
15. Bouzigon R, Grappe F, Ravier G, Dugue B. Whole- and partial-body cryostimulation/cryotherapy: current technologies and practical applications. J Therm Biol. 2016;61:67–81. https://pubmed.ncbi.nlm.nih.gov/27712663/
16. Haq A. An evaluation of the effects of whole body cryotherapy treatment for sports recovery and performance. 2021.
17. Dugue B, Bernard JP, Bouzigon R, de Nardi M, Douzi W, Feirreira JJ, et al. Whole body cryotherapy/cryostimulation, 39th informatory note on refrigeration technologies. IIF-IIR; 2020. https://iifiir.org/fr/fridoc/la-cryotherapie-corps-entiercryostimulation-39-lt-sup-gt-e-lt-sup-gt-note-142805
18. Louis J, Theurot D, Filliard JR, Volondat M, Dugué B, Dupuy O. The use of whole-body cryotherapy: time- and dose-response investigation on circulating blood catecholamines and heart rate variability. Eur J Appl Physiol. 2020;120(8):1733–43. https://pubmed.ncbi.nlm.nih.gov/32474683/

19. Polidori G, Elfahem R, Abbes B, Bogard F, Legrand F, Bouchet B, et al. Preliminary study on the effect of sex on skin cooling response during whole body cryostimulation (−110 °C): modeling and prediction of exposure durations. Cryobiology. 2020;97:12–9.

20. Cuttell S, Hammond L, Langdon D, Costello J. Individualising the exposure of −110 °C whole body cryotherapy: the effects of sex and body composition. J Therm Biol. 2017;65:41–7.

21. Hausswirth C, Schaal K, Le Meur Y, Bieuzen F, Filliard JR, Volondat M, et al. Parasympathetic activity and blood catecholamine responses following a single partial-body Cryostimulation and a whole-body Cryostimulation. PLoS One. 2013;8(8):e72658. https://doi.org/10.1371/journal.pone.0072658.

22. Hammond LE, Cuttell S, Nunley P, Meyler J. Anthropometric characteristics and sex influence magnitude of skin cooling following exposure to whole body cryotherapy. Biomed Res Int. 2014;2014:1.

23. Choi JK, Miki K, Sagawa S, Shiraki K. Evaluation of mean skin temperature formulas by infrared thermography. Int J Biometeorol. 1997;41(2):68–75. https://pubmed.ncbi.nlm.nih.gov/9429341/

24. Elfahem R, Abbes B, Bouchet B, Murer S, Bogard F, Moussa T, et al. Whole-body Cryostimulation: new insights in Thermo-Aeraulic fields inside chambers. Inventions. 2023;8(4):81.

25. Aguilella-Arzo M, Alcaraz A, Aguilella VM. Heat loss and hypothermia in free diving: estimation of survival time under water. Am J Phys. 2003;71(4):333–7.

26. Polidori G, Cuttell S, Hammond L, Langdon D, Legrand F, Taiar R, et al. Should whole body cryotherapy sessions be differentiated between women and men? A preliminary study on the role of the body thermal resistance. Med Hypotheses. 2018;120:60–4.

27. Schlich E, Schumm M, Schlich M. 3D-body-scan als Anthropometrisches Verfahren zur Bestimmung der Spezifischen Körperoberfläche. Ernahrungs Umschau. 2010;57(4):178–83.

Future Perspectives

Paolo Capodaglio, Benoit Dugué, Giovanni Lombardi,
Guillaume Polidori, Jacopo Maria Fontana,
and Raffaella Cancello

P. Capodaglio (✉)
Research Laboratory in Biomechanics, Rehabilitation and Ergonomics, IRCCS Istituto
Auxologico Italiano, Piancavallo (Verbania), Italy

Physical Medicine and Rehabilitation, Department of Surgical Sciences, University of Torino,
Torino, Italy
e-mail: p.capodaglio@auxologico.it; paolo.capodaglio@unito.it

B. Dugué
Laboratory Mobilité, Vieillissement, Exercice (MOVE), Faculty of Sports Sciences,
University of Poitiers, Poitiers, France
e-mail: benoit.dugue@univ-poitiers.fr

G. Lombardi
Laboratory of Experimental Biochemistry and Molecular Biology, IRCCS Istituto Ortopedico
Galeazzi, Milan, Italy

Department of Athletics, Strength and Conditioning, Poznań University of Physical
Education, Poznań, Poland
e-mail: giovanni.lombardi@grupposandonato.it; lombardi@awf.poznan.pl

G. Polidori
Structure Fédérative de Recherche CAP Santé, University of Reims Champagne Ardennes,
Reims, France
e-mail: guillaume.polidori@univ-reims.fr

J. M. Fontana
Research Laboratory in Biomechanics, Rehabilitation and Ergonomics, IRCCS Istituto
Auxologico Italiano, Piancavallo (Verbania), Italy
e-mail: j.fontana@auxologico.it

R. Cancello
Obesity Unit and Laboratory of Nutrition and Obesity Research, Department of Endocrine
and Metabolic Diseases, IRCCS Istituto Auxologico Italiano, Milan, Italy
e-mail: r.cancello@auxologico.it

P. Capodaglio (ed.), *Whole-Body Cryostimulation*,
https://doi.org/10.1007/978-3-031-18545-8_19

Spasticity

The application of local cryotherapy to temporarily reduce spasticity is a widespread clinical practice. Treatment approaches to manage spasticity associated with upper motor neuron lesion disorders include also the use of oral neuropharmacological agents, injectable materials such as botulinum toxin, surgical treatment, contracture reduction, orthosis, topical anaesthesia application using various massage techniques, strengthening the antagonist musculature with electrical stimulation. The tissue-based effects promoted by the application of cold therapy include post-injury reduction of swelling and oedema, an increase in the local circulation, lowering of the acute inflammation that follows tissue damage, muscle spasm reduction and pain inhibition. Muscle contraction can be facilitated by using cold therapy and this can be used to improve muscle contraction to increase joint ranges of motion after injury. Another effect of cold is a time-related reduction in spasticity once the cold has been applied for some time. The results of a study on children with spastic cerebral palsy [1] indicate that local cold therapy is an effective method when combined with physical and occupational therapy in reducing spasticity and improving hand function. After assessing that no defective skin sensation was present, a cold gel pack was applied over a wet towel to the skin of the treated area and, after checking that no abnormal reactions were present, the cold pack was applied for 20 min. Immediately after cold application all children received a physical and occupational programme for 2 h three times per week for a successive 3 months. Spasticity, range of motion and hand function evaluated before and after the treatment by using the Modified Ashworth Scale, the electronic goniometer and the Peabody Developmental Motor Scale improved more in the group where cold packs had been applied as compared to the one undergoing only the physical and occupational programme. A dated study [2] on the efficacy of local cryotherapy in reducing spasticity of the calf in 25 subjects with clinical signs of spasticity secondary to traumatic brain injury, spinal cord injury and stroke showed a statistically significant reduction in spasticity during cryotherapy, but equivocal results post-cryotherapy, leading to the conclusion that dichotomous results are possible. This may well reflect the complex nature of spasticity coupled with the variable nature of central nervous system injuries as well as uncontrolled variables associated with the clinical method of ice pack application [2, 3]. Nevertheless, ice pack applications appeared in most cases to provide temporary reduction of spasticity when the initial level of spasticity was 'clinically significant' [2]. Subsequent and long-term cold applications have been shown to induce prolonged inhibitory effects on clonus in patients with upper motor neuron involvement and sustained clonus [4]. A recent original study suggested that topical application of cold could be a novel and simple-to-use therapeutic strategy for stroke patients. Their results suggested that application of menthol to paw derma attenuated infarct volumes and ameliorated sensorimotor deficits in stroke mice induced by middle cerebral artery occlusion [5]. The benefits were associated with reductions in oxidative stress, neuroinflammation and infiltration of monocytes and macrophages in ischaemic brains, through the activation of peripheral cold receptors

(TRPM8) expressed in the derma tissue of limbs. Major approaches developed to treat acute ischaemic stroke fall into two categories: reperfusion therapy (thrombolysis or mechanical removal of thrombi) and neuroprotection. There is a huge unmet clinical need for neuroprotective strategies able to improve the outcomes of stroke patients. Huang et al. (2022) found that topically cold stimulus was neuroprotective by reducing the oxidative stress in the infarcted cortex, suppressing astrogliosis and microgliosis, and reducing the infiltration of monocytes after stroke, thus opening a perspective on a novel supplemental therapeutic strategy of cold-based therapies for stroke patients.

Pain

Cold-induced analgesia is achieved by lowering the skin temperature. The attainment of a clinically optimal physiologic response by using cold therapy requires the skin tissue to be cooled effectively. A number of studies have been performed to establish the critical level of tissue cooling required for specific effects. Localised analgesia requires a skin temperature that is below 13.6 °C, and the explanation for this analgesic effect is that the cold reduces the nerve conduction velocity [6]. A painless period of up to 2 h has been observed following one visit to whole-body cryostimulation (WBC) [7]. In a randomised controlled trial, Hirvonen et al. [8] reported that WBC (−110 °C) seems to relieve pain more effectively than other cryotherapies (WBC −60 °C, local cold air −30 °C, cold packs locally) in regard to active rheumatoid arthritis. Exposure to cryogenic temperatures in patients with low back pain (LBP) reduced significantly pain, slightly increased the release of β-endorphins, the plasma level of cortisol and adrenaline, although the latter difference was statistically insignificant [9]. Cold-induced analgesia seems to work via a number of mechanisms including: decreased receptor sensitivity [10] decreased receptor firing rate [11], decreased nerve conduction velocity (NCV), reduced muscle spasm as a counter irritant to pain [12]. Evidence shows that cooling skin temperature to between 10 °C and 13 °C and a 10–33% reduction in NCV result in localised analgesia [6, 13]. This is currently regarded as the threshold for optimally inducing analgesia in the clinical setting [14]. Theoretical guidelines from animal models suggest tissue temperature windows between 5 °C and 15 °C should be achieved; however, such large reductions seem difficult to attain. Future research must clarify what the optimal tissue temperature reduction should be, and the subsequent effect on treatment outcome.

Obesity and Diabetes

The transdifferentiation property of adipose organ allows prospecting a therapeutic strategy: browning of obese adipose organ (see Chap. 9). The most physiologic way to reach WAT-BAT conversion is chronic cold exposure and it has been recently showed that people living in cold exposed areas have large amounts of

BAT even in visceral areas of adipose organ usually composed by WAT. Chronic cold exposure or treatments mimicking the chronic cold exposure, through WAT-BAT transdifferentiation and BAT activation, could represent the perspective therapies for obesity and type 2 diabetes, but larger studies are needed. The gold standard of detection of BAT activation is 18F-fluorodeoxyglucose positron emission tomography (PET) with computed tomography (CT). However, a major limitation of PET/CT as a tool for human BAT studies is the clinically significant doses of ionising radiation. To allow non-invasive, quantitative measures of BAT mass and activity with lower costs, several other imaging methods, including the infrared thermography (IRT)/thermal imaging have been developed. IRT is a safe, rapid and inexpensive technique for detecting BAT in humans. Further research focusing on patients with varying degrees of BMI and also undergoing treatments other than those used in current studies will be needed to shed light on factors that may influence individual responses to cryogenic exposure. This would support the definition of personalised gender-specific protocols and development of guidelines on its clinical use. Changes in response to WBC may differ between overweight and different classes of obesity because adipose tissue is an effective insulator and may act as a barrier to heat loss. Subjects with higher BMI show higher mean skin temperature drop with faster cooling of the skin. Other than the relative amount of fat, also the distribution of fat pads represents a variable that should be taken into account [15]. However, besides the obesity state, the cardiorespiratory fitness (CF) might be considered (see Chap. 4). According to previous researches, equally obese subjects experienced different humoral effects depending on CF. Indeed, when exposed to WBC, obese patients with a low-CF experienced a greater improvement in circulating inflammatory mediators, and in the potential activation of adipose tissue browning (i.e. release of irisin from the skeletal muscle) than their high-CF counterpart [16, 17]. For these reasons, future studies with larger cohorts and control groups are needed to investigate the effects of more WBC sessions than those used in current studies.

Autonomic Dysfunction

The autonomic nervous system (ANS) is designed to maintain physiologic homeostasis. Its widespread connections make it vulnerable to disruption by many disease processes such as neurodegenerative disorders resulting in numerous symptoms involving the cardiovascular, gastrointestinal and urogenital systems. The degree to which dysautonomia contributes to a patient's overall disability can be quite variable. Constipation, urinary urgency and incontinence, heat intolerance and orthostatic hypotension are frequent problems that contribute significantly to morbidity and mortality, especially in the elderly (Table 19.1). Primary neurodegenerative disorders such as Parkinson and several systemic diseases such as diabetes mellitus, autoimmune conditions and paraneoplastic syndromes can impact the ANS. Examples of diseases in which secondary dysautonomia can occur include

Table 19.1 Possible symptoms of dysautonomia that could be treated with WBC

Balance problems	Fainting, loss of consciousness	Fatigue
Weakness	Migraine or frequent headaches	Difficulty swallowing
Ongoing tiredness	Noise/light sensitivity	Mood swings
Nausea and vomiting	Dizziness, vertigo, lightheadedness	Brain "fog"/forgetfulness/lack of focus and mental clarity
GI problems (costipation)	Visual disturbances (blurred vision)	Sleeping problems
Abnormally fast or slow heart rate	Dehydration	Frequent urination/incontinence
Anxiety	Low blood sugar (hypoglycemia)	Erectile dysfunction
Excessive sweating or not being able to sweat (hyperhidrosis and hypohidrosis)	Shortness of breath	Exercise intolerance (shortness of breath)

also sarcoidosis, Crohn's disease, ulcerative colitis, celiac disease, Charcot-Marie-Tooth disease, Chiari malformation, amyloidosis, Guillain-Barre syndrome, Ehlers-Danlos syndrome, Lambert-Eaton syndrome, vitamin B and E deficiencies and HIV. The aforementioned disorders are frequently associated with peripheral and/or cardiac denervation. Hausswirth et al. reported significant increases in norepinephrine concentrations in the immediate stages after WBC compared to resting controls [18]. They found similar between-group differences in resting vagal-related heart-rate variability indices (the root-mean-square difference of successive normal R–R intervals and high-frequency band). An interesting caveat was that the magnitude of these effects was reduced when participants substituted WBC for a partial body cryostimulation that did not involve head cooling. WBC showed the largest influence on parasympathetic reactivation, which is currently considered to be an important indicator of systemic recovery, as compared against active, passive and contrast water-therapy conditions. It has nevertheless to be remembered that much of the knowledge of the sympathetic/parasympathetic balance after cold exposure stems from heart rate variability studies which is informative for the regulation of the heart but may not be relevant on other organs. It could be advisable to study the effects of cold on other organs and skin. Experiments could therefore be designed to study the effects of cold exposure on the pupillary light reflex, the baroreceptor reflex and the electric resistance of the skin in order to get a clearer picture on the effects of cold on the human body. Interestingly, a recent preliminary work on the impact of regular cold exposure on electrodermal activity in older patients with joint degenerative diseases has been presented [19]. This work showed that the use of daily WBC combined with physical exercise induced physiological adaptations, lowered the sympathetic nervous activity and reduced stress level in these patients. These adaptations also seem to depend on gender and age.

Intestinal Syndromes

The autonomic nervous system, which is the primary pathway involved in brain-gut communication, plays an important role in functional bowel disorders. Communications along the brain-gut axis involve neural pathways as well as immune and endocrine mechanisms. The two branches of the autonomic nervous system are integrated anatomically and functionally with visceral sensory pathways, and are responsible for the homeostatic regulation of gut function. The autonomic nervous system is also a major mediator of the visceral response to central influences such as psychological stress and other central factors. There have been a growing number of reports demonstrating disordered autonomic function in subgroups of functional bowel patients [20–22]. Given the 'training effect' of WBC on the autonomic system, a possible impact on gastrointestinal disorders can be expected, but no studies are available so far.

Capsulitis and Joint Stiffness

Flexibility is an intrinsic property of body tissues, which among other factors determines the range of motion (ROM). The latter is associated with tendon and neuro-muscular factors. Increased ROM would therefore result from either an increased tendon ability to mechanically tolerate stretch loads or a decreased neural activation resulting in greater muscle elongation under the same load. An increase in neural activation of the muscle has been linked to suppressed muscle flexibility. One of the most common manipulations to reduce neural activation and affect ROM is the use of thermal agents. Warm-up prior to exercise is known to affect elastic properties of the muscle-tendon system, but also application of cold agents can reduce neural activity and affect ROM. It has been shown that local cryotherapy decreases nerve conduction velocity and also limits the presence of pain [13]. Bleakely and Costello suggest, in their systematic review, that cryotherapy could have beneficial effects on ROM, but the evidence is sometimes conflicting and warrants further research [23]. A decrease in neural activation of the muscle has been linked with greater ROM and cryotherapy is an effective technique to reduce neural activation. A randomised controlled trial on 30 patients with adhesive capsulitis showed that the addition of WBC to modalities and joint manipulation proved to be more effective in improvement of ROM of the shoulder, pain and function than mobilisation alone [24]. It is possible that WBC produced a local analgesia, or acted as a counterirritant to pain, which facilitated mobilisation. Results from a study on the acute effects of WBC on sit-and-reach amplitude in women and men support the hypothesis that ROM is increased immediately after a single session of WBC [25].

Ageing

A 2021 review [26] explored the effects of WBC from the perspective of applications with age with subjects over the age of 55 years old. Blood-based factors such as erythropoietin and IL-3 increased after WBC; in older subjects with Mild

Cognitive Impairment a significant improvement of short-term memory was noted with reduced levels of IL-6. They concluded that WBC appears to be an exciting non-pharmacological treatment with pleiotropic action. In the ageing period, oxidative stress increases as a result of the reduction in the systemic antioxidant defence and excessive production of reactive oxygen species (ROS). Reduction in antioxidant capacity is one of the causes of cell dysfunction in the ageing process. It has been found that oxidative stress is one of the pathogenic factors of obesity, diabetes, dyslipidaemia and cardiovascular diseases [27, 28]. Oxidative stress is also increased in neurodegenerative diseases such as multiple sclerosis, Parkinson's disease, Alzheimer's disease and also in the pathogenesis of stroke [29, 30]. A significant increase in ROS concentration was also found in the course of neoplastic diseases or rheumatoid arthritis [31].

In a study by Wojciak cryogenic temperatures acutely increased blood levels of Sirtuin1 (Sirt1) in the blood serum increased in older men undertaking high levels of physical activity [32]. The repeated use of WBC increased the concentration of both Sirt1 and Sirt3 and the antioxidant defence systems; however, this effect depends on age, performed level of physical activity and number of applied treatments. They concluded that WBC treatments could be used as an adjunct therapy for healthy ageing. Elderly, who are more likely to be malnourished or have frailty syndrome, not only can be negatively impacted by dietary interventions and restrictions but also have poor compliance with these methods. In this context, a short duration of cold exposure may be more feasible than long-term dietary modifications in such patients. Indirect support for the association between lower body temperature and longer lifespans comes from numerous studies on caloric restriction in animals. In these studies, various animal species maintained on diets with 30–40% fewer calories than normal showed both lower body temperatures and lifespans extended by up to 50% compared to those on regular diets [33, 34]. Although limited in number and scale, there are indications that a similar phenomenon may occur in humans. Preliminary results from a randomised clinical trial involving 150 human participants, testing the effects of a 25% calorie reduction, showed a significant reduction in core body temperature of approximately 0.4 °F after 6 months (Redman). This association between lower body temperature and increased lifespan due to caloric restriction has prompted researchers to use lower body temperature as a 'biomarker' of extended survival not only in studies directly related to caloric restriction but also in the emerging field of 'calorie restriction mimetics' (Ingram). As this area of research is still developing, further investigation is needed to fully understand the implications of lower body temperature and its potential role in extending human lifespans. Caloric restriction and its mimetics are central goals of longevity research, offering promising avenues for understanding the fundamental mechanisms of ageing and age-related diseases.

A relevant aspect of the ageing frail phenotype is represented by the dysfunctional locomotor apparatus characterised by bone and skeletal muscle mass and strength loss. A dysfunctional locomotor apparatus means increased risk of fall and fracture but also, being skeletal muscle and bone two organs of absolute relevance in the management of the energy substrates (i.e. they are the largest organs and use and store high amount of carbohydrates and lipids), it also means metabolic alterations that could hesitate into metabolic diseases (e.g. metabolic syndrome, diabetes) [35]. There is evidence, although still limited, that WBC may stimulate pro-anabolic functions (or inhibit catabolism) in these organs. In the case of bone, the anti-inflammatory effect of WBC has an impact on the osteoimmune RANK-RANKL-OPG axis and sees an increase in the relative amount of the osteogenic mediators, OPG, in professional rugby players submitted to high-volume training [36]. Further, WBC seems to modify the mechanosensing function of bone (i.e. sclerostin) and the metabolic activity (CTx-I) depending on the physical activity level of the subject [37]. About skeletal muscle, there are evidences that WBC improves muscle metabolism [38, 39], decreases myostatin, the main catabolic factor for muscles, and increases strength [38] in young subjects.

Sleep Disorders

Whole-body cryotherapy at −60 °C and, to a lesser extent, local cryotherapy seems to be a treatment option for restless legs syndrome in addition to conventional pharmacological treatment, as assessed by several questionnaires regarding symptoms, sleep and quality of life [40]. Moreover, whole-body and partial-body cryotherapy have been reported to improve sleep quality in physically active men after training in the evening and after training in professional soccer players [41, 42]. As exposure to cold (e.g. winter swimming, cold-water immersion, WBC) has been shown to reduce inflammation, oxidative stress, endothelial dysfunction and to improve sleep quality, it has been hypothesised that WBC might also have a beneficial effect in the alleviation of the consequences of sleep apnoea (OSA) [42]. Specifically, it has been proposed that cooling therapies could be included as an adjunct therapy to help patients with central sleep apnoea syndrome who do not respond to continuous positive airway pressure (CPAP) treatment—which is supposed to increase air pressure in the pharynx, preventing thereby the collapse of upper airways. WBC has been shown to determine local adipose tissue reduction and redistribution [43]. A reduction in local adipose tissue around the neck might be beneficial on sleep apnoea severity by reducing the upper airway collapsibility. Also, it has been shown that WBC impacts the sympatho-vagal balance by increasing parasympathetic activity [44], which might have an effect on sleep disordered breathing with related hypoxia and their associated cardiovascular consequences. However, to our knowledge, up to now, no studies have investigated the role of WBC as an adjunct to OSA therapy. Only recently an RCT (NCT05206916) has been proposed by researchers of the Sohag University to evaluate the role of cryotherapy in OSA patients. Noteworthy, there are no studies published investigating the effects of cold on the expression of clock genes and on the circadian rhythm of mediators of sleep.

Microbiota

Modifying gut microbiota may significantly impact human health, especially concerning cognitive performance [45]. Among others, a possible way of influencing gut microbiota could be exposure to WBC. Animal studies have indeed suggested that exposure to cold temperatures can impact the gut microbiota composition and influence metabolic processes. Some studies have shown that cold exposure can lead to changes in the abundance and diversity of gut microbial communities. One such study, published in the journal *Cell Reports* in 2015 [46], investigated the effects of cold exposure on the gut microbiota of mice. The researchers found that cold exposure altered the composition of the gut microbiota, leading to an increase in the abundance of certain bacteria, which has been associated with metabolic benefits. The changes in the gut microbiota were also linked to improved glucose metabolism and increased energy expenditure in mice. Another study, published in the journal *Cell* in 2019 [47], demonstrated that microbiota depletion via treatment with different cocktails of antibiotics or in germ-free mice impaired the thermogenic capacity of BAT by blunting the increase in the expression of uncoupling protein 1 (UCP1) and reducing the browning process of WAT. Gavage of the bacterial metabolite butyrate increased the thermogenic capacity of ABX-treated mice, reversing the deficit. These results indicate that gut microbiota contribute to upregulated thermogenesis in cold environments/stress and that this may be partially mediated via butyrate [47]. Intestinal microbiota seems to play a pivotal role both in the healthy functioning of the central nervous system and in pathology development. The study conducted by Rymaszewska et al. showed that 10 daily WBC sessions caused a significant improvement in cognitive functioning in people with mild cognitive impairments, especially memory processes (immediate episodic memory, delayed recall, logical memory, semantic knowledge, anterograde memory and phonemic verbal fluency) [48]. WBC caused a significant increase in plasma NO level, BDNF concentration and a reduction of IL-6. WBC-induced alterations in gut microbiota decrease in the inflammatory response and insulin resistance may impact key metabolic features of dementia. Although the metabolic consequences of cold exposure are similar to those observed in caloric restriction, the former method may be preferable in the case of the population at risk of developing dementia. Recognising subgroups of patients with specific alterations in the gut microbiota, metabolic dysregulation and aberrant immune-inflammatory processes may provide bases for developing personalised treatment strategies. While these animal studies provide valuable insights into the potential effects of cold exposure on the gut microbiota and metabolism, it's essential to approach the findings with caution when extrapolating them to human physiology. Human studies in this area are limited, and further research is needed to fully understand the implications of cold exposure on the gut microbiota and its metabolic effects in humans.

Resting Energy Expenditure

Whole-body cryotherapy (WBC) has attracted significant interest concerning its potential impact on resting energy expenditure (REE), which refers to the number of calories needed by the body at rest in a fasted state. While the available research on this topic is not yet extensive, some studies suggest that exposure to extreme cold temperatures during WBC may lead to a temporary increase in REE. When the body is exposed to extreme cold, it naturally generates heat to maintain its core temperature, which could result in an elevated metabolic rate. However, the precise magnitude and duration of this effect require further investigation, as ongoing research continues to explore these aspects.

Cold-induced thermogenesis has been proposed as a potential strategy to raise REE in patients living with obesity [49]. A study demonstrated that both single and multiple WBC sessions significantly increased REE in lean and obese women, although the effectiveness varied between the two groups. To gain a better understanding of the metabolic effects over extended periods, longitudinal studies are needed, focusing on the duration of the REE increase obtained after WBC sessions. As the evidence in this area is still in its early stages, further evaluations involving repeated WBC therapy sessions in people with obesity are advisable to establish its potential role as a strategy to significantly augment REE in this specific patient population. Numerous studies have examined the effects of acclimation to mild cooling on energy expenditure, revealing both increases and declines in response. A decline in energy expenditure during mild cooling is characteristic of a habituation response. The idea behind habituation to cold stress is that it benefits the organism by conserving energy that would otherwise be expended in responding to non-lethal stimuli. For a comprehensive review of the human habituation response to cold stress, Yurkevicius et al. provide valuable insights. Several experimental studies have reported decreases in metabolic rate during mild cooling conditions, such as 12 °C water immersion. However, more severe or repeated exposure to cold is more likely to induce a hypermetabolic response [50]. The range of metabolic responses to mild cooling conditions appears to vary widely across different study locations. Previous work among populations outside circumpolar regions have documented a significant correlation between BAT metabolic activity and change in energy expenditure after cooling suggesting that BAT plays a mechanistic role in non-shivering thermogenesis [51–54]. Despite evidence for a significant relationship between BAT metabolic activity and cold-induced energy expenditure, the tissue-specific metabolic rate of BAT is estimated to contribute less than 12 kcal/100 g/day to total energy expenditure [52]. BAT may contribute to cold-induced energy expenditure through its action as an endocrine organ by triggering an increase in metabolism within other tissues during NST (Bal et al. 2017) [55]. For instance, BAT secretes interleukin-6, 3-methyl-2-oxovaleric acid, 5-oxoproline, β-hydroxyisobutyric acid and 12,13-diHOME which upregulate oxidative metabolism in skeletal muscle [55–58]. Deep muscles that co-locate with BAT, such as levator scapulae, exhibit an increase in metabolism during non-shivering thermogenesis [53]. Therefore, additional research is necessary to investigate the factors influencing hypo- versus hypermetabolic responses to WBC.

Personalised WBC

Personalised protocols for WBC require answers to several questions in order to optimise the physiological response. Key considerations include determining the optimal temperature and duration of exposure to elicit the desired effects. To achieve this, further research is needed to explore various factors, such as the number of WBC sessions, the temperature settings in the cryogenic chamber, the duration of exposure to cryogenic cold and how mean skin temperature variation affects individual responses. These considerations should also be taken in the context of individual factors like body fat, gender, physiological profile and duration of the anti-inflammatory and metabolic benefits associated with a WBC cycle. Given that gender differences may play a role in the response to WBC, they must be carefully accounted for in the development of personalised protocols. According to the 39th Informatory Note on Refrigeration Technologies by the International Institute of Refrigeration Working group (October 2020) [59], several issues need to be investigated: differences in the working temperature of cryochambers, consideration of body composition and individual cooling potential, dose effects of treatments, safety issues. Indeed, it is well established that body composition (i.e. fat mass) is the main variable affecting the decrease in body (skin and core) temperature. At clinical level, the main question to be answered is: what is the optimal temperature and duration to elicit the required physiological response? Further studies are needed regarding the number of WBC sessions, the temperature in the cryogenic chamber, the duration of exposure to cryogenic cold and the mean skin temperature variation, also in relation to individual body fat, gender, physiological profile and the duration of the anti-inflammatory and metabolic beneficial effects (anti-inflammatory, antidepressant, metabolic, analgesics) elicited by a WBC cycle. To develop predictive equations for WBC protocols, researchers will need to draw upon experimental cellular, molecular and clinical-functional data lakes. This comprehensive approach will allow for a deeper understanding of the physiological mechanisms underlying WBC and its potential effects on various aspects of health, including anti-inflammatory, antidepressant, metabolic and analgesic benefits. By leveraging this wealth of data, scientists can design protocols that are tailored to individual needs and goals, ensuring the safe and effective use of WBC as a therapeutic intervention. Overall, personalised WBC protocols hold great promise for maximising the benefits of this treatment and advancing its potential as a valuable tool in improving health and well-being. However, to achieve this, continued research and collaboration between disciplines will be essential in unlocking the full potential of WBC therapy.

Conclusive Remarks

Altogether, the chapters included in this book summarise a big share of the published and ongoing WBC research. We tried to describe the cutting-edge studies and the evidence provided so far on the clinical use of WBC. Most findings will have to be consolidated at clinical level by larger, randomised controlled studies and gaps in knowledge about molecular/cellular mechanisms will have to be filled. Hopefully, this chapter will serve researchers to plan future studies on the clinical application of WBC in different conditions that have not been investigated so far: the wide range of conditions with sympathetic overdrive, post-stroke spasticity and sleep apnoea, to cite a few. In the wish list, studies on BAT activation, effects on skin and cold receptors, electrodermal activity, microbiota, effects of cold stimulus in adipose-derived stromal human cells in vitro that are able to differentiate into adipocytes, osteocytes and myocytes, and cellular in vitro models that will allow to unveil molecular pathways in terms of gene expression and secretory activity (metabolomics) under acute and chronic cold stimulation could consolidate scientific evidences and further proceed towards personalised protocols in the frame of precision medicine, a paradigm shift from a 'one-size-fits-all' approach to an optimised strategy for treatment of diseases for each person.

References

1. Abd El-Maksoud GM, Sharaf MA, Rezk-Allah SS. Efficacy of cold therapy on spasticity and hand function in children with cerebral palsy. J Adv Res. 2011;2:319–25.
2. Price R, Lehmann JF, Boswell-Bessette S, Burleigh A, deLateur BJ. Influence of cryotherapy on spasticity at the human ankle. Arch Phys Med Rehabil. 1993;74:300–4.
3. Urbscheit N, Johnston R, Bishop B. Effects of cooling on the ankle jerk and H-response in hemiplegic patients. Phys Ther. 1971;51:983–90.
4. Boyraz I, Oktay F, Celik C, Akyuz M, Uysal H. Effect of cold application and tizanidine on clonus: clinical and electrophysiological assessment. J Spinal Cord Med. 2009;32:132–9.
5. Huang S-S, Su H-H, Chien S-Y, Chung H-Y, Luo S-T, Chu Y-T, Wang Y-H, MacDonald IJ, Lee H-H, Chen Y-H. Activation of peripheral TRPM8 mitigates ischemic stroke by topically applied menthol. J Neuroinflammation. 2022;19:192.
6. Bugaj R. The cooling, analgesic, and rewarming effects of ice massage on localized skin. Phys Ther. 1975;55:11–9.
7. Metzger D, Zwingmann C, Protz W, Jäckel WH. Whole-body cryotherapy in rehabilitation of patients with rheumatoid diseases—pilot study. Rehabilitation. 2000;39:93–100.
8. Hirvonen HE, Mikkelsson MK, Kautiainen H, Pohjolainen TH, Leirisalo-Repo M. Effectiveness of different cryotherapies on pain and disease activity in active rheumatoid arthritis. A randomised single blinded controlled trial. Clin Exp Rheumatol. 2006;24:295–301.
9. Barłowska-Trybulec M, Zawojska K, Szklarczyk J, Góralska M. Effect of whole body cryotherapy on low back pain and release of endorphins and stress hormones in patients with lumbar spine osteoarthritis. Reumatologia. 2022;60:247–51.
10. Kunesch E, Schmidt R, Nordin M, Wallin U, Hagbarth KE. Peripheral neural correlates of cutaneous anaesthesia induced by skin cooling in man. Acta Physiol Scand. 1987;129:247–57.
11. Mense S. Effects of temperature on the discharges of muscle spindles and tendon organs. Pflugers Arch. 1978;374:159–66.
12. Saeki Y. Effect of local application of cold or heat for relief of pricking pain. Nurs Health Sci. 2002;4:97–105.
13. Algafly AA, George KP. The effect of cryotherapy on nerve conduction velocity, pain threshold and pain tolerance. Br J Sports Med. 2007;41:365–9; discussion 369
14. Bleakley CM, Hopkins JT. Is it possible to achieve optimal levels of tissue cooling in cryotherapy? Phys Ther Rev. 2010;15:344–50.
15. Cholewka A, Stanek A, Sieroń A, Drzazga Z. Thermography study of skin response due to whole-body cryotherapy. Skin Res Technol. 2012;18:180–7.

16. Dulian K, Laskowski R, Grzywacz T, Kujach S, Flis DJ, Smaruj M, Ziemann E. The whole body cryostimulation modifies irisin concentration and reduces inflammation in middle aged, obese men. Cryobiology. 2015;71:398–404.
17. Ziemann E, Zembroñ-Lacny A, Kasperska A, Antosiewicz J, Grzywacz T, Garsztka T, Laskowski R. Exercise training-induced changes in inflammatory mediators and heat shock proteins in young tennis players. J Sports Sci Med. 2013;12:282–9.
18. Hausswirth C, Schaal K, Le Meur Y, Bieuzen F, Filliard J-R, Volondat M, Louis J. Parasympathetic activity and blood catecholamine responses following a single partial-body cryostimulation and a whole-body cryostimulation. PLoS One. 2013;8:e72658.
19. Machnia M, Douzi W, Jdidi H, Miller E, Dugué B. Impact of regular cold exposure on electrical skin resistance in patients with joint degenerative diseases. Clin Physiol Funct Imaging. 2023. https://doi.org/10.1111/cpf.12862. Epub ahead of print. PMID: 37861346.
20. Spaziani R, Djuric V, Kamath M, Armstrong D, Fallen E, Upton A, Tougas G. A low resting vagal tone predicts response to acid perfusion in patients with esophageal symptoms. Gastroenterology. 1996;110:A762.
21. Aggarwal A, Cutts TF, Abell TL, Cardoso S, Familoni B, Bremer J, Karas J. Predominant symptoms in irritable bowel syndrome correlate with specific autonomic nervous system abnormalities. Gastroenterology. 1994;106:945–50.
22. Jørgensen LS, Christiansen P, Raundahl U, Ostgaard S, Christensen NJ, Fenger M, Flachs H. Autonomic nervous system function in patients with functional abdominal pain. An experimental study. Scand J Gastroenterol. 1993;28:63–8.
23. Bleakley CM, Costello JT. Do thermal agents affect range of movement and mechanical properties in soft tissues? A systematic review. Arch Phys Med Rehabil. 2013;94:149–63.
24. Ma S-Y, Je HD, Jeong JH, Kim H-Y, Kim H-D. Effects of whole-body cryotherapy in the management of adhesive capsulitis of the shoulder. Arch Phys Med Rehabil. 2013;94:9–16.
25. De Nardi M, La Torre A, Benis R, Sarabon N, Fonda B. Acute effects of whole-body cryotherapy on sit-and-reach amplitude in women and men. Cryobiology. 2015;71:511–3.
26. Kujawski S, Newton JL, Morten KJ, Zalewski P. Whole-body cryostimulation application with age: a review. J Therm Biol. 2021;96:102861.
27. Matsuda M, Shimomura I. Increased oxidative stress in obesity: implications for metabolic syndrome, diabetes, hypertension, dyslipidemia, atherosclerosis, and cancer. Obes Res Clin Pract. 2013;7:e330–41.
28. Panth N, Paudel KR, Parajuli K. Reactive oxygen species: a key hallmark of cardiovascular disease. Adv Med. 2016;2016:1. https://doi.org/10.1155/2016/9152732.
29. Jiang T, Sun Q, Chen S. Oxidative stress: a major pathogenesis and potential therapeutic target of antioxidative agents in Parkinson's disease and Alzheimer's disease. Prog Neurobiol. 2016;147:1–19.
30. Ohl K, Tenbrock K, Kipp M. Oxidative stress in multiple sclerosis: central and peripheral mode of action. Exp Neurol. 2016;277:58–67.
31. Valko M, Leibfritz D, Moncol J, Cronin MTD, Mazur M, Telser J. Free radicals and antioxidants in normal physiological functions and human disease. Int J Biochem Cell Biol. 2007;39:44–84.
32. Wojciak G, Szymura J, Szygula Z, Gradek J, Wiecek M. The effect of repeated whole-body cryotherapy on Sirt1 and Sirt3 concentrations and oxidative status in older and young men performing different levels of physical activity. Antioxidants (Basel). 2020;10(1):37. https://doi.org/10.3390/antiox10010037. PMID: 33396247; PMCID: PMC7823702
33. Rikke BA, Johnson TE. Lower body temperature as a potential mechanism of life extension in homeotherms. Exp Gerontol. 2004;39:927–30.
34. Rikke BA, Yerg JE III, Battaglia ME, Nagy TR, Allison DB, Johnson TE. Strain variation in the response of body temperature to dietary restriction. Mech Ageing Dev. 2003;124:663–78.
35. Gerosa L, Malvandi AM, Malavolta M, Provinciali M, Lombardi G. Exploring cellular senescence in the musculoskeletal system: any insights for biomarkers discovery? Ageing Res Rev. 2023;88:101943.

36. Galliera E, Dogliotti G, Melegati G, Corsi Romanelli MM, Cabitza P, Banfi G. Bone remodelling biomarkers after whole body cryotherapy (WBC) in elite rugby players. Injury. 2013;44:1117–21.

37. Straburzyńska-Lupa A, Cisoń T, Gomarasca M, Babińska A, Banfi G, Lombardi G, Śliwicka E. Sclerostin and bone remodeling biomarkers responses to whole-body cryotherapy (− 110 °C) in healthy young men with different physical fitness levels. Sci Rep. 2021;11:16156.

38. Jaworska J, Rodziewicz-Flis E, Kortas J, Kozłowska M, Micielska K, Babińska A, Laskowski R, Lombardi G, Ziemann E. Short-term resistance training supported by whole-body Cryostimulation induced a decrease in Myostatin concentration and an increase in isokinetic muscle strength. Int J Environ Res Public Health. 2020;17:5496.

39. Jaworska J, Micielska K, Kozłowska M, Wnorowski K, Skrobecki J, Radzimiński L, Babińska A, Rodziewicz E, Lombardi G, Ziemann E. A 2-week specific volleyball training supported by the whole body Cryostimulation protocol induced an increase of growth factors and counteracted deterioration of physical performance. Front Physiol. 2018;9:1711.

40. Happe S, Evers S, Thiedemann C, Bunten S, Siegert R. Whole body and local cryotherapy in restless legs syndrome: a randomized, single-blind, controlled parallel group pilot study. J Neurol Sci. 2016;370:7–12.

41. Douzi W, Dupuy O, Tanneau M, Boucard G, Bouzigon R, Dugué B. 3-min whole body cryotherapy/cryostimulation after training in the evening improves sleep quality in physically active men. Eur J Sport Sci. 2019;19:860–7.

42. Douzi W, Dupuy O, Theurot D, Boucard G, Dugué B. Partial-body cryostimulation after training improves sleep quality in professional soccer players. BMC Res Notes. 2019;12:141.

43. Loap S, Lathe R. Mechanism underlying tissue cryotherapy to combat obesity/overweight: triggering thermogenesis. J Obes. 2018;2018:5789647.

44. Louis J, Theurot D, Filliard J-R, Volondat M, Dugué B, Dupuy O. The use of whole-body cryotherapy: time- and dose-response investigation on circulating blood catecholamines and heart rate variability. Eur J Appl Physiol. 2020;120:1733–43.

45. Łuc M, Misiak B, Pawłowski M, Stańczykiewicz B, Zabłocka A, Szcześniak D, Pałęga A, Rymaszewska J. Gut microbiota in dementia. Critical review of novel findings and their potential application. Prog Neuro-Psychopharmacol Biol Psychiatry. 2021;104:110039.

46. Chevalier C, Stojanović O, Colin DJ, et al. Gut microbiota orchestrates energy homeostasis during cold. Cell. 2015;163:1360–74.

47. Li B, Li L, Li M, et al. Microbiota depletion impairs thermogenesis of Brown adipose tissue and Browning of white adipose tissue. Cell Rep. 2019;26:2720–2737.e5.

48. Rymaszewska J, Lion KM, Stańczykiewicz B, Rymaszewska JE, Trypka E, Pawlik-Sobecka L, Kokot I, Płaczkowska S, Zabłocka A, Szcześniak D. The improvement of cognitive deficits after whole-body cryotherapy - a randomised controlled trial. Exp Gerontol. 2021;146:111237.

49. De Nardi M, Bisio A, Della Guardia L, Facheris C, Faelli E, La Torre A, Luzi L, Ruggeri P, Codella R. Partial-body Cryostimulation increases resting energy expenditure in lean and obese women. Int J Environ Res Public Health. 2021;18:4127.

50. Yurkevicius BR, Alba BK, Seeley AD, Castellani JW. Human cold habituation: physiology, timeline, and modifiers. Temp Austin Tex. 2022;9:122–57.

51. Chondronikola M, Volpi E, Børsheim E, et al. Brown adipose tissue activation is linked to distinct systemic effects on lipid metabolism in humans. Cell Metab. 2016;23:1200–6.

52. Muzik O, Mangner TJ, Leonard WR, Kumar A, Janisse J, Granneman JG. 15O PET measurement of blood flow and oxygen consumption in cold-activated human brown fat. J Nucl Med Off Publ Soc Nucl Med. 2013;54:523–31.

53. u Din M, Raiko J, Saari T, et al. Human brown adipose tissue [15O]O2 PET imaging in the presence and absence of cold stimulus. Eur J Nucl Med Mol Imaging. 2016;43:1878–86.

54. van der Lans AAJJ, Hoeks J, Brans B, et al. Cold acclimation recruits human brown fat and increases nonshivering thermogenesis. J Clin Invest. 2013;123:3395–403.

55. Bal NC, Maurya SK, Pani S, Sethy C, Banerjee A, Das S, Patnaik S, Kundu CN. Mild cold induced thermogenesis: are BAT and skeletal muscle synergistic partners? Biosci Rep. 2017;37:BSR20171087.

56. Shamsi F, Wang C-H, Tseng Y-H. The evolving view of thermogenic adipocytes — ontogeny, niche and function. Nat Rev Endocrinol. 2021;17:726–44.
57. Stanford KI, Lynes MD, Takahashi H, et al. 12,13-diHOME: an exercise-induced Lipokine that increases skeletal muscle fatty acid uptake. Cell Metab. 2018;27:1111–1120.e3.
58. Whitehead A, Krause FN, Moran A, et al. Brown and beige adipose tissue regulate systemic metabolism through a metabolite interorgan signaling axis. Nat Commun. 2021;12:1905.
59. International Institute of Refrigeration Working Group Whole body cryotherapy/cryostimulation, 39th Informatory Note on Refrigeration Technologies. 2020. https://doi.org/10.18462/iif.NItec39.09.2020.

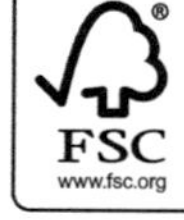